Histopathologic Diagnosis of Mycotic Diseases

Written by one of the very few pathologists who has real expertise in this field, this book is a comprehensive key for the identification of fungal infections in tissues. With updated terminology and presentation, all invasive mycoses types are covered, detailing their epidemiology, pathology, histomorphology of fungal elements, and differential diagnoses. Each of the separate fungal groups has a good combination of text and high-quality illustrations, which is a critical feature for clinicians to state the mycopathological diagnoses.

Key Features

1. Elaborates on the histological observations of both the pathological reaction and the histomorphology of fungal elements, guiding the reader in the right direction for obtaining a diagnosis of the infection.
2. Includes key observations that can be a game changer for infectious diseases specialists and histopathologists studying the combination of fungal morphology and host response.
3. Follows a logical layout, structure, and organization with a wealth of high-quality illustrations of the various fungi in tissues elucidated by different stains.

Histopathologic Diagnosis
of Invasive Mycoses

Henrik Elvang Jensen
Professor of Pathology
Section for Pathobiology
Faculty of Health and Medical Sciences
University of Copenhagen, Denmark

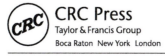

CRC Press
Taylor & Francis Group
Boca Raton New York London

CRC Press is an imprint of the
Taylor & Francis Group, an **informa** business

First edition published 2023
by CRC Press
6000 Broken Sound Parkway NW, Suite 300, Boca Raton, FL 33487-2742

and by CRC Press
4 Park Square, Milton Park, Abingdon, Oxon, OX14 4RN

CRC Press is an imprint of Taylor & Francis Group, LLC

© 2023 Henrik Elvang Jensen

Library of Congress Cataloging-in-Publication Data

Names: Jensen, Henrik Elvang, author.
Title: Histopathologic diagnosis of invasive mycoses / by Henrik Elvang Jensen.
Description: First edition. | Boca Raton, FL : Taylor & Francis, 2023. | Includes bibliographical references and index.
Identifiers: LCCN 2022042619 (print) | LCCN 2022042620 (ebook) | ISBN 9781032306704 (paperback) | ISBN 9781032306711 (hardback) | ISBN 9781003306177 (ebook)
Subjects: MESH: Invasive Fungal Infections | Mycoses--diagnosis | Mycoses--physiopathology | Diagnosis, Differential
Classification: LCC RA644.M92 (print) | LCC RA644.M92 (ebook) | NLM WC 450 | DDC 616.9/69--dc23/eng/20220919
LC record available at https://lccn.loc.gov/2022042619
LC ebook record available at https://lccn.loc.gov/2022042620

ISBN: 978-1-032-30671-1 (hbk)
ISBN: 978-1-032-30670-4 (pbk)
ISBN: 978-1-003-30617-7 (ebk)

DOI: 10.1201/9781003306177

Typeset in Minion
by KnowledgeWorks Global Ltd.

Contents

Preface

For nearly 40 years, I have had the privilege of receiving fungal infection cases from all over the world for diagnostic consultation. Therefore, I have been able to collect several cases covering almost every type of invasive fungal infection in humans and animals. Moreover, I have delivered annual lectures and courses on the histomorphological diagnosis of mycoses in several countries and arranged pre-congress workshops at different world congresses including the International Society for Human and Animal Mycology (ISHAM) congresses in Berlin (2012), Melbourne (2015), and Amsterdam (2018). I have also published more than 100 peer-reviewed papers and chapters in textbooks and co-authored international guidelines for the histopathological diagnosis of invasive mycoses. As I see it, the major problem for pathologists and clinicians is that they are not regularly confronted with fungal infections (in contrast to bacterial and viral infections) unless they are working in regions where these infections are endemic. Moreover, most invasive mycoses are symptomatically and clinically non-specific. Therefore, many invasive mycotic infections are not diagnosed until a tissue sample has been collected and processed for histopathology, at which time it is crucial to obtain trustworthy data based on the pathology and histomorphology of the fungal elements present in the sample (i.e., to reach the correct diagnosis, which is needed for appropriate therapy). In recent years, several new molecular techniques have been developed to diagnose mycoses in tissue samples; however, these techniques do not differentiate between colonization, dormancy, or contamination with fungi and true tissue invasion. Therefore, confirming that results from molecular techniques are consistent with the pathology and fungal histomorphology of the tissue is paramount. Histopathology remains the gold standard for obtaining trustworthy diagnoses of invasive mycoses.

The text of this book is separated into 32 chapters and supplemented by approximately 300 histological figures (i.e., photographs) that illustrate the mycoses described in each chapter. Following an introduction to invasive mycoses, there are five chapters describing invasive mycoses from the pathological viewpoint: 1) Histopathological classification of invasive mycoses, 2) Histopathological staining of invasive fungi, 3) Pathomorphological identification of invasive fungi, 4) Identification of invasive fungi using *in situ* techniques, and 5) Glossary of medical mycology. Next, the particular invasive mycoses and lesions caused by each pathogen are described in separate chapters. Each of these chapters has an updated list of references, which are cited in the text. The text of each chapter has been separated into the following sections: 1) Introduction, 2) Epidemiology, 3) Pathology, 4) Histomorphology of fungi and related pathogens, 5) Differential diagnoses, and 6) References.

I hope that the book, which is dedicated to the histopathological diagnosis of invasive mycoses and lesions of related pathogens, will be not only of value for both medical and veterinary pathologists and clinicians in general but also a guide to a variety of specialists in different medical disciplines, especially those working on infectious diseases, haematology, oncology, and in critical care units.

Finally, I would like to express my very special thanks to Dennis Brok for his enthusiasm in the editing and layout of the many photomicrographs. I am grateful for the skilful assistance provided by laboratory technicians Betina G. Andersen and Elisabeth W. Petersen. Thanks also go to Benedicte Kragh and Nicole L. Henriksen for their editorial work.

Henrik Elvang Jensen
Professor of Pathology
University of Copenhagen, Denmark

About the author

Professor Henrik Elvang Jensen has served as a pathologist for nearly 40 years and has had the privilege of receiving fungal infection cases from all over the world for diagnostic consultation. Therefore, he has been able to collect several cases of almost all kinds of invasive fungal infections in humans and animals. Moreover, he has, on a yearly basis, given lectures and courses on the histomorphological diagnosis of mycoses in several countries and arranged pre-congress workshops at different world congresses including the ISHAM congresses in Berlin (2012), Melbourne (2015), and Amsterdam (2018) on the same topic. During the years, he has published more than 100 peer-reviewed papers and several chapters in textbooks and is a co-author of more international guidelines, all dealing with the histopathological diagnosis of invasive mycoses.

1

Introduction

Invasive mycoses (i.e., invasive fungal infections) are becoming more common in the human population worldwide for many reasons (1, 2). In particular, more people are at risk of acquiring opportunistic fungal infections due to ageing populations, immunosuppression associated with transplantation, cancer therapy, immunosuppressive diseases, and metabolic diseases such as diabetes mellitus (1). Coronavirus disease 2019 (COVID-19) has contributed to a rise in mucormycosis cases, especially in India. Here, the predisposing factors include uncontrolled diabetes and systemic corticosteroid treatments, which reduce the inflammation in the lungs of COVID-19 patients (2). In India, mucormycosis has become known as "black fungus" due to the colonization of blood vessels following invasive infection by the fungi, which results in thrombosis and tissue death (infarct formation) and typically turns the tissue black. Notably, however, the disease termed "black fungus" is caused by hyaline fungi (i.e., members of the Mucorales; Fig. 1.1) and not by the black fungi (dematiaceous/phaeoid fungi), which are the cause of phaeohyphomycosis and chromoblastomycosis (Fig. 1.2).

Ideally, a fungal pathogen is diagnosed from typical clinical symptoms by identifying the fungus within lesions accompanied by a host reaction and subsequently by identifying the infectious agent from culture or by molecular techniques (3). Unfortunately, this is rarely achieved, especially for invasive mycoses. Moreover, patients with fungal infections frequently have other diseases, which may mask fungal-related symptoms. Due to the non-specific nature of clinical symptoms including radiological observations, a trustworthy diagnosis usually depends on clinical and laboratory tests like mycological cultivation, diverse molecular techniques, and the application of histopathology. These tests may include detecting the following: 1) fungal antigens in fluids such as serum, spinal fluid, bronchoalveolar lavage, and urine; 2) anti-fungal antibodies; 3) fungal metabolites such as D-arabinitol; and 4) cell wall markers such as (1, 3)-β-D-glucan and galactomannan (4). In recent years, several molecular techniques have been developed to diagnose invasive mycoses, which may identify fungi rapidly and accurately (1, 4). In particular, polymerase chain reaction (PCR)-based techniques may be used for the non-culture-based diagnosis of fungal infections in blood and other clinical specimens, including fresh and formalin-fixed tissue specimens. Due to the risk of false negative and false positive results from the cultures as well as the non-culture-based diagnostic tests for mycotic infections, an examination should always be complemented by histopathology when diagnosing fungal infections. This is especially important for invasive mycoses caused by opportunistic pathogenic fungi. The diagnosis and management of invasive mycoses still rely on recognizing the interactions between fungi, related pathogens, and the host (1).

Many non-culture-based techniques are not applicable for unusual or rare fungal pathogens, and molecular and non-culture-based laboratory techniques will only identify the targets that they have been designed to detect. Isolation of fungi from tissues may also be problematic, and several weeks may be needed to obtain results for some pathogens (e.g., *Histoplasma* and *Paracoccidioides*). Moreover, when a mycosis is not suspected clinically (often, they are mistaken for inflammation due to non-mycotic agents or neoplasms), the whole biopsy specimen may be fixed in formalin and embedded in paraffin wax when used for pathological examination. Therefore, portions are not available for culture (5). In these cases, histopathological and immunohistological techniques together with *in situ* hybridization may be the only means of establishing an aetiological diagnosis in the absence of new biopsies. However, for some fungal pathogens, the formalin-fixed and paraffin-embedded tissue may be used to identify fungi using PCR techniques (4, 6). As described above, samples sent for histopathology may not be suspected of exhibiting a fungal infection. However, mycoses should always be considered a possibility for susceptible (e.g., immunosuppressed) patients or patients from locations linked to pathogenic fungi, such as coccidioidomycosis in the southwest United States or *Cryptococcus gattii* in southwest Canada on Vancouver Island (1). Although the morphology of fungal elements within tissues may provide a tentative diagnosis, it may be impossible to provide an unambiguous diagnosis based on morphological details alone. This is due to the morphological similarities among tissue forms of several fungal genera or the presence of sparse or atypical fungal elements (Fig. 1.3) (7, 8).

Histopathological examinations may complement the diagnosis of diseases caused by fungi and related pathogens.

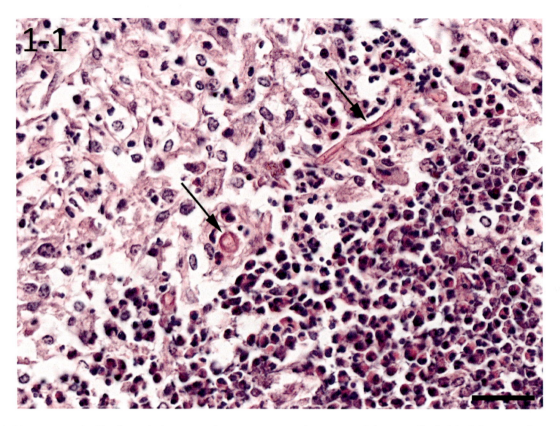

Figure 1.1 Mucormycosis. The fungal elements of mucormycosis, the cause of the so-called "black fungus" disease in India, are hyaline (arrows) within tissues when stained by haematoxylin and eosin. HE. Bar = 60 μm.

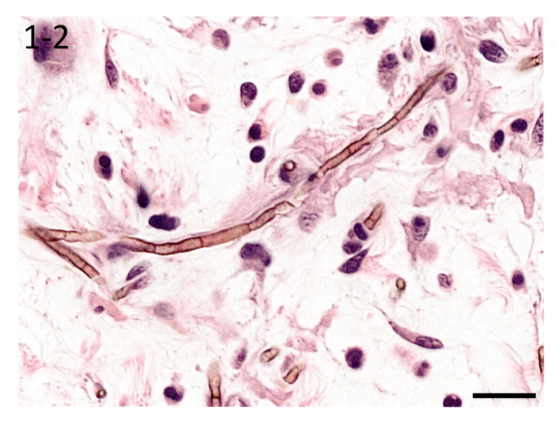

Figure 1.2 The cause of phaeohyphomycosis and chromoblastomycosis is coloured fungi (dematiaceous/phaeoid fungi), which appear brown/black in haematoxylin and eosin-stained sections. HE. Bar = 35 μm.

For some pathogens, a generic or specific aetiological diagnosis may be obtained within 24 hours by the unequivocal identification of characteristic fungal elements in tissue sections (9–11). Histological identification of the aetiological agent is the only reliable way of diagnosing particular fungi and related infectious agents, such as the aetiology of lacaziosis, rhinosporidiosis, and pneumocystosis (Figs. 1.4–1.6), because these pathogens cannot be cultured on media, or only in cell cultures. In addition, recent research has shown that *Rhinosporidium seeberi* (Fig. 1.5), which causes rhinosporidiosis, is not a fungus, and the organism has now been assigned to the order mesomycetozoans, a heterogeneous group at the boundary of animals and fungi (12). However, within tissues, *R. seeberi* resembles a mycotic infection, and because it has traditionally been included in the medical mycology/mycopathology literature, it has been included in this book together with the algoses.

As described above, the aetiological significance of results obtained by cultivating an organism or by molecular techniques can usually only be confirmed by histopathological evaluation (13). Moreover, the clinical dilemma of whether a fungal isolate is truly pathogenic, merely a superficial colonizer, a component of the normal mycobiota (e.g., *Candida albicans*), or an environmental contaminant (e.g., *Aspergillus* spp. (Figs. 1.7 and 1.8) or a member of the class Mucorales) is solved only by histological documentation of tissue invasion together with a typical host reaction (14). Within the upper respiratory airways and the lungs, histological evaluation of the inflammatory reaction and the distribution of fungal elements in a tissue section can also determine whether the disease is an invasive infection or an allergic reaction (e.g., invasive versus allergic bronchopulmonary aspergillosis). Histopathological evaluation of invasive mycoses may also be used to assess the efficacy of anti-fungal therapy in pre- and post-treatment biopsy specimens (13). Finally, histopathological studies may sometimes confirm the presence of multiple infections (e.g., the simultaneous bacterial and fungal infections or multiple mycotic infections that occur in patients with acquired immune deficiency syndrome [AIDS]) or exclude a fungal disease by revealing another process that accounts for the clinical observations. Accurate diagnoses are essential for optimal therapies, accurate prognoses, and a better understanding of the pathological and epidemiological aspects of different mycoses (5).

Thus, histopathology remains the gold standard for determining whether a fungus identified by cultivation or molecular techniques represents contamination, colonization (especially in the gastrointestinal tract and airways), or a true invasive infection (15).

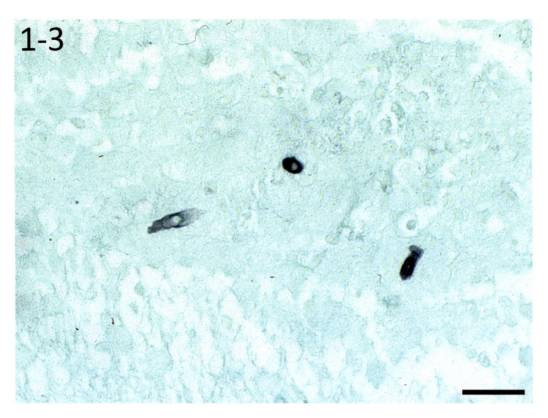

Figure 1.3 When only sparse or atypical fungal elements are present, it is not possible to provide an unambiguous diagnosis based on morphological details; however, the diagnosis "invasive mycosis" can be stated. GMS. Bar = 40 μm.

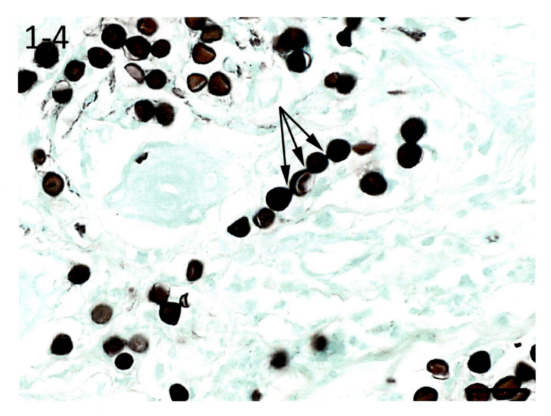

Figure 1.4 Histological demonstration of the aetiological agent is the only reliable method for diagnosing particular fungal infections, for example, lacaziosis (caused by *Lacazia loboi*), in which characteristic chains like a string of pearls are present (arrows). GMS. Bar = 25 μm.

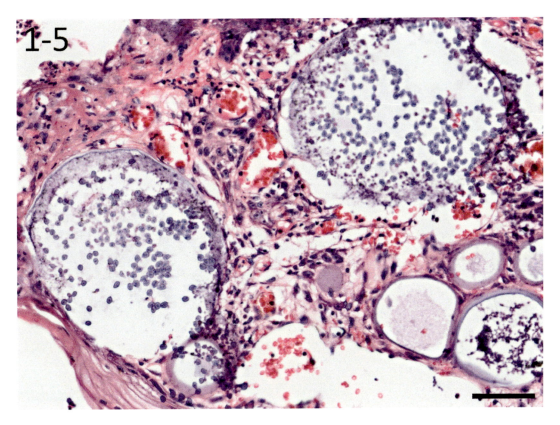

Figure 1.5 *R. seeberi*, which causes rhinosporidiosis, is not a fungus and has been assigned to the order mesomycetozoans, a heterogeneous group at the boundary of animals and fungi. HE. Bar = 75 μm.

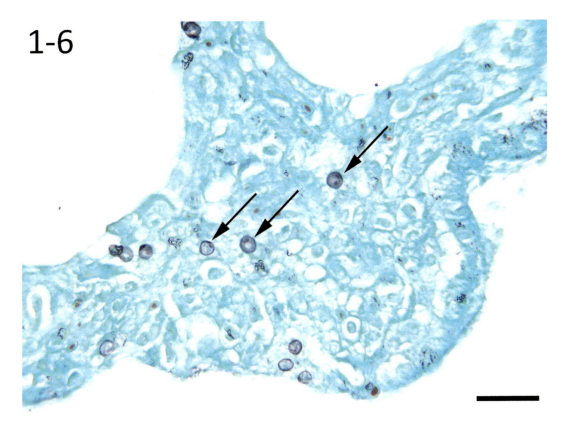

Figure 1.6 *Pneumocystis jirovecii* (arrows), which causes pneumocystosis, cannot be cultured on media. However, it may be transferred to cell cultures *in vitro*. GMS. Bar = 20 μm.

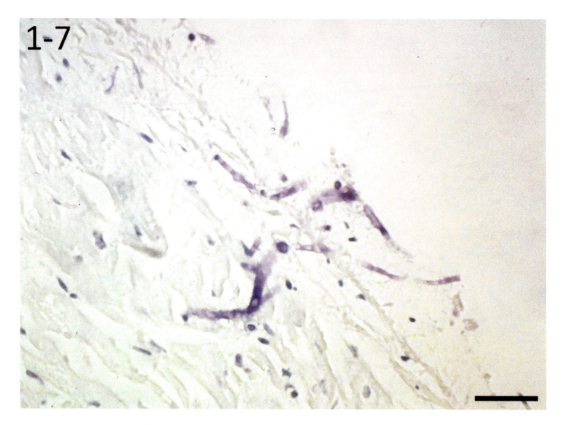

Figure 1.7 Postmortem ingrowth of *Aspergillus* hyphae from the surface of a heart. The presence of hyphae within the myocardial tissue is not accompanied by any host reaction. HE. Bar = 50 μm.

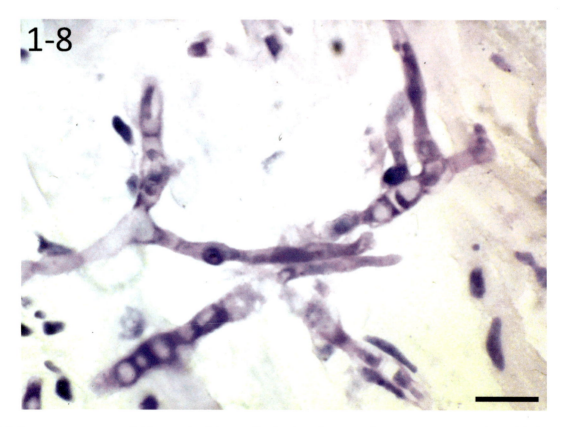

Figure 1.8 Postmortem myocardial ingrowth of *Aspergillus* hyphae due to surface contamination. The viable hyphae are present with vacuoles and septation but have not induced an inflammatory reaction or necrosis. HE. Bar = 15 μm.

REFERENCES

1. Hospenthal DR. 2015. Approach to patients with suspected fungal infections. In: Diagnosis and Treatment of Fungal Infections. 2nd ed. Hospenthal DR, Rinaldi MG, Eds. Springer. pp 3–7.

2. Hoenigl M, Seidel D, Carvalho A, Rudramurthy SM, Arastehfar A et al. 2021. The emergence of COVID-19 associated mucormycosis: Analysis of cases from 18 countries. Lancet, 33, doi: 10.2139/ssrn.3844587.

3. Jensen HE, Chandler FW. 2007. Histopathological diagnoses of mycoses. In: Topley and Wilson's Microbiology & Microbial Infections. Medical Mycology. 10th ed. Merz WG, Hay RJ, Eds. Hodder Arnold. pp 121–143.

4. Reiss E, Obayashi T, Orle K, Yoshida M, Zancopé-Oliveira RM. 2000. Non-culture based diagnostic tests for mycotic infections. Med Mycol, 38, 147–159.

5. Jensen HE. 1994. Systemic bovine aspergillosis and zygomycosis in Denmark with reference to pathogenesis, pathology, and diagnosis. APMIS, 102, 1–48.

6. Jensen HE. 2021. Histopathology in the diagnosis of invasive fungal diseases. Cur Fungal Infect Rep, 15, 23–31.

7. Chandler FW, Kaplan W, Ajello L. 1980. A Colour Atlas and Textbook of the Histopathology of Mycotic Diseases. Wolfe Medical Publications, Inc.

8. Jensen HE, Schønheyder HC, Hotchi M, Kaufman L. 1996. Diagnosis of systemic mycoses by specific immunohistochemical tests. APMIS, 104, 241–258.

9. Baker RD, Angulo OA, Barroso-Tobila C, Carbonell LM, Cespedes R et al. 1971. The Pathologic Anatomy of Mycoses: Human Infection with Fungi, Actinomycetes and Algae. Springer.

10. Anthony PP. 1973. A guide to the histological identification of fungi in tissues. J Clin Pathol, 26, 828–831.

11. Schwarz J. 1982. The diagnosis of deep mycoses by morphologic methods. Human Pathol, 13, 519–533.

12. Mendoza L, Taylor JW, Ajello L. 2002. The class Mesomycetozoea: A heterogeneous group of microorganisms at the animal-fungal boundary. Annu Rev Microbiol, 56, 315–344.

13. Chandler FW, Watts JC. 1987. Pathologic Diagnosis of Fungal Infections. ASCP Press.

14. Hoog GS, de Guého E. 1985. A plea for the preservation of opportunistic fungal isolates. Diagn Microbiol Infect Dis, 3, 369–372.

15. Guarner J, Brandt ME. 2011. Histopathologic diagnosis of fungal infections in the 21st century. Clin Microbiol Rev, 24, 247–280.

2

Histopathological classification of invasive mycoses

Mycoses may be classified in a number of different ways. For example, they may be classified according to their preferred location (i.e., whether they are superficial or deep-seated/invasive mycoses). Further, deep-seated mycoses may be classified according to whether they cause predominantly systemic infections or local invasive lesions of subcutaneous tissues, following penetration of the skin or mucous membranes (especially in the gastrointestinal tract and airways). Mycoses may also be classified based on fungal pathogenicity (e.g., opportunistic pathogenic, facultative pathogenic, or obligate pathogenic fungi). Classification can also be based on the predominant morphology of the fungal elements observed in tissues. For example, the mycoses may be caused by yeasts or filamentous fungi. Moreover, filamentous structures (hyphae) may be hyaline (non-pigmented) or coloured (dematiaceous/phaeoid). In addition, an overall classification may be based on geographical distribution, with particular mycoses being endemic or restricted to specific locations. An epidemiological classification may be used based on how the mycoses are transmitted. For example, some mycoses are transmitted by inhalation, whereas others are acquired by skin penetration (i.e., implantation). Finally, mycoses may be classified based on their *in vitro* morphological characteristics (1–7). For pathologists, who fundamentally are morphologists, it seems natural to base the classification of invasive mycoses primarily on morphology and features of the fungal elements within tissues, together with the pathological response observed in haematoxylin and eosin (HE) stained sections, because HE is the standard stain used in most histopathological laboratories. Based on this stipulation, mycoses may be classified histopathologically as follows: A) mycoses due to the presence of fungi with clear or light-coloured (hyaline) septate hyphae (Fig. 2.1; Table 2.1); B) mycoses due to the presence of coloured fungal elements (dematiaceous/phaeoid fungi; Fig. 2.2; Table 2.2); C) mycoses and non-mycoses with similar clinicopathological lesions: for example, mycetomas, which are invasive cutaneous or subcutaneous lesions (containing coloured grains) that are caused by hyaline or dematiaceous fungi (eumyotic mycetomas) and bacterial agents (actinomycotic mycetomas; Fig. 2.3; Table 2.3); D) mycoses involving predominantly yeast-like cells (Fig. 2.4; Table 2.4); E) mycoses due to the presence of large spherules (Fig. 2.5; Table 2.5); and F) sporadic and rare mycoses, which may be present in all of the patterns described above, and the algoses (Fig. 2.6; Table 2.6), which are traditionally included in mycopathology (2, 3, 7). Therefore, the mycoses described in the following chapters have been classified according to fungal pathomorphological observations from HE-stained histological slides. However, mycetomas are classified clinicopathologically. Importantly, some fungi may cause more than one type of mycosis. For example, fungi that cause phaeohyphomycoses or hyalohyphomycoses may also cause mycetomas.

Within the different classes, it is crucial to characterize the observed elements as precisely as possible. For example, within the broad category of yeast-like cells, further defining features include the size and shape of individual cells; the thickness of the cell wall; the number and shape of blastoconidia (i.e., buds); how the buds are attached to the parent cells; pigmentation; encapsulation; the number of nuclei; and the presence of pseudohyphae, hyphae (with presence or absence of septation), or arthroconidia (2, 3).

A. MYCOSES DUE TO THE PRESENCE OF FUNGI WITH CLEAR OR LIGHT-COLOURED (HYALINE) SEPTATE HYPHAE

1. Aspergillosis
2. Fusariosis
3. Scedosporiosis/lomentosporiosis
4. Mucormycosis
5. Entomophthoromycosis
6. Pythiosis
7. Hyalohyphomycosis, minor

B. MYCOSES DUE TO THE PRESENCE OF COLOURED FUNGAL ELEMENTS (DEMATIACEOUS FUNGI)

1. Phaeohyphomycosis
2. Chromoblastomycosis

DOI: 10.1201/9781003306177-2

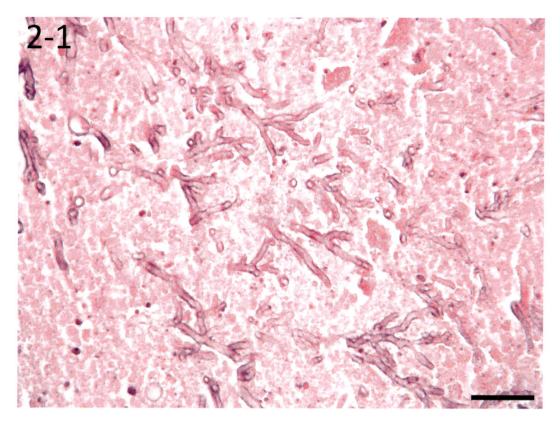

Figure 2.1 *A. fumigatus*. In haematoxylin and eosin-stained sections, the outlines of hyaline and septate hyphae are usually identifiable. HE. Bar = 40 μm.

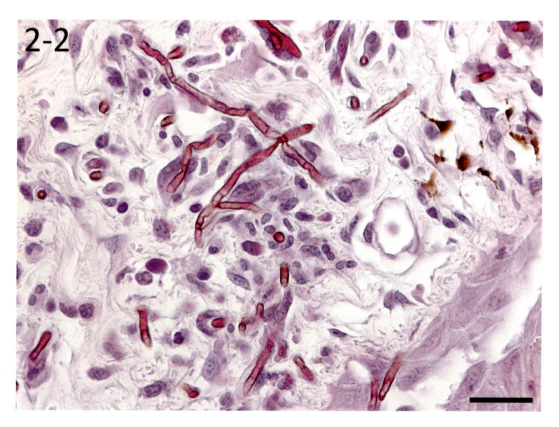

Figure 2.2 *Cladophialophora* elements appear coloured, as do other dematiaceous/phaeoid fungi, in haematoxylin and eosin-stained sections. HE. Bar = 60 μm.

Table 2.1 Characteristics of fungi occurring as hyaline hyphae in invasive lesions (hyalohyphomycoses)

Mycosis	Aspergillosis	Fusariosis	Scedosporiosis and lomentosporiosis	Mucormycosis	Entomophthoromycosis	Pythiosis	Hyalohyphomycosis, minor
Aetiology	*Aspergillus* spp.	*Fusarium* spp.	*Scedosporium apiospermum* (asexual state of *Pseudallescheria boydii*), *S. boydii*, *S. aurantiacum*, and *Lomentospora prolificans* (which may contain melanin)	*Mucor, Rhizopus, Lichtheimia, Rhizomucor, Cunninghamella,* and others	*Basidiobolus* spp., *Conidiobolus* spp.	*Pythium insidiosum*	*Paecilomyces, Purpureocillium, Gliomastix, Scopulariopsis, Penicillium, Trichoderma, Sarocladium, Acremonium, Schizophyllum, Geotrichum candidum,* and others
Width (µm)	3–6	3–8	2–5	6–25	6–12 (up to 30)	5–10	2–10
Contours	Parallel	Parallel	Parallel	Irregular	Irregular	Irregular	Irregular and parallel. Genus dependent
Pattern of branching	Dichotomous	Dichotomous or right angle	Dichotomous and/or haphazard	Haphazard	Haphazard	Haphazard	Dichotomous, haphazard, and at right angles. Genus dependent
Orientation of branches	Parallel or radial	Random and parallel	Random and parallel	Random	Random	Random and radial	Parallel, radial, and random. Genus dependent
Frequency of septation	Frequent	Frequent	Frequent	Infrequent	Frequent	Infrequent	Frequent or infrequent. Genus dependent

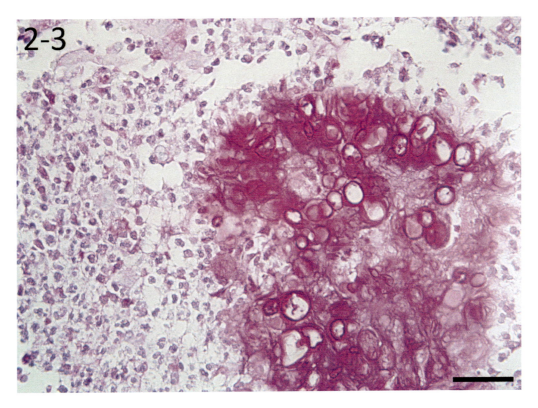

Figure 2.3 For mycetomas, defined clinicopathologically, the aetiology may vary considerably. Lesions may be caused by hyaline or dematiaceous fungi (hyphae or yeasts: i.e., eumycotic mycetomas, as shown here) or bacteria (i.e., actinomycotic mycetomas). However, the lesions can be classified by the granules they contain, which are surrounded by a pyogranulomatous inflammation. HE. Bar = 60 μm.

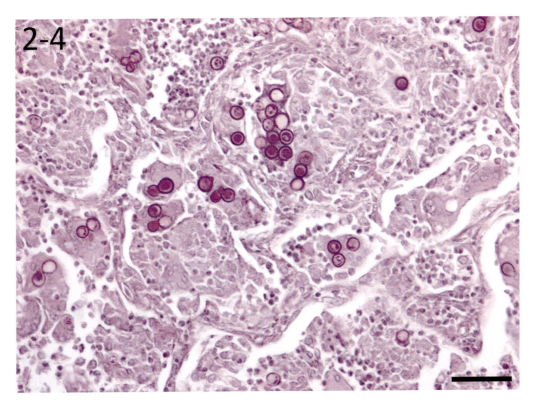

Figure 2.4 A major characteristic of some invasive mycoses is the growth of yeast-like cells, which may vary in terms of their shape, the number of buds, the attachment of buds, the thickness of the cell wall, the presence of simultaneous pseudohyphae and/or true hyphae. However, all contain unicellular elements, as shown here for *B. dermatitidis*. PAS. Bar = 50 μm.

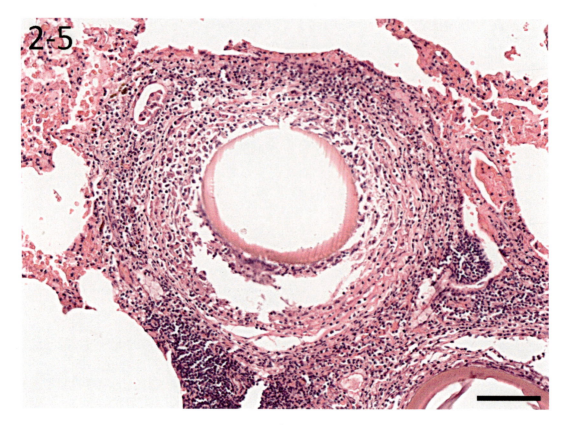

Figure 2.5 In tissue sections, invasive elements can be classified as spherules, which are large spherical elements with endospores in the lesions. Adiaspiromycosis is shown here. HE. Bar = 150 μm.

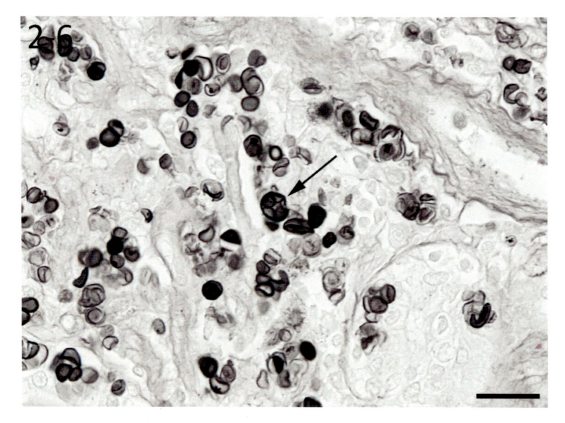

Figure 2.6 Sporadic and rare mycoses may vary considerably in size, shape, and colour. However, algal infections, which are often enclosed in mycopathology, show a characteristic pattern in histological slides. Intracellular cleavage (arrow) may not be visible in haematoxylin and eosin-stained sections. GMS. Bar = 60 μm.

Table 2.2 Features of lesions due to phaeohyphomycosis and chromoblastomycosis

Mycoses due to dematiaceous fungi	Dematiaceous fungal pathogens	
Phaeohyphomycosis	*Cladophialophora bantiana*, *Bipolaris spicifera*, *Exophiala jeanselmei*, and other phaeoid fungi	Dominated by phaeoid, often branched hyphae with a width of 2–6 µm. Often with constrictions at the site of septation and vesicle formation. Yeast-like phaeoid elements may be present
Chromoblastomycosis	May be caused by more than 150 fungal species from a variety of genera. These genera include *Fonsecaea*, *Cladophialophora*, *Phialophora*, *Rhinocladiella*, and *Exophiala*	Thick-walled, large (6–12 µm), often spherical, dark-brown, sclerotic cells with septation in one or two planes

Table 2.3 Clinicopathological features and pathogens of the lesions associated with mycetomas

Mycetomatous pathogens		
Eumycotic Caused by true fungi	*Acremonium* spp., *Aspergillus* spp., *Curvularia geniculata*, *Exophiala jeanselmei*, *Leptosphaeria senegalensis*, *Madurella grisea*, *M. mycetomatis*, *Neotestudina rosatii*, *Pseudallescheria boydii*, *Pyrenochaeta romeroi*, and others	Granules, 0.2 mm to several mm in diameter, composed of broad (2–6 µm), hyaline or phaeoid, and septate hyphae that often branch and form chlamydoconidia
Actinomycotic Caused by bacteria	*Actinomadura madurae*, *A. pelletieri*, *Nocardia* spp., *Nocardiopsis dassonvillei*, *Streptomyces somaliensis*, and others	Granules, less than 0.1 to several mm in diameter, composed of delicate gram-positive filaments, 1 µm wide, which are often branched and beaded

C. MYCOSES: EUMYCOTIC MYCETOMAS AND ACTINOMYCOTIC MYCETOMAS

1. Mycetomas

D. MYCOSES DUE TO THE PRESENCE OF YEAST-LIKE CELLS

1. Candidosis
2. Trichosporonosis
3. Cryptococcosis
4. Blastomycosis
5. Histoplasmosis capsulati
6. Histoplasmosis duboisii
7. Paracoccidioidomycosis
8. Sporotrichosis

9. Talaromycosis
10. Pneumocystosis
11. Lacaziosis

E. MYCOSES DUE TO THE PRESENCE OF LARGE SPHERULES

1. Coccidioidomycosis
2. Adiaspiromycosis
3. Rhinosporidiosis (Order mesomycetozoans)

F. RARE MYCOSES AND ALGOSES

1. Rare mycoses
2. Algoses

Table 2.4 Features of fungi that mainly occur as yeast-like cells in tissue

Feature	Candidosis		Trichosporonosis	Cryptococcosis	Blastomycosis	Histoplasmosis capsulati	Histoplasmosis duboisii	Paracoccidioidomycosis	Sporotrichosis	Talaromycosis	Pneumocystosis	Lacaziosis
	Candida spp.	Candida glabrata	Trichosporon spp.	Cryptococcus neoformans and C. gattii	Blastomyces dermatitidis	Histoplasma capsulatum var. capsulatum	H. capsulatum var. duboisii	Paracoccidioides brasiliensis and P. lutzii	Sporothrix schenckii spp. complex	Talaromyces (Penicillium) marneffei	Pneumocystis jirovecii	Lacazia (Loboa) loboi
Size (µm)	3–6	2–5	3–8	2–20	7–15*	2–4	6–12	5–60	2–10	2.5–5	2–10	5–12
Shape	Spherical or oval	Spherical or oval	Rectangular or oval	Pleomorphic	Spherical	Spherical or oval	Oval	Spherical	Pleomorphic cigar-shaped cells are characteristic	Spherical, oval, or elongated	Spherical, oval, or concentric	Spherical
Number of buds	Single; chains	Single	Single	Single and rarely multiple	Single	Single	Single	Multiple; "steering wheel" forms	Single and rarely multiple	None	None	Multiple; chains
Attachment of buds	Narrow	Narrow	Narrow	Narrow	Very broad	Narrow	Narrow	Narrow	Narrow	-NA-	-NA-	Narrow; tubular
Schizogony	–	–	–	–	–	–	–	–	–	+	+	–
Thickness of cell wall	Thin	Thin	Thin	Thin	Thick	Thin	Thick	Variable	Thin	Thin	Thick in cysts Thin in the trophic form	Thick
Pseudohyphae and/or hyphae	Characteristic	Absent	Characteristic	Rare	Rare	Rare	Absent	Rare	Rare	Absent	Absent	Absent
Number of nuclei	Single	Single	Single	Single	Multiple	Single	Single	Multiple	Single	Single	Multiple in cysts, single in the trophic form	Multiple
Mucicarmine reaction	–	–	–	+**	+/–	–	–	+/–	–	–	–	–

* Microforms, 2–4 µm in diameter, may also occur in the tissue.
** Some strains may be capsule deficient and non-carminophilic.
-NA- : not applicable

Table 2.5 Features of fungi and fungal-like elements (order mesomycetozoans) present as large spherules

	Coccidioides immitis and C. posadasii	Emmonsia crescens (Chrysosporium parvum var. crescens) and E. parva (C. parvum var. parvum)	Rhinosporidium seeberi (Order mesomycetozoans)
External diameter of spherule (µm)	20–200	200–400	100–400
Thickness of spherule wall (µm)	5–8	22–25	3–5
Diameter of endospores	2–5	None	6–10
Hyphae or arthroconidia	Rare	None	None
Special stain reactions			
Grocott's methenamine silver	+	+	+
Mucicarmine	–	–	+

Table 2.6 Features of rare mycoses and algoses

Mycoses and algoses	Pathogens	Typical morphology
Rare mycoses	Malassezia, Sporobolomyces, Rhodotorula, Pseudozyma (renamed Moesziomyces), Saccharomyces, Saprochaete, Kodamaea, the invasive forms of Alternaria and Phialemonium, Emergomyces spp., and others	Depending on the species, these mycoses may have any form described under classifications A–E. A diagnosis should only be made after histopathological verification of tissue invasion by fungi with corresponding morphology, obtained by repeated cultivation and/or molecular evidence
Algoses	Primarily due to the achlorophyllic algae Prototheca ciferrii (genotype 1), P. bovis (serotype 2), and P. blaschkeae (serotype 3), which were formerly named P. zopfii; and P. wickerhamii. In rare cases, chlorophyllic algae (Chlorella spp.) may cause invasive infections	Spherical, oval, or polyhedric cells are surrounded by a 2–3 µm clear halo, often measuring between 7 and 30 µm. The cells are surrounded by a thick capsule. Because algae reproduce by fission (intracellular cleavage) to produce endospores, intracellular septations are typically observed together with morula-like structures

REFERENCES

1. Hospenthal DR. 2015. Approach to patients with suspected fungal infections. In: Diagnosis and Treatment of Fungal Infections. 2nd ed. Hospenthal DR, Rinaldi MG, Eds. Springer. pp 3–7.
2. Jensen HE, Chandler FW. 2007. Histopathological diagnoses of mycoses. In: Topley and Wilson's Microbiology & Microbial Infections. Medical Mycology. 10th ed. Merz WG, Hay RJ, Eds. Hodder Arnold. pp 121–143.
3. Jensen HE. 2021. Histopathology in the diagnosis of invasive fungal diseases. Curr Fungal Infect Rep, 15, 23–31.
4. Chandler FW, Kaplan W, Ajello L. 1980. A Colour Atlas and Textbook of the Histopathology of Mycotic Diseases. Wolfe Medical Publishers, Inc.
5. Chandler FW, Watts JC. 1987. Pathologic Diagnosis of Fungal Infections. ASCP Press.
6. Guarner J, Brandt ME. 2011. Histopathologic diagnosis of fungal infections in the 21st century. Clin Microbiol Rev, 24, 247–280.
7. Salfelder K. 1990. Atlas of Fungal Pathology. Kluwer Academic Publishers.

3

Histopathological staining of invasive fungi

Haematoxylin and eosin (HE) is a versatile stain that enables pathologists to evaluate the host's inflammatory response, detect Splendore–Hoeppli material (asteroid bodies), and determine whether a fungus is hyaline (colourless) or phaeoid (naturally pigmented/dematiaceous (Figs. 3.1–3.3) (1). Many fungi, such as *Aspergillus* spp. and the moulds that cause mucormycosis, are readily detected by HE, but some fungi are not stained or stained poorly (e.g., *Candida* spp.). However, even poor staining may reveal the outline of fungal elements. Moreover, pathologists should always examine a granulomatous or pyogranulomatous inflammation carefully for fungal elements (Fig. 3.2) (2). It may be difficult to distinguish fungal elements from tissue components in HE-stained sections, particularly the thin blood vessels in brain and lung tissue, and when fungi are sparse or weakly stained, they are easily overlooked (Figs. 3.3 and 3.4). Therefore, particular stains are usually applied to adequately reveal the presence and morphology of fungal pathogens in tissue sections (3–6).

Gomori's/Grocott's methenamine silver (GMS) stain (Fig. 3.5), the periodic acid-Schiff stain (PAS) (Fig. 3.6), and Gridley's stain for fungi (GF) (Fig. 3.7) are preferred to demonstrate fungal elements in tissue sections. These procedures are based on the principle that adjacent hydroxyl groups of complex polysaccharides in fungal cell walls are oxidized to aldehydes by chromic acid or periodic acid. In the GMS procedure, the aldehydes reduce the methenamine silver nitrate complex; fungal cell walls stain brown/black because reduced silver is deposited where aldehydes are located. In the PAS and GF procedures, the aldehydes react with Schiff's reagent, colouring the fungi magenta. All three procedures stain the cell walls of fungal elements but tend to obscure the internal details of these cells. This is a major disadvantage of using these stains, because the innate colour of fungal elements is masked, making it impossible to determine whether a fungus is hyaline or phaeoid. Consequently, it may be difficult to determine whether a mycosis is caused by pigmented fungi (e.g., phaeohyphomycosis, chromoblastomycosis, or black-grain eumycotic mycetomas) (3, 4). Therefore, duplicate HE-stained and unstained sections should always be examined for pigmentation of fungal elements. Another limitation of the fungal stains is that they do not show the host's reaction to fungal invasion. However, colocalization may be observed in HE-stained sections, or the GMS-stained section may be counterstained with HE (Fig. 3.8) (7). Another disadvantage of using the silver stains is that normal structures in tissues also stain positive. These structures include basement membranes, collagen bundles, melanin, and neurosecretory granules (Fig. 3.4) (7–9). The GMS stain is excellent for detecting fungi in tissue sections because it provides better contrast for screening and, in most instances, it will stain old and non-viable organisms that may be refractory to the PAS and GF procedures (7).

Stains for mucin, such as Alcian blue and Mayer's or Southgate's mucicarmine procedures, readily demonstrate the mucopolysaccharide capsule of *Cryptococcus* spp. (Fig. 3.9). This staining reaction usually will differentiate typical cryptococci from non-encapsulated yeast-form pathogens of similar size and appearance. However, capsule-deficient cryptococci (so-called "dry" variants) may not stain positive for mucin. In addition, mucin stains are not specific for *Cryptococcus* spp. because the cell walls of *Blastomyces dermatitidis*, *Paracoccidioides brasiliensis*, and *Rhinosporidium seeberi* are also coloured by these stains (7).

The cell walls of cryptococci contain silver-reducing substances (melanin-like substances derived from dihydroxyphenylalanine), which react positively with a modified Fontana–Masson stain for melanin (10–12). Because this reaction does not depend on the presence of a mucinous capsule, it can be used to identify capsule-deficient cryptococci (13). If the pathogens that cause phaeohyphomycosis are non-pigmented or lightly pigmented in tissue sections, stains for melanin can be used to highlight their cell walls (Fig. 3.10) (3, 14).

Modified Gram stains (Fig. 3.11), such as the Brown and Brenn, and MacCallum–Goodpasture procedures, highlight the filaments of the pathogens that cause actinomycosis, nocardiosis, streptomycosis, and actinomycotic mycetomas. The GMS procedure can also be used to highlight these pathogens, but staining may be sporadic and weak. The HE, PAS, and Gridley procedures do not stain the actinomycetes, although the granules associated with actinomycosis and actinomycotic mycetomas stain well (7). Modified Gram stains are also needed to detect bacteria other than actinomycetes that may complicate a mycotic or

DOI: 10.1201/9781003306177-3

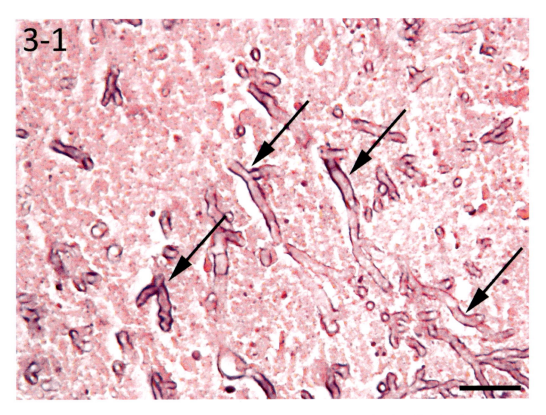

Figure 3.1 In haematoxylin and eosin-stained tissue sections, the cytoplasm and walls of hyaline fungi are often pink. In the present case of acute myocardial aspergillosis due to *A. fumigatus*, dichotomous branching of the hyphae is clearly visible (arrows). HE. Bar = 20 μm.

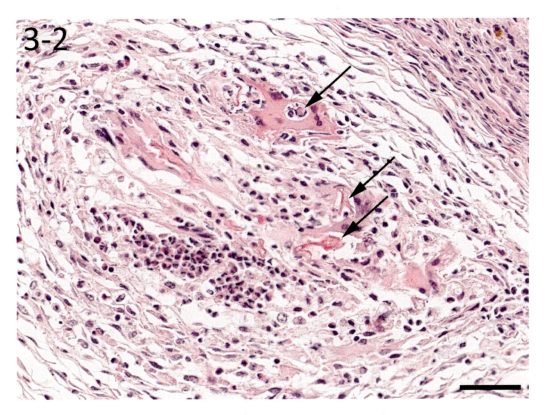

Figure 3.2 In haematoxylin and eosin-stained tissue sections, the outline of fungal elements may also be preserved in chronic lesions, as in the present case where the elements of mucormycosis are visible within multinucleate giant cells (arrows). HE. Bar = 75 μm.

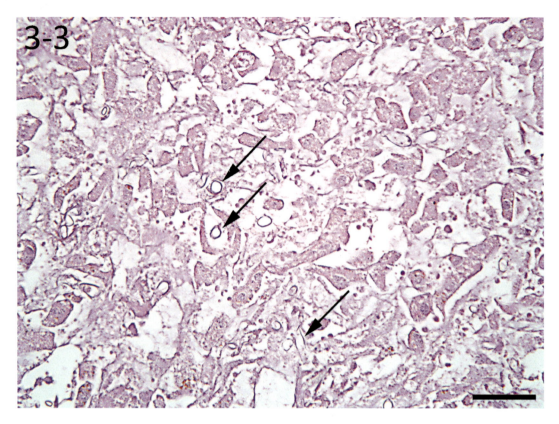

Figure 3.3 In haematoxylin and eosin-stained tissue sections, necrosis may be so advanced that the outline of fungal elements is difficult to identify, as in this liver biopsy that exhibits mucormycosis (arrows). HE. Bar = 40 μm.

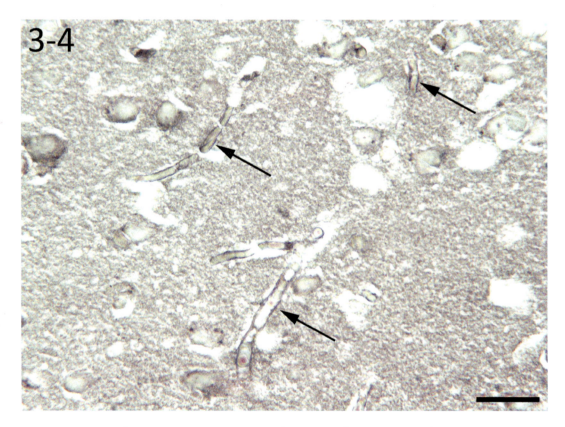

Figure 3.4 In tissue sections, silver stains (e.g., Grocott's methenamine silver stain) may also stain normal structures, such as basement membranes, around small vessels/capillaries (arrows). These may be mistaken for hyphae. GMS. Bar = 35 μm.

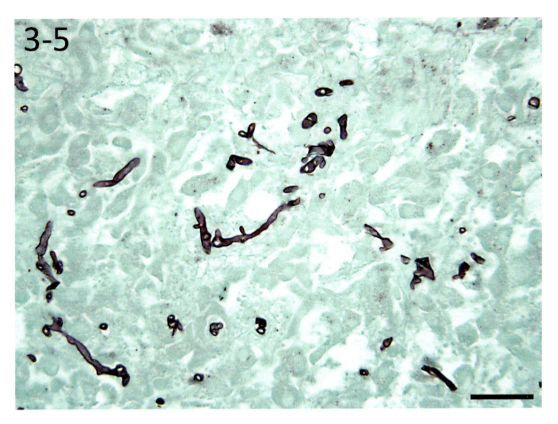

Figure 3.5 If mycosis is suspected, fungal stains should be applied (e.g., Gomori's/Grocott's methenamine silver stain). In most cases, this will highlight the fungal elements (same liver biopsy as in Fig. 3.3). GMS. Bar = 40 µm.

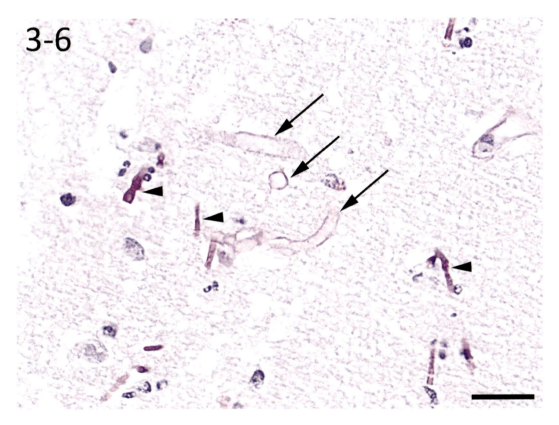

Figure 3.6 Together with the silver stains, the periodic acid-Schiff stain is also widely used to highlight fungal elements, as in this case of cerebral candidosis due to *Candida albicans* (arrowheads). Note that the basement membrane of vessels is faintly stained (arrows) and may be mistaken for hyphae. PAS. Bar = 40 µm.

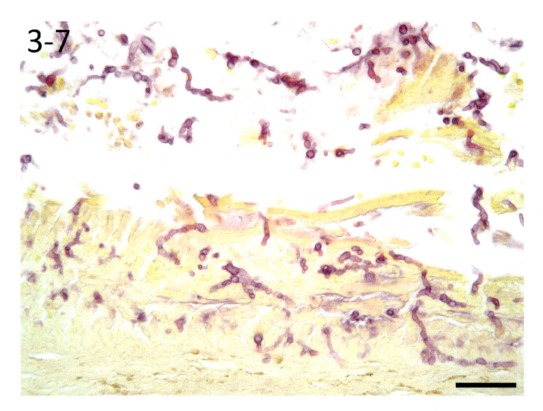

Figure 3.7 Gridley's stain for fungi (GF) may also be used as a standard procedure to visualize fungi. As in the present case of invasive dermal aspergillosis caused by *A. fumigatus*, the fungal elements stain purple/red on a yellow background. GF. Bar = 35 μm.

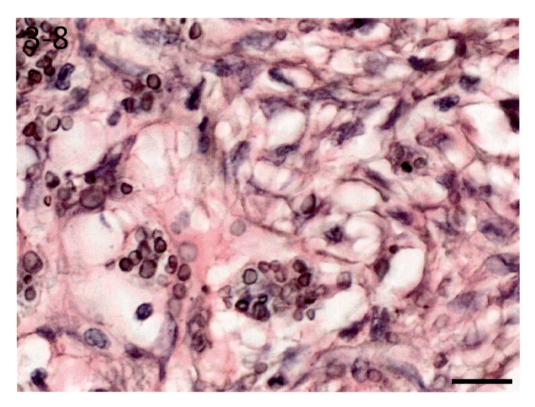

Figure 3.8 Because silver stains may mask the host reaction and the location of fungal elements, optimal visualization may be achieved by counterstaining the silver-stained sections with haematoxylin and eosin. In the present case, pulmonary cryptococcosis was first stained with Grocott's methenamine silver stain and then stained with haematoxylin and eosin. GMS and HE. Bar = 15 μm.

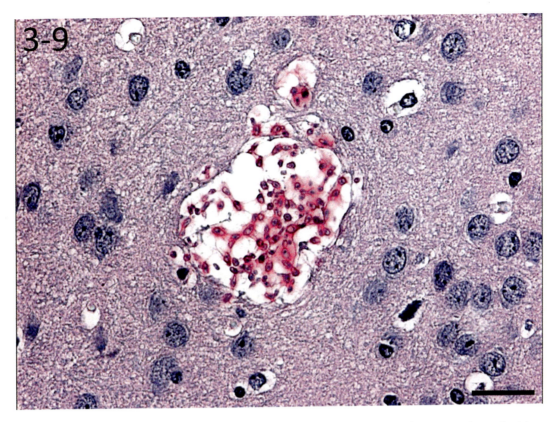

Figure 3.9 Stains for mucin, such as Mayer's mucicarmine (MM), are used to visualize the mucopolysaccharide capsule of *Cryptococcus* spp., as in the present case of cerebral cryptococcosis. MM. Bar = 20 μm.

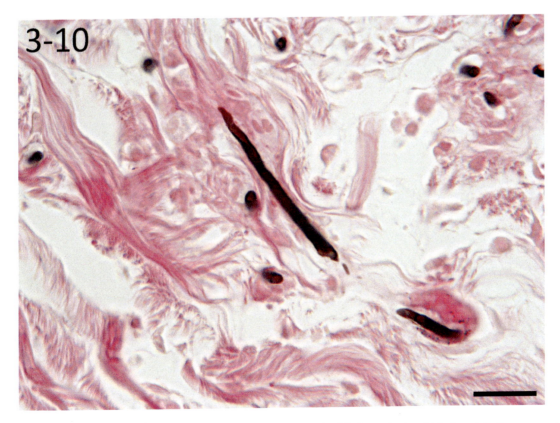

Figure 3.10 The Fontana-Masson (FM) staining procedure is used to highlight melanin within fungi. In the present case of phaeohyphomycosis, the hyphae are stained black by this procedure. FM. Bar = 35 μm.

actinomycotic infection, or that might be the primary cause of the disease (e.g., botryomycosis) (3). Some fungi are usually Gram-positive, especially the yeast forms of *Candida* spp. and the conidia of *Aspergillus* spp.

Because *Nocardia* spp. are weakly acid-fast and non-alcohol-fast in tissue sections, these filamentous bacteria can be distinguished from the non-acid-fast pathogens that cause actinomycosis. In tissue, organisms stain red and blue when acid and non-acid fast, respectively (Fig. 3.12). The cytoplasm of some fungi with yeast-like tissue forms may also be acid-fast, especially *B. dermatitidis* and *Histoplasma capsulatum* var. *capsulatum* (15).

The staining properties and limitations of the most frequently used histological stains are listed in Table 3.1.

Some fungi in paraffin-embedded or freshly frozen tissue sections can be stained using optical brighteners that have a diaminostilbene backbone structure and fluorescence under ultraviolet light. Brighteners such as Calcofluor White M2R, Blankophor, and Uvitex 2B are often used (2, 16). Most of these fluorescent brighteners have an affinity for particular glycosidic linkages in the polysaccharide fungal cell wall. However, whitening agents do not always highlight fungi; therefore, only positive results from these compounds can be used for a definitive diagnosis of "mycosis" (Figs. 3.13 and 3.14). There is no advantage in using whitening agents compared with the rapid methenamine silver techniques to detect fungi in tissue sections (17).

Cytological specimens may be used to discover fungal elements in invasive mycoses. These specimens include bronchoalveolar lavage fluid, cerebrospinal fluid, sputum, and fine-needle aspirates (7). Smears may be examined without any staining. However, a 20 min treatment with 10% KOH can destroy tissue cells and reveal fungi. KOH treatment is generally used for superficial mycoses. Staining with Indian ink is only used on smears, especially spinal fluid containing *Cryptococcus* spp., which appear as brilliant white halos on a black background.

Cytological specimens are often stained using traditional stains, such as Giemsa, Wright, and May-Grunwald stains. However, stains that have been traditionally used on tissue sections may also be applied, such as PAS and GMS.

Staining procedures are described in standard manuals and textbooks of histochemistry and histological techniques (5, 6).

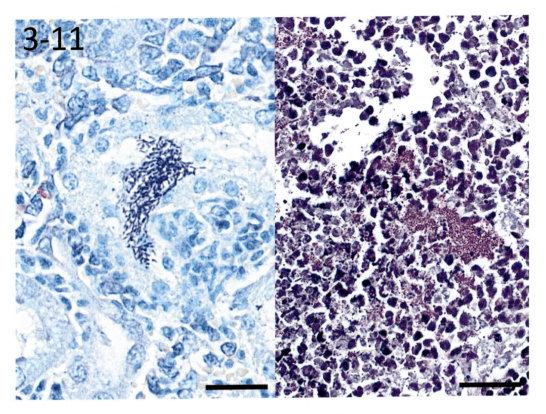

Figure 3.11 The Gram stains are used to differentiate Gram-positive and Gram-negative bacteria in tissue sections. In the present cases, Gram-positive bacteria (purple/blue) are visible on the left, within the lumen of a kidney tubule. On the right, Gram-negative bacteria are visible in the neutrophilic exudate. Gram. Bar = 15 μm.

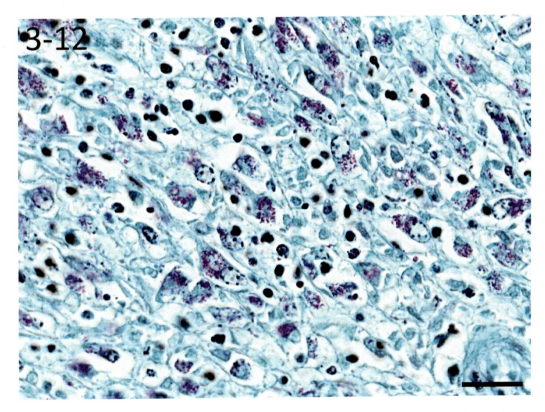

Figure 3.12 The acid-fast stains (e.g., Ziehl-Neelsen [ZN]) are primarily used to differentiate acid-fast and non-acid-fast bacteria in tissue sections. In the present case of paratuberculosis, acid-fast bacteria (red) are visible within macrophages. ZN. Bar = 20 μm.

Table 3.1 Properties and limitations of frequently used histological stains

Histological stain	Result	Limitations
Haematoxylin and eosin (HE) (Figs. 3.1–3.3)	Many fungi show pink cytoplasm and blue nuclei; tissue reaction visible; innate colour of fungus visible; shows Splendore–Hoeppli material	Not all fungal cells stain; some stain poorly. Natural pigment visible
Gomori's/Grocott's methenamine silver stain (GMS) (Figs. 3.4, 3.5, and 3.8)	Fungi brown/black; old and non-viable fungi stain also; filaments of *Actinomyces* spp. and *Nocardia* spp. stain positive; combined GMS and HE very useful	Innate fungal colour not visible; tissue response and internal details of fungi not visible
Periodic acid-Schiff (PAS) (Fig. 3.6)	Fungi stain pink/red with blue nuclei	Some polysaccharides in the tissue will also be stained
Gridley's stain for fungi (GF) (Fig. 3.7)	Fungi stain purple/red	Innate fungus colour not visible
Fontana–Masson (FM) (Fig. 3.10)	Stains melanin in fungi and tissues	Dematiaceous fungi and *Cryptococcus* spp. are stained dark brown to black
Mucicarmine (Mayer or Southgate) (MM) (Fig. 3.9)	Stains mucopolysaccharides, special stain for *Cryptococcus* spp. (mucoid capsule stains red; Alcian blue can also be used, and then the capsule is stained blue)	*Cryptococcus* spp. without capsule may not stain; one layer of *R. seeberi* stains
Gram stains (Brown and Brenner, MacCallum and Goodpasture, Weigert) (Gram) (Fig. 3.11)	Many fungi are stained or partly stained; *Actinomyces* spp. and *Nocardia* spp. and other bacteria stain positive; pathogens that cause botryomycosis stain positive	Most fungal elements are not stained selectively; *Candida* spp. stain purple/blue
Acid-fast stains (Kinyoun, Fite-Faraco, Ziehl-Neelsen) (ZN) (Fig. 3.12)	*Nocardia* spp. mostly positive; valuable for *Mycobacterium tuberculosis*, *Mycobacterium* subspecies, and *M. leprae*	Fungi are generally not acid-fast. Pathogens that cause blastomycosis and histoplasmosis may stain red (partly acid-fast)
Fluorescent brighteners (Calcofluor White 2R, Blankophor, Uvitex 2B) (Figs. 3.13 and 3.14)	Depending on the filters used in the fluorescence microscopic analysis, fungi are stained green or blue	Because fluorescent brighteners have an affinity for polysaccharides, some polysaccharides in tissue may also be stained

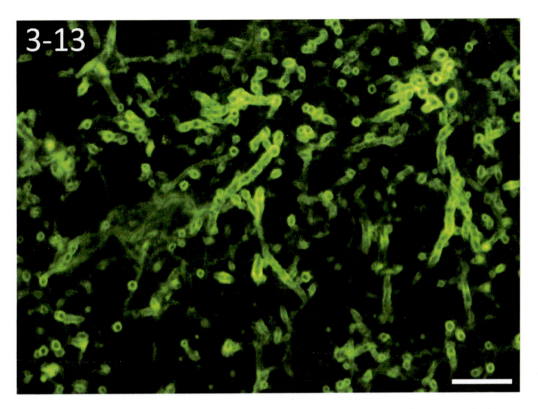

Figure 3.13 Fluorescent staining of fungi in tissue sections using an optical brightener. The stains, which are not specific, are used to screen clinical specimens and tissue sections for fungal elements. This section is derived from a case of chronic pulmonary aspergillosis caused by *A. fumigatus*. Fluorescence. Bar = 20 μm.

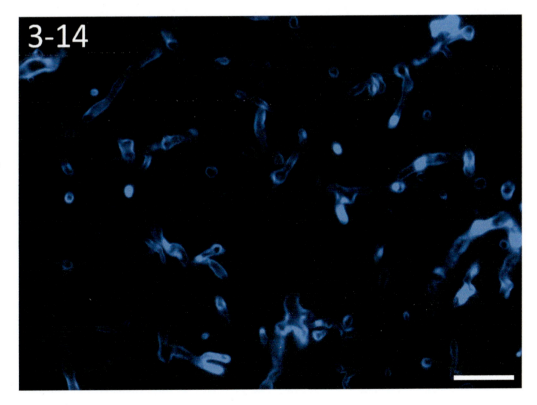

Figure 3.14 Fluorescent staining of fungi in tissue sections using an optical brightener. The stains, which are not specific, are used to screen clinical specimens and tissue sections for fungal elements. This section is derived from a case of chronic mucormycotic nephritis caused by *Lichtheimia corymbifera*. Fluorescence. Bar = 20 μm.

REFERENCES

1. Matsumoto T, Ajello L, Matsuda T, Szaniszlo PJ, Walshet TJ. 1994. Developments in hyalohyphomycosis and phaeohyphomycosis. J Med Vet Mycol, 32, Suppl. 1, 329–349.

2. Jensen HE. 1994. Systemic bovine aspergillosis, and zygomycosis in Denmark with reference to pathogenesis, pathology, and diagnosis. APMIS, 102, Suppl. 42, 1–48.

3. Chandler FW, Watts JC. 1987. Pathologic Diagnosis of Fungal Infections. ASCP Press.

4. Salfelder K. 1990. Atlas of Fungal Pathology. Kluwer Academic Publishers.

5. Suvarna SK, Layton C, Bancroft JD (Eds). 2019. Bancroft's Theory and Practice of Histological Techniques. 8th ed. Elsevier.

6. Wick MR (Ed). 2008. Diagnostic Histochemistry. Cambridge University Press.

7. Jensen HE, Chandler FW. 2007. Histopathological diagnoses of mycoses. In: Topley and Wilson's, Microbiology & Microbial Infections. Medical Mycology. 10th ed. Merz WG, Hay RJ, Eds. Hodder Arnold. pp 121–143.

8. Jensen HE. 2021. Histopathology in the diagnosis of invasive fungal diseases. Curr Fungal Infect Rep, 15, 23–31.

9. Guarner J, Brandt, ME. 2011. Histopathologic diagnosis of fungal infections in the 21st century. Clin Microbiol Rev, 24, 247–280.

10. Kwon-Chung KJ, Hill WB, Bennett JE. 1981. New, special stain for histopathological diagnosis of cryptococcosis. J Clin Microbiol, 13, 383–387.

11. Wheeler MH, Bell AA. 1987. Melanins and their importance in pathogenic fungi. Curr Topics Med Mycol, 2, 338–387.

12. Dixon DM, Szaniszlo PJ, Polak A. 1991. Dihydroxynaphthalene (DHN) melanin and its relationship with virulence in the early stages of phaeohyphomycosis. In: The Fungal Spore and Disease Initiation in Plants and Animals. Cole GT, Hoch HC, Eds. Plenum Press. pp 297–318.

13. Ro JY, Lee SS, Ayala AG. 1987. Advantage of Fontana–Masson stain in capsule-deficient cryptococcal infection. Arch Pathol Lab Med, 111, 53–57.

14. Wood C, Russel-Bell B. 1983. Characterization of pigmented fungi by melanin staining. Am J Dermatopathol, 5, 77–81.

15. Wages DS, Wear DJ. 1982. Acid-fastness of fungi in blastomycosis and histoplasmosis. Arch Pathol Lab Med, 106, 440–441.

16. Monheit JE, Cowan DF, Moore DG. 1984. Rapid detection of fungi in tissues using calcofluor white and fluorescence microscopy. Arch Pathol Lab Med, 108, 616–618.

17. Shimono LH, Harman B. 1986. A simple and reliable rapid methenamine silver stain for *Pneumocystis carinii* and fungi. Arch Pathol Lab Med, 110, 855–856.

4

Pathomorphological identification of invasive fungi

Due to their relatively large size, polysaccharide content, and morphological characteristics, fungal elements are often readily detected in tissue sections; in other cases, they may be identified by conventional light microscopy (1, 2). As described in the chapter on histopathological classification of invasive mycoses, fungi and related pathogens identified in tissue sections may be grouped as follows: A) fungi with clear or light-coloured (hyaline) septate hyphae; B) the presence of coloured fungal elements (dematiaceous/phaeoid fungi); C) the presence of similar characteristic clinicopathological lesions that are caused by both fungi and bacteria, that is, mycetomas caused by hyphae or yeasts (eumycotic mycetomas) or by bacteria (actinomycotic mycetomas); D) the presence of predominantly yeast-like cells; E) the presence of large spherules; and F) the sporadic and rare mycoses, which may be present in any of the patterns described above, as well as the algoses, which are traditionally included in mycopathology.

In pathology, grouping mycoses into broad morphological categories is useful for histopathological differential diagnoses of invasive mycoses. When fungal elements are correctly grouped, an infection may be identified at the genus or even species level by its defining morphology, tinctorial features, and the accompanying host reaction (1, 3). However, some yeast-like pathogens and hyphal tissue forms appear similar in tissue sections. Moreover, the appearance of hyphae in sections is often influenced by steric orientation, the age of the hyphae, the type of infected tissue, and the host response (4). For some mycoses, techniques such as immunohistochemistry, *in situ* hybridization, or polymerase chain reaction (PCR) are necessary to make a diagnosis. Such techniques are often needed to differentiate between, for example, aspergillosis, fusariosis, and scedosporiosis (Figs. 4.1–4.3) (5, 6).

For several invasive mycoses, it is crucial to obtain a reliable diagnosis as quickly as possible to implement the most appropriate therapy and understand the prognostic implications (6, 7). For some invasive mycoses, pathogens can be identified in tissue sections based on their morphological characteristics. If a sufficient number of typical elements are identified, an overall etiological diagnosis may be obtained. This is feasible for diseases such as adiaspiromycosis, blastomycosis, coccidioidomycosis, cryptococcosis, histoplasmosis

capsulati, histoplasmosis duboisii, lacaziosis, paracoccidioidomycosis, talaromycosis marneffei, rhinosporidiosis, sporotrichosis species, sporotrichosis luriei, and pneumocystosis (1, 3, 5, 6). When screening sections with yeast-like elements, the size, shape, number of buds (if present), attachment of buds, presence of schizogony, thickness of the cell wall, presence of pseudohyphae and/or hyphae, number of nuclei within cells, and mucicarmine reaction should be noted (Fig. 4.4). For other invasive mycoses, lesions may be caused by several members of a genus that are morphologically similar in tissue specimens. Diseases caused by these fungi include candidosis and trichosporonosis, two diseases that are difficult to distinguish (1, 6). Obtaining a reliable diagnosis based solely on histopathological observations is extremely difficult for fungi that form hyaline hyphae. The width, contours, pattern of branching, orientation of branches, and septation frequency must be noted when screening sections with hyaline hyphae (Fig. 4.5). Obviously, the characteristics of fungal elements in aspergillosis, fusariosis, scedosporiosis, lomentosporiosis, and the rarely observed pathogens that cause hyalohyphomycoses cannot be reliably differentiated pathomorphologically (3, 6). Moreover, aspergillosis, fusariosis, and scedosporiosis may be difficult to differentiate and in some cases be misinterpreted as mucormycosis or candidosis (8). Some transversely sectioned hyphae may appear yeast-like (Fig. 4.6). In such cases, it may be necessary to melt the tissue out of the paraffin block, reposition the tissue before embedding it again, and cut it at an angle that is perpendicular to the original cut. Necrotic and chronic lesions may contain atypical and bizarre fungal elements due to hypoxia, necrosis, or antifungal therapy. These elements may render a reliable diagnosis impossible, apart from confirming the presence of an invasive mycosis (Fig. 4.7) (3). If morphological structures cannot be identified, the disease may be classified at a particular level (e.g., chromoblastomycosis, hyalohyphomycosis, or phaeohyphomycosis). In such cases, the application of immunohistochemical techniques, specific probes for *in situ* hybridization, or samples may be taken from a paraffin block for PCR to make a more specific diagnosis (5, 8, 9). The possibility of dual fungal infections may be resolved by identifying each pathogen using immunohistochemistry and/or *in situ* hybridization (Figs. 4.8–4.10) (5, 8).

DOI: 10.1201/9781003306177-4

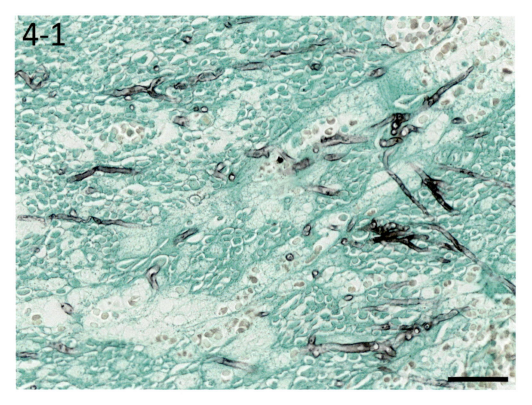

Figure 4.1 The form of hyphae found in tissues affected by aspergillosis, fusariosis, and scedosporiosis is similar. Compare the hyphae from this case of aspergillosis with those from cases of fusariosis (Fig. 4.2) and scedosporiosis (Fig. 4.3). GMS. Bar = 50 μm.

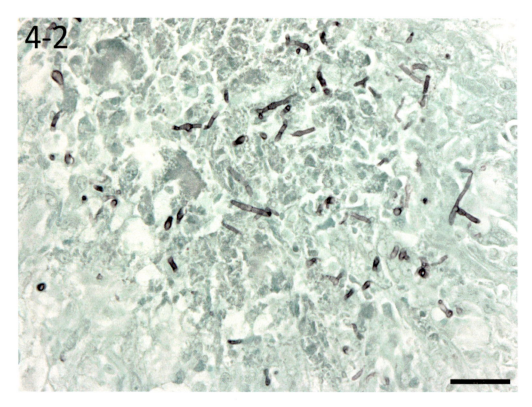

Figure 4.2 The form of hyphae found in tissues affected by aspergillosis, fusariosis, and scedosporiosis is similar. Compare the hyphae from this case of fusariosis with those from cases of aspergillosis (Fig. 4.1) and scedosporiosis (Fig. 4.3). GMS. Bar = 50 μm.

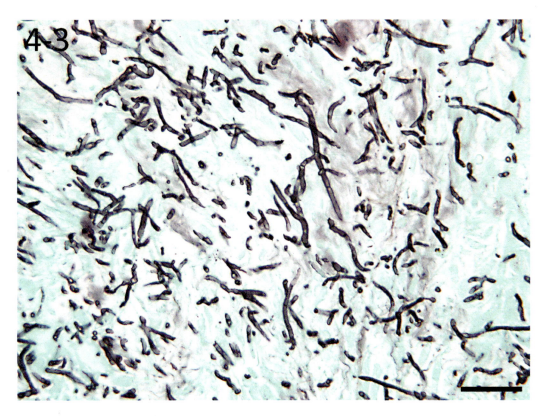

Figure 4.3 The form of hyphae found in tissues affected by aspergillosis, fusariosis, and scedosporiosis is similar. Compare the hyphae from this case of scedosporiosis with those from cases of aspergillosis (Fig. 4.1) and fusariosis (Fig. 4.2). GMS. Bar = 50 μm.

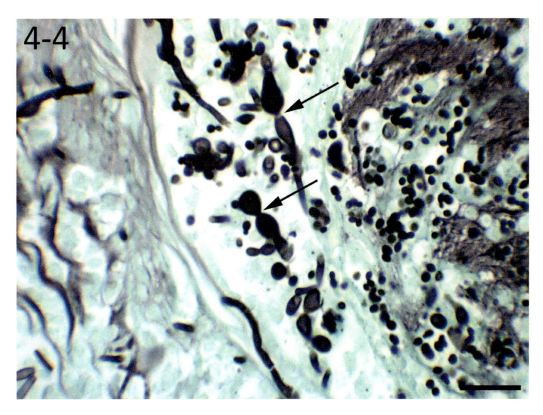

Figure 4.4 Pseudohyphae are elongated chains of buds that fail to separate (arrows). These are exhibited by various fungal genera, as in the present case of candidosis due to *C. albicans*. GMS. Bar = 35 μm.

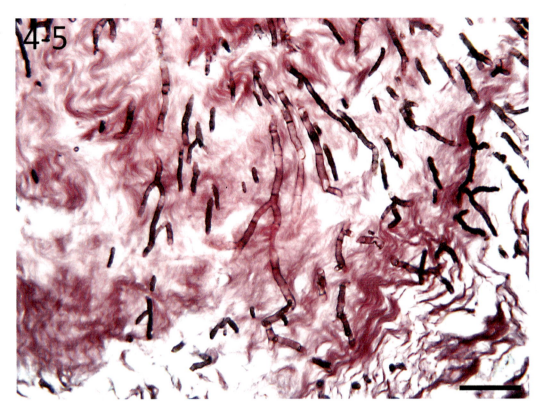

Figure 4.5 When screening sections with hyaline hyphae, the width, contours, pattern of branching, orientation of branches, and septation frequency should be noted. An aspergillosis case due to *A. fumigatus* with characteristic hyphal features is shown. GMS and HE. Bar = 30 μm.

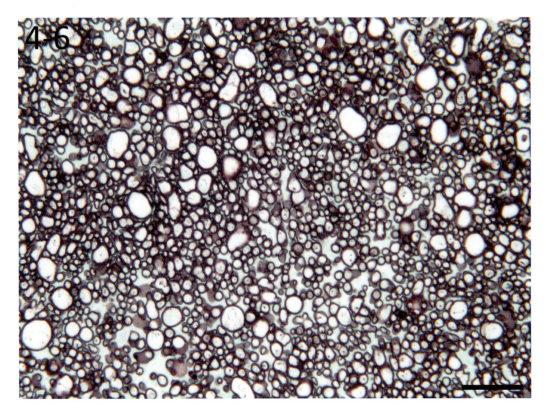

Figure 4.6 Cross-sectioned hyphae may be similar to yeast-like elements, as in this case of pulmonary aspergillosis caused by *A. fumigatus*. GMS. Bar = 30 μm.

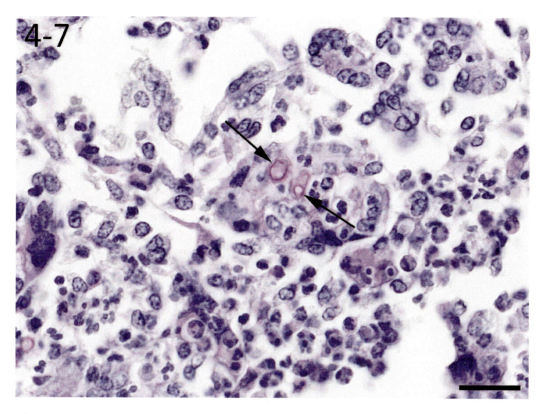

Figure 4.7 In chronic lesions, atypical unidentifiable fungal forms (arrows) are often present, as in this case of pulmonary aspergillosis. PAS. Bar = 25 μm.

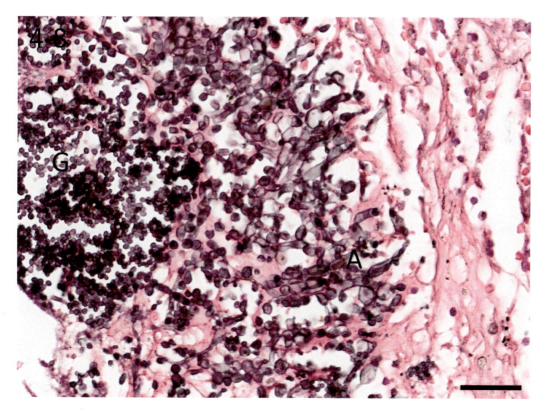

Figure 4.8 The presence of different fungi within the same lesion should be determined by immunohistochemistry and/or *in situ* hybridization. In this case of intestinal candidosis, elements of both *C. albicans* (A) and *C. glabrata* (G) are visible. Compare with Fig. 4.9. GMS and HE. Bar = 25 μm.

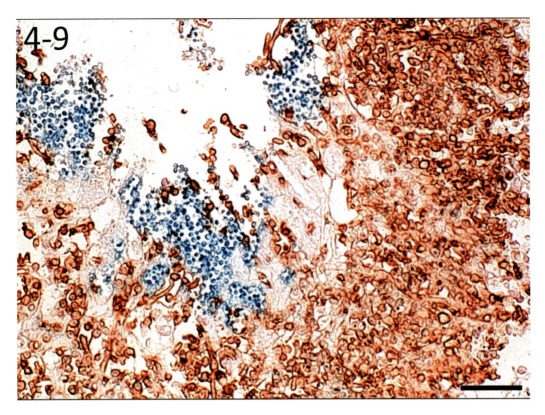

Figure 4.9 Immunohistochemical identification of *C. albicans* (3,3'-diaminobenzidine, brown) and *C. glabrata* (5-bromo-4-chloro-3-indolyl β-D-galactopyranoside, blue) within the same intestinal candidosis lesion as shown in Fig. 4.8. IHC. Bar = 20 µm.

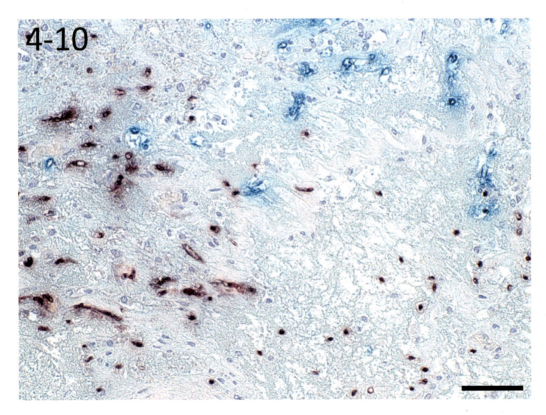

Figure 4.10 A dual infection of aspergillosis (brown stained hyphae) and mucormycosis (blue stained hyphae) as demonstrated immunohistochemically by two different chromogens: brown (3,3'-diaminobenzidine) and blue (5-bromo-4-chloro-3-indolyl β-D-galactopyranoside). IHC. Bar = 40 µm

Conidial heads are sometimes formed in solid organs, especially those accessible to air in the upper respiratory tract (sinus system) and within cavities of the lung (Fig. 4.11). Fungal species may be identified from the morphology of these conidial heads (fructification bodies) (1). In lesions, deposits of calcium oxalate crystals, which are birefringent, may be used to identify *Aspergillus niger* (1). In other cases, infection with *A. niger* may cause generalized oxalosis (1).

Mycetomas constitute a distinct type of disease that is characterized by clinicopathological lesions that are caused by either fungi (eumycotic mycetomas) or bacteria (actinomycotic mycetomas) (1). Regardless of the cause, mycetomas contain granules of various colours. Studying these granules in appropriately stained sections should reveal whether the pathogen is an actinomycete (i.e., a branched, filamentous bacterium) or a eumycete (i.e., a true fungus) and, if a eumycete, whether it is hyaline (white grained) or phaeoid (black grained). The microscopic architecture, size, shape, and colour of the granules are correlated with the pathogen, and each species, with a few exceptions, forms its own distinctive type of granule (10). Therefore, the gross and microscopic appearance of granules may provide specialists with insight into the identity of the organisms involved. Although morphological appearance may indicate a particular etiological diagnosis for the mycetoma, definitive identification of invasive pathogens should, whenever possible, be based on microbiological culture (3).

As shown in Table 4.1, mycoses are grouped according to the histomorphological features of the common pathogenic fungi and related microorganisms in order to facilitate differential diagnoses. Because diseases caused by algae are traditionally included in medical mycology, these are described too.

Although particular patterns of inflammation, such as acute necrosis with or without suppuration, abscess formation, granuloma formation, and pyogranulomatous inflammatory reactions (Figs. 4.12–4.14), may suggest a fungal infection, there are no clear histological criteria for making an etiological diagnosis based only on the host response. In addition, inflammatory patterns are often atypical and unreliable in immunodeficient patients. Furthermore, the travel history of a patient may help to resolve diagnoses because the geographic distribution of some pathogenic fungi is limited (11).

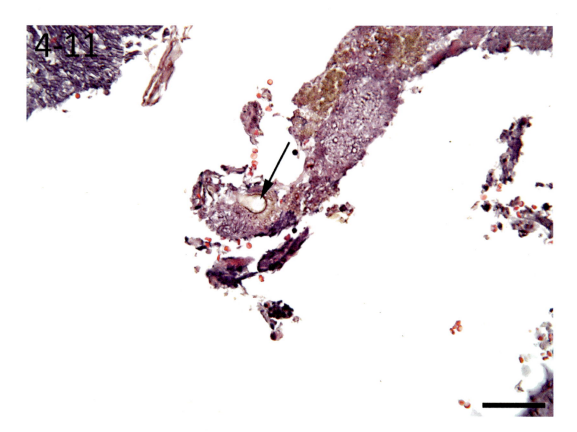

Figure 4.11 The morphology of conidial heads (fructification/fruiting bodies [arrow]) may be used to identify fungal species, as in the present case of A. *fumigatus* sinusitis. HE. Bar = 100 μm.

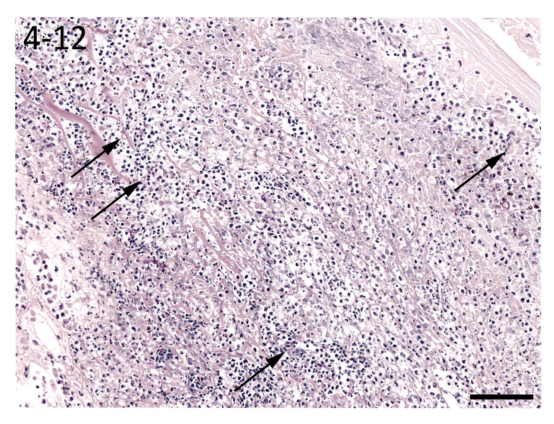

Figure 4.12 Acute, necrotizing, and suppurative inflammation may be due to numerous infectious etiologies including fungi (arrows). This case of panophthalmitis was caused by *F. solani*. HE. Bar = 125 μm.

Table 4.1 Histomorphological features of fungi and related pathogens in tissue sections

A. Presence of fungi with clear or light-coloured (hyaline) septate hyphae		
Mycosis	**Pathogen(s)**	**Typical morphology in tissue**
Aspergillosis	A. fumigatus, A. flavus, A. niger, and others	Septate, dichotomously branched hyphae of uniform width (3–6 μm); conidial heads sometimes formed in cavity lesions with access to air. Calcium oxalate crystals may be present in the case of A. niger
Fusariosis	Fusarium solani, F. oxysporum, F. verticillioides (moniliforme), and others	The width of Fusarium hyphae is 3–8 μm, and these often have constrictions that are involved in the formation of septa and may contain local vesicles within the hyphae
Scedosporiosis/lomentosporiosis	Scedosporium apiospermum (asexual state of Pseudallescheria boydii), S. boydii, S. aurantiacum, Lomentospora prolificans, and others	Septate, randomly branched hyphae, 2–5 μm wide; conidia of scedosporium type may be formed in cavity lesions. Hyphae of Lomentospora may appear melanized
Mucormycosis	Mucor, Rhizopus, Lichtheimia, Rhizomucor, Cunninghamella, and others	Broad, thin-walled, aseptate or infrequently septate hyphae, 6–25 μm wide, with non-parallel contours and random branches. Sporangia sometimes formed in cavity lesions with access to air
Entomophthoromycosis	Basidiobolus spp., Conidiobolus spp.	Frequently septate, 6–12 (up to 30) μm irregular, random and haphazard branching, moderate to thick-walled hyphae. Often covered with Splendore-Hoeppli material
Pythiosis	Pythium insidiosum	Infrequently septate, 5–10 μm irregular, random and radial, and haphazard branching with moderate to thick-walled hyphae. Often covered with Splendore-Hoeppli material
Hyalohyphomycosis, minor	Pathogenic members of the genera Paecilomyces, Purpureocillium, Gliomastix, Scopulariopsis, Penicillium, Trichoderma, Schizophyllum, Geotrichum candidum, and others	Septate, branched, hyaline hyphae, 2–10 μm wide, usually dichotomous with irregular contours, and random branches. Genus dependent, and other forms may apply too
B. Presence of coloured fungal elements (dematiaceous/phaeoid fungi)		
Mycosis	**Pathogen(s)**	**Typical morphology in tissue**
Phaeohyphomycosis	Bipolaris spicifera, Cladophialophora bantiana, Exophiala jeanselmei, Phialophora parasitica, and other phaeoid fungi	Phaeoid (brown) hyphae, 2–6 μm wide, may be branched and are often constricted at their frequent and prominent septations; phaeoid yeast forms and chlamydoconidia sometimes present.
Chromoblastomycosis	C. carrionii, Fonsecaea compacta, F. pedrosoi, P. verrucosa, Rhinocladiella aquaspersa, and others	Large, 6–12 μm in diameter, spherical to polyhedral, thick-walled, dark-brown, muriform cells (sclerotic bodies) with septations along one or two planes; phaeoid hyphae sometimes present

(Continued)

Table 4.1 Histomorphological features of fungi and related pathogens in tissue sections (Continued)

C. Presence of mycetomas

Mycosis/actinomycosis	Pathogen(s)	Typical morphology in tissue
Eumycotic mycetomas (eumycetomas) due to true fungi	Acremonium spp., Aspergillus spp., Curvularia geniculata, E. jeanselmei, Leptosphaeria senegalensis, Madurella grisea, M. mycetomatis, Neotestudina rosatii, P. boydii, Pyrenochaeta romeroi, and others	Granules, 0.2 mm to several millimetres in diameter, composed of broad (2–6 μm), hyaline or phaeoid, and septate hyphae that often branch and form chlamydoconidia
Actinomycotic mycetomas (actinomycetomas) due to filamentous bacterial pathogens	Actinomadura madurae, A. pelletieri, Nocardia spp., Nocardiopsis dassonvillei, Streptomyces somaliensis, and others	Granules, 0.1 to several mm in diameter, composed of delicate Gram-positive filaments, less than 0.1 μm wide, which are often branched and beaded

D. Presence of yeast-like cells

Mycosis	Pathogen(s)	Typical morphology in tissue
Candidosis	Candida albicans, C. guilliermondii, C. krusei, C. parapsilosis, C. pseudotropicalis (kefyr), C. tropicalis, and others	Spherical to oval, budding, yeast-like cells (blastoconidia), 3–6 μm in diameter; pseudohyphae; and septate hyphae
	C. glabrata	Spherical to oval yeast-like cells 2–5 μm in diameter
Trichosporonosis	Trichosporon asahii, T. inkin	Pleomorphic yeast-like cells, 3–8 μm in diameter; septate hyphae; and, rarely, arthroconidia
Cryptococcosis	Cryptococcus neoformans spp. and C. gattii	Pleomorphic yeast-like cells, 2–20 μm in diameter, with mucin-positive capsules and single or, rarely, multiple narrow-based buds; some strains are capsule deficient and their capsular material may not be detected with mucin stain
Blastomycosis	Blastomyces dermatitidis	Spherical, multinucleate, yeast-like cells, 7–15 μm in diameter, with thick walls and single, broad-based buds. Microforms of 2–4 μm may be formed
Histoplasmosis capsulati	Histoplasma capsulatum var. capsulatum	Spherical to oval, uninucleate, yeast-like cells, 2–4 μm in diameter; often clustered because of growth within mononuclear phagocytes
Histoplasmosis duboisii	H. capsulatum var. duboisii	Spherical to oval, uninucleate, yeast-like cells, 6–12 μm diameter, which have thick walls and bud by a narrow base, creating typical "hour-glass" or "figure-of-eight" forms
Paracoccidioidomycosis	Paracoccidioides brasiliensis and P. lutzii	Large, spherical, yeast-like cells, 5–60 μm in diameter, with multiple buds attached by narrow necks ("steering wheel" forms)
Sporotrichosis	Sporothrix schenckii spp. complex	Pleomorphic, spherical to oval, and, at times, "cigar"-shaped yeast forms, 2–10 μm in diameter, which produce single and, rarely, multiple buds
	Sporothrix luriei	Hyaline, large (10–20 μm), thick-walled yeast forms together with the typical "eyeglass" configuration of incompletely separated cells

(Continued)

Table 4.1 Histomorphological features of fungi and related pathogens in tissue sections (Continued)

Mycosis	Pathogen(s)	Typical morphology in tissue
Talaromycosis	Talaromyces (Penicillium) marneffei	Spherical to oval or elongated yeast-like cells, 2.5–5 μm in diameter, with a single transverse septum; short hyphal forms and elongated, curved "sausage" forms with one or more septa may be formed in necrotic and cavity lesions
Pneumocystosis	Pneumocystis jirovecii (P. carinii in animals)	Thin-walled spherical, oval trophic form is 2–10 μm in diameter; cysts are thick walled, 4–6 μm in diameter
Lacaziosis	Lacazia (Loboa) loboi	Spherical, budding, yeast-like cells, 5–12 μm in diameter, that form chains of cells, each connected by a narrow tube-like isthmus; secondary budding is sometimes present
E. Presence of large spherules		
Mycosis	**Pathogen(s)**	**Typical morphology in tissue**
Adiaspiromycosis	Chrysosporium parvum var. crescens	Large adiaconidia, 200–400 μm in diameter, with thick (22–25 μm) walls; budding and endosporulation do not occur
Coccidioidomycosis	Coccidioides immitis and C. posadasii	Spherical, thick-walled, endosporulating spherules, 20–200 μm in diameter; mature spherules contain small, 2–5 μm in diameter, uninucleate endospores; septate hyphae and chains of arthroconidia sometimes occur in necrotic nodules
Rhinosporidiosis	Rhinosporidium seeberi	Large sporangia, 100–400 μm in diameter, with thin walls (3–5 μm) that enclose numerous sporangiospores, 6–10 μm in diameter
F. Rare mycoses and algoses		
Mycosis	**Pathogen(s)**	**Typical morphology in tissue**
Rare mycoses	Malassezia, Sporobolomyces, Rhodotorula, Pseudozyma (renamed Moesziomyces), Saccharomyces, Saprochaete, Kodamaea, the invasive forms of Alternaria and Phialemonium, Emergomyces spp., and others	Depending on the species, these may take any form described in classifications A–E of the chapter on the histopathological classification of invasive mycoses. A diagnosis should only be made after histopathological verification of tissue invasion by fungi, with morphology confirmed by repeated cultivation and/or molecular evidence
Algoses	Prototheca wickerhamii, P. ciferrii, P. bovis, and P. blaschkeae (the last three formerly known as P. zopfii)	Spherical, oval, or polyhedral sporangia, 7–30 μm in diameter with 2–3 μm halos, that, when mature, contain 2–20 sporangiospores

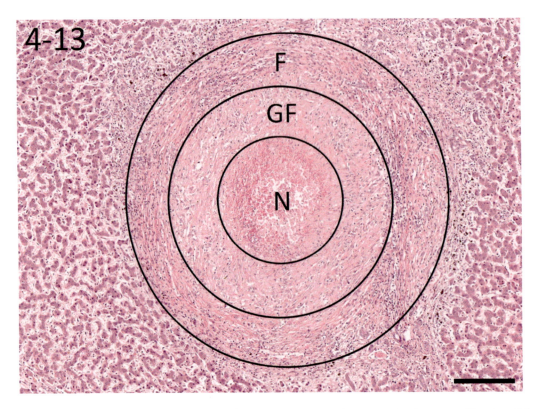

Figure 4.13 Abscesses are usually caused by pyogenic bacteria. However, they may also be caused by *Candida* spp., as in the present case of chronic apostematous hepatic candidosis. Around the necrotic centre (N), there is a rim of epithelioid cells and macrophages intermingled with collagen and fibroblasts. A granulomatous-fibrotic reaction (GF) and fibrous tissue (F) are also shown. HE. Bar = 150 μm.

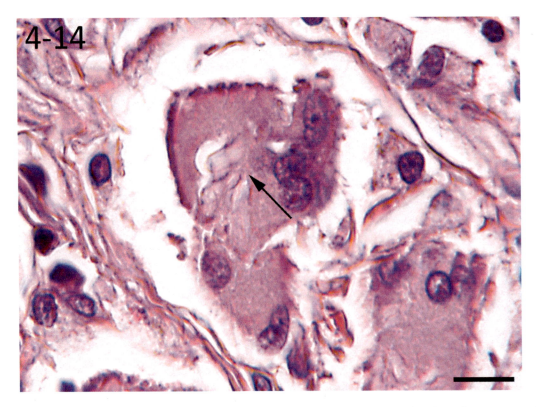

Figure 4.14 Granulomatous inflammation containing macrophages, epithelioid cells, and multinucleate giant cells may develop in several chronic mycoses. In the present case of pythiosis, fungal elements of *P. insidiosum* (arrow) have been phagocytosed by a multinucleate giant cell. HE. Bar = 15 μm.

REFERENCES

1. Salfelder K. 1990. Atlas of Fungal Pathology. Kluwer Academic Publishers.
2. Schwarz J. 1982. The diagnosis of deep mycoses by morphologic methods. Human Pathol, 13, 519–533.
3. Jensen HE, Chandler FW. 2007. Histopathological diagnoses of mycoses. In: Topley and Wilson, Medical Mycology. 10th ed. Merz WG, Hay RJ, Eds. Hodder Arnold. pp 121–143.
4. Jensen HE, Schønheyder H. 1989. Immunofluorescence staining of hyphae in the histopathological diagnosis of mycoses in cattle. J Med Vet Mycol, 27, 33–44.
5. Jensen HE. 2021. Histopathology in the diagnosis of invasive fungal diseases. Curr Fungal Infect Rep, 15, 23–31.
6. Guarner J, Brandt ME. 2011. Histopathologic diagnosis of fungal infections in the 21st century. Clin Microbiol Rev, 24, 247–280.
7. Hospenthal DR. 2015. Approach to patients with suspected fungal infections. In: Diagnosis and Treatment of Fungal Infections. 2nd ed. Hospenthal DR, Rinaldi MG, Eds. pp. 3–7.
8. Jensen HE, Salonen J, Ekfors TO. 1997. The use of immunohistochemistry to improve sensitivity and specificity in the diagnosis of systemic mycoses in patients with haematological malignancies. J Pathol, 181, 100–105.
9. Jensen HE, Schønheyder HC, Hotchi M, Kaufman L. 1996. Diagnosis of systemic mycoses by specific immunohistochemical tests. APMIS, 104, 241–258.
10. Chandler FW, Watts JC.1987. Pathologic Diagnosis of Fungal Infections. ASCP Press.
11. Warnock DW, Dupont B, Kauffman CA, Sirisanthana T. 1998. Imported mycoses in Europe. Med Mycol, Suppl. 1, 36, 87–94.

5

Identification of invasive fungi using
in situ techniques

To specifically identify fungi within a tissue, and thereby make a diagnosis, the pathogen must in many cases be cultured and/or identified by real-time polymerase chain reaction (PCR) assays. However, cultivation and PCR methods do not guarantee a successful diagnosis. These techniques may also provide misleading results due to contamination, even if the material has been collected by laser capture microdissection methods. Ideally, fungi should be identified using *in situ* techniques. However, as described in previous chapters, this may not always be possible based on morphological criteria. Therefore, several *in situ* diagnostic techniques have been developed. These are based on *in situ* recognition of specific fungal antigens (immunohistochemistry) or DNA/RNA sequences (*in situ* hybridization).

IMMUNOHISTOCHEMISTRY

Immunohistochemistry (IHC) techniques detect antigens (epitopes) within tissue sections. These techniques rely on access to primary reagents that are fully characterized in terms of their sensitivity and, in particular, specificity (1). Both direct and indirect protocols are used to obtain immunohistochemical diagnoses of mycoses. To visualize specific reactions, different labelling techniques may be used (e.g., fluorochromes, gold-silver complexes, and enzyme labelling) (1–3). In addition, avidin–biotin enzyme complex (ABC) methods may also be applied (4). Enzyme-labelled techniques are preferred to fluorochrome techniques because the former procedures allow the host's reaction to the fungi to be evaluated simultaneously with the immunoreactivity (1, 4, 5). Furthermore, enzyme-labelled techniques provide permanent slides which can be stored, and fluorescence microscopes are not needed.

Immunohistochemical and/or *in situ* hybridization techniques are the only procedures capable of generating an accurate *in situ* etiological diagnosis for formalin-fixed tissue sections in cases with no morphological markers (4). When the histomorphology of fungal elements within a single lesion or within different organ lesions from the same patient suggests different mycoses, the fungal elements are analyzed to determine whether these are derived from the same genus and species. In such cases, dual/multiple immunostaining and/or *in situ* hybridization may be used to obtain a reliable diagnosis (Fig. 5.1) (4, 5). For example, different *Cryptococcus neoformans* serotypes may be separated within tissues by these techniques, when different specific primary reagents are used (6).

Unfortunately, many of the specific reagents required for immunohistochemistry are not commercially available because these are based on polyclonal reagents and heterologous absorption with cross-reacting antigens may be needed to render them specific (Figs. 5.2 and 5.3) (4). However, specific and highly sensitive monoclonal antibodies are available for the most frequently occurring invasive mycoses, such as candidosis (Fig. 5.4), aspergillosis (Figs. 5.5–5.7), fusariosis (Figs. 5.8 and 5.9), and mucormycosis (Fig. 5.10) (5, 7).

The immunohistochemical methods that are used to identify fungi causing invasive infections are listed in Table 5.1.

IN SITU HYBRIDIZATION

In situ hybridization (ISH) can accurately identify several species of fungi that cause invasive mycoses. This method uses oligonucleotide probes to target specific complementary sequences in the nucleic acids within the fungi (8). Both DNA and RNA sequences can be detected (9). Due to the natural amplification of ribosomal RNA (rRNA) molecules, *in situ* techniques are usually based on probes that target rRNA (10, 11). The rRNA of fungi is highly conserved among species, as it is in other microorganisms. However, the level of sequence variation is sufficient to identify species. When specific probes are available, simple hybridization procedures may be completed inexpensively in only a few hours (12, 13). Because rRNA is fragile and rapidly disintegrates when irreversibly damaged, especially viable cells are targeted. The probes used for *in situ* hybridization are designed to be very specific for the target organism; therefore, unknown species will be negative (14). Universal (pan-fungal) probes may be used initially to screen sections for fungal elements (10, 15). However, standard histochemical stains, such as periodic acid-Schiff and Grocott's methenamine silver, exhibit greater sensitivity in detecting fungi (8).

DOI: 10.1201/9781003306177-5

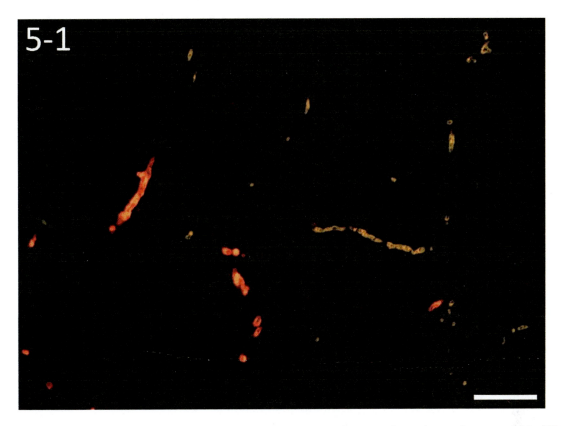

Figure 5.1 Concomitant pulmonary aspergillosis and mucormycosis. Dual immunohistochemical staining with differently labelled specific antibodies towards *Aspergillus* spp. and members of the order Mucorales. The hyphae of aspergillosis are stained green, whereas those of mucormycosis are orange. IHC. Bar = 90 μm.

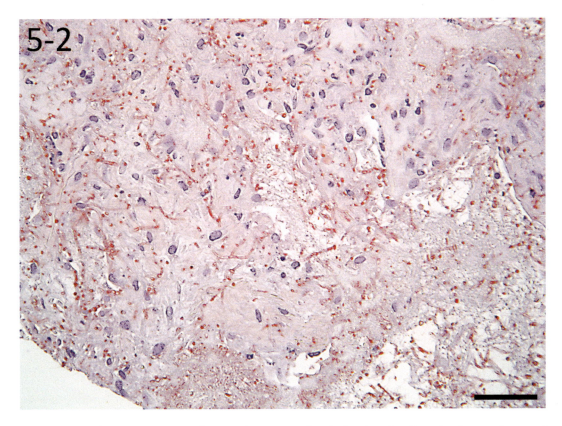

Figure 5.2 Pulmonary scedosporiosis. Heterologous absorption of polyclonal antibodies raised towards somatic antigens of *S. apiospermum* identifies *Scedosporium* hyphae. IHC. Bar = 100 μm.

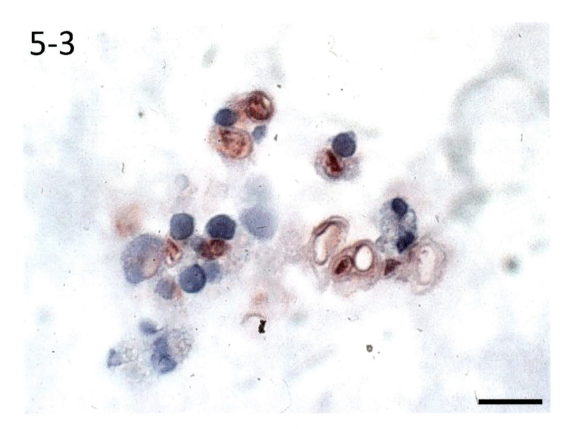

Figure 5.3 Mammary protothecosis. Heterologous absorption of polyclonal antibodies raised towards somatic antigens of *P. bovis* are used to identify the algae. IHC. Bar = 30 μm.

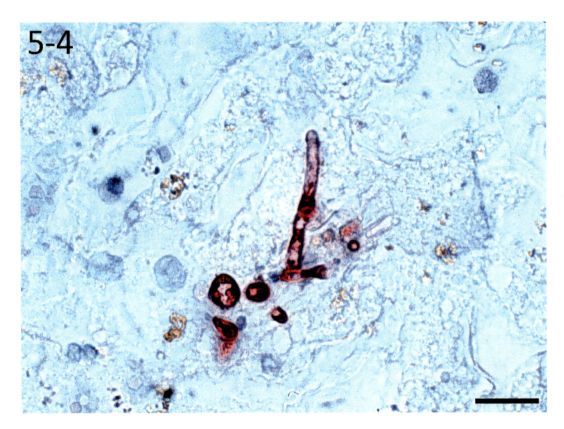

Figure 5.4 Pulmonary candidosis. Specific monoclonal antibodies are suitable for *in situ* identification of *Candida* spp. in tissues. In the present case, *C. albicans* was cultured. IHC. Bar = 10 μm.

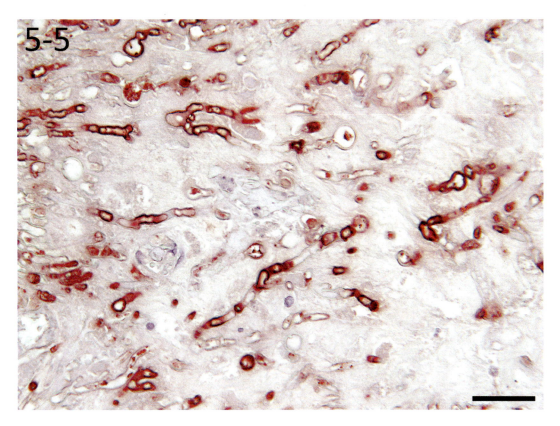

Figure 5.5 Pulmonary aspergillosis. Commercially available monoclonal antibodies can specifically identify hyphae of *Aspergillus* spp. *in situ*. IHC. Bar = 30 μm.

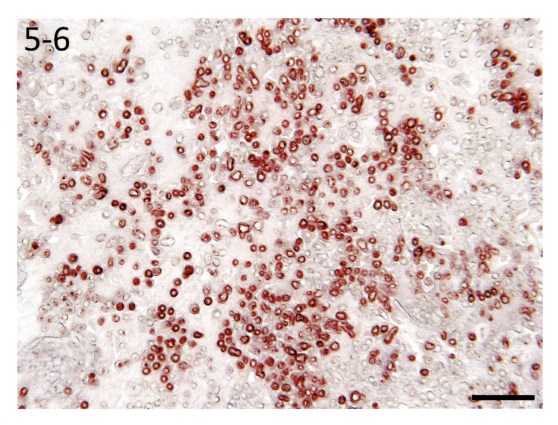

Figure 5.6 Pulmonary aspergillosis. Immunostaining of *Aspergillus* hyphae by specific, commercially available monoclonal antibodies is also valuable when only cross-sectioned hyphae are present. IHC. Bar = 30 μm.

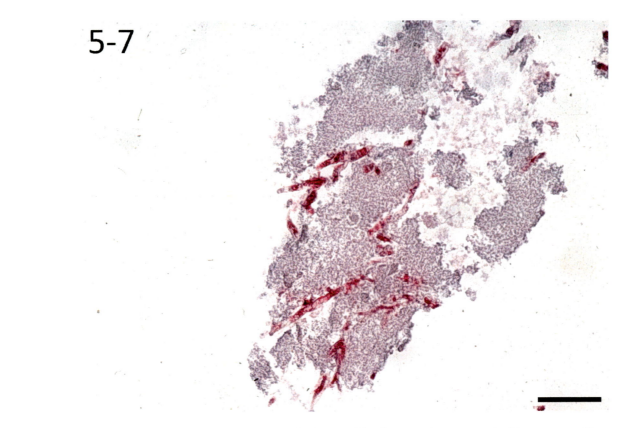

Figure 5.7 Cerebral aspergillosis. In biopsies, only a few atypical hyphae may be present. In this case, specific commercially available monoclonal antibodies towards *Aspergillus* spp. were used to obtain a correct diagnosis *in situ*. IHC. Bar = 50 μm.

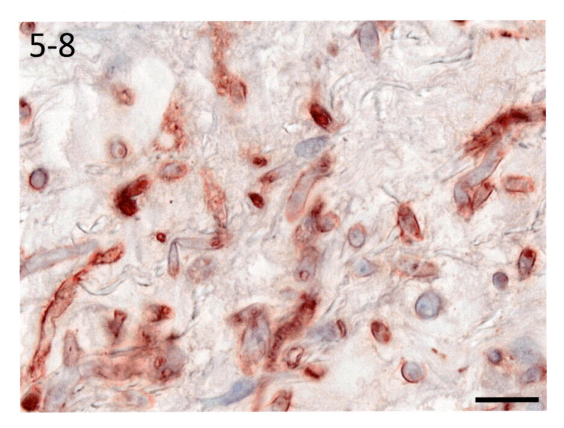

Figure 5.8 Cerebral fusariosis. *In situ* techniques may be used to distinguish *Fusarium* hyphae from those of other organisms, such as *Aspergillus* and *Scedosporium*. IHC. Bar = 20 μm.

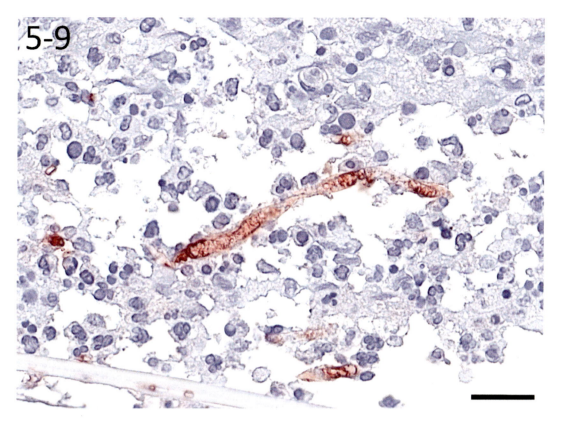

Figure 5.9 Ocular fusariosis. In lesions containing only a few fungal elements, specific *in situ* immunostaining of single hyphae may be necessary to diagnose fusariosis. IHC. Bar = 20 μm.

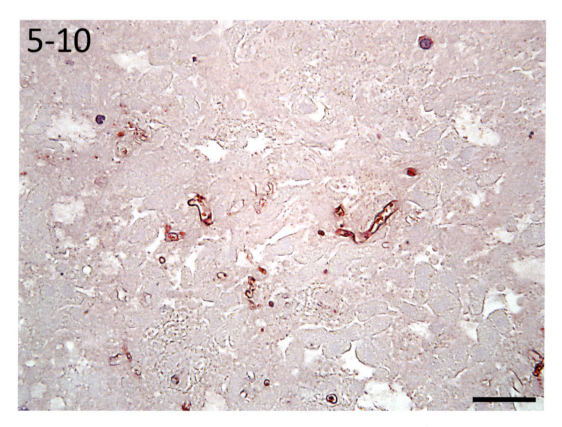

Figure 5.10 Cerebral mucormycosis. For mucormycosis, hyphae may be immunostained *in situ* using commercially available specific monoclonal antibodies. IHC. Bar = 45 μm.

Table 5.1 *In situ* staining methods for invasive fungi

Disease	Targets	*In situ* techniques
Aspergillosis	*Aspergillus* spp. (including *A. fumigatus*, *A. terreus*, *A. niger*, *A. nidulans*, *A. flavus*, and others)	Immunohistochemistry (8, 20–23) *In situ* hybridization (24, 25)
Fusariosis	*Fusarium solani*, *F. oxysporum*, *F. anthophilum*	Immunohistochemistry (8, 22, 23, 26) *In situ* hybridization (19, 24, 27)
Scedosporiosis/ lomentosporiosis	*Scedosporium prolificans*, *S. apiospermum* (*Pseudallescheria boydii*)	Immunohistochemistry (8, 22, 28) *In situ* hybridization (24, 29)
Trichosporonosis	*Trichosporon beigelii*	Immunohistochemistry (23, 26, 30) *In situ* hybridization (31)
Mucormycosis	*Rhizopus microspores*, *R. arrhizus*, *R. oryzae*, *Mucor* spp., *Lichtheimia* spp.	Immunohistochemistry (8, 21, 23, 32) *In situ* hybridization (11, 16)
Pythiosis	*Pythium insidiosum*	Immunohistochemistry (33–45)
Phaeohyphomycosis	*Alternaria* spp., *Bipolaris* spp., *Cladosporium* spp., *Phoma betae*	Immunohistochemistry (46, 47) *In situ* hybridization (16)
Mycetomas	*Curvularia* spp., *Madurella* spp., *S. apiospermum*, *A. fumigatus*	Immunohistochemistry (8, 20–22) *In situ* hybridization (24, 48)
Candidosis	*Candida* spp. (including *C. albicans*, *C. glabrata*, and others)	Immunohistochemistry (8, 23, 30, 47–53) *In situ* hybridization (11, 25, 54, 55)
Cryptococcosis	*C. neoformans*, *C. gattii*	Immunohistochemistry (7, 23, 26, 56–58) *In situ* hybridization (55)
Blastomycosis	*Blastomyces dermatitidis*	Immunohistochemistry (59) *In situ* hybridization (55)
Histoplasmosis capsulati	*Histoplasma capsulatum*	Immunohistochemistry (60. 61) *In situ* hybridization (55)
Histoplasmosis duboisii	*H. capsulatum* var. *duboisii*	Immunohistochemistry (61, 62) *In situ* hybridization (55)
Paracoccidioidomycosis	*Paracoccidioides brasiliensis* and *P. lutzii*	Immunohistochemistry (63) *In situ* hybridization (64)
Sporotrichosis	*Sporothrix schenckii*	Immunohistochemistry (23, 65–67) *In situ* hybridization (55)
Talaromycosis	*Talaromyces marneffei*	Immunohistochemistry (68) *In situ* hybridization (69)
Pneumocystosis	*Pneumocystis jirovecii/P. carinii*	Immunohistochemistry (70, 71) *In situ* hybridization (72, 73)
Coccidioidomycosis	*Coccidioides immitis*	Immunohistochemistry (74) *In situ* hybridization (55)
Algoses/protothecosis	*Prototheca* spp.	Immunohistochemistry (75) *In situ* hybridization (76)

For fluorescence *in situ* hybridization (FISH), the classical DNA probes consist of fluorochrome-labelled oligonucleotide probes or polynucleotides, targeting a specific sequence of fungal rRNA. Peptide nucleic acid (PNA) probes are also used for *in situ* identification of fungi (16). PNA probes are oligomers of single bases linked by a peptide backbone. Compared to the classical probes, PNA probes have a high affinity for their complementary sequences and are less susceptible to degradation (16, 17). The binding of enzyme-labelled probes can be evaluated microscopically immediately after hybridization. For indirectly labelled probes, an enzyme or reporter molecule is bound to the probe and this will often generate a stronger signal. Different fungal species may be identified within the same tissue by labelling each probe with reporter molecules that generate different coloured signals (e.g., fluorophores).

Several types of probes have been successfully used to detect and identify fungi. These include oligonucleotide DNA probes, PNA probes (peptide nucleic acids; DNA mimics with a peptide backbone) (16), and locked nucleic acid (LNA) probes (a mix of DNA and locked nucleic acid (LNA)-modified nucleotides in which the 2′ oxygen and the 4′ carbon are linked via a methylene unit) (18, 19). PNA and LNA nucleotides are particularly useful because these hybridize strongly with their complementary RNA and DNA nucleotides, forming temperature stable hybrids. In recent years, probes targeting the most important invasive fungi and related pathogens have been developed and evaluated on tissue specimens obtained from both experimental and spontaneous infections, and the probe sequences have been published (Figs. 5.11 and 5.12; Table 5.1).

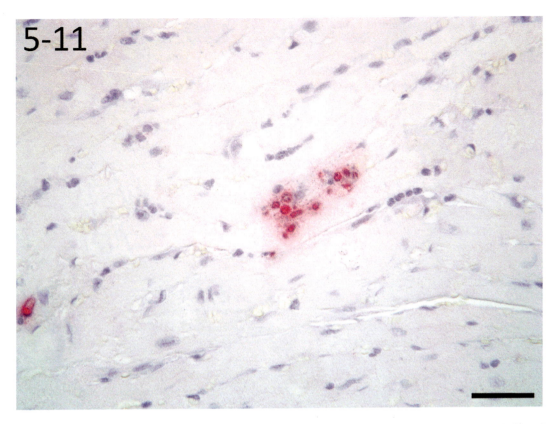

Figure 5.11 Myocardial candidosis due to *C. albicans. In situ* hybridization may be used to identify *Candida* at the genus or species level. ISH. Bar = 30 µm.

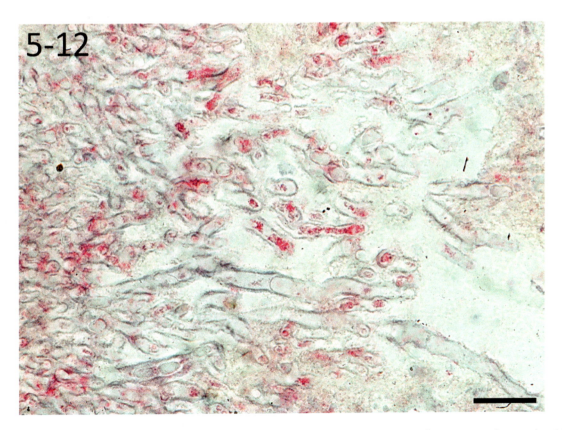

Figure 5.12 Pulmonary aspergillosis due to *A. fumigatus.* Several *in situ* hybridization techniques may be used to identify *Aspergillus* hyphae. Some species may also be distinguished. ISH. Bar = 20 µm.

In addition to their applications in tissue sections, both immunohistochemical and *in situ* hybridization methods can usually be applied to identify fungi and related pathogens in other specimens, including bronchoalveolar lavage fluid, bone marrow, exudate smears, cerebrospinal fluid, and sputum.

REFERENCES

1. Jensen HE. 1994. Systemic bovine aspergillosis, and zygomycosis in Denmark with reference to pathogenesis, pathology, and diagnosis. APMIS, 102, 1–48.

2. El Nageeb S, Hay RJ. 1981. Immunoperoxidase staining in the recognition of *Aspergillus* infections. Histopathology, 5, 437–444.

3. Kaufman L. 1992. Immunohistochemical diagnosis of systemic mycoses: An update. Eur J Epidemiol, 8, 377–382.

4. Jensen HE, Schønheyder H, Hotchi M, Kaufman L. 1996. Diagnosis of systemic mycoses by specific immunohistochemical tests. APMIS, 104, 241–258.

5. Jensen HE, Chandler FW. 2007. Histopathological diagnoses of mycoses. In: Topley and Wilson's Microbiology & Microbial Infections. Medical Mycology. 10th ed. Merz WG, Hay RJ, Eds. Hodder Arnold. pp 121–143.

6. Krockenberger MB, Canfield PJ, Kozel TR, Shinoda T, Ikeda R et al. 2001. An immunohistochemical method that differentiates *Cryptococcus neoformans* varieties and serotypes in formalin-fixed paraffin-embedded tissues. Med Mycol, 39, 523–533.

7. Jensen HE, Salonen J, Ekfors TO. 1997. The use of immunohistochemistry to improve sensitivity and specificity in the diagnosis of systemic mycoses in patients with haematological malignances. J Pathol, 181, 100–105.

8. Guarner J, Brandt ME. 2011. Histopathologic diagnosis of fungal infections in the 21st century. Clin Microbiol Rev, 24, 247–280.

9. Levsky JM, Singer RH. 2003. Fluorescence in situ hybridization: Past, present and future. J Cell Sci, 116, 2833–2838.

10. Rickerts V, Khot PD, Myerson D, Ko DL, Lambrecht E et al. 2011. Comparison of quantitative real time PCR with sequencing and ribosomal RNA-FISH for the identification of fungi in formalin fixed, paraffin-embedded tissue specimens. BMC Infect Dis, 11, 1–12.

11. Rickerts V, Smith IM, Mousset S, Kommedal O, Fredricks DN. 2013. Deciphering the aetiology of a mixed fungal infection by broad-range PCR with sequencing and fluorescence in situ hybridisation. Mycoses, 56, 681–686.

12. Moter A, Gobel UB. 2000. Fluorescence in situ hybridization (FISH) for direct visualization of microorganisms. J Microbiol Methods, 41, 85–112.

13. Wagner M, Haider S. 2012. New trends in fluorescence in situ hybridization for identification and functional analyses of microbes. Curr Opin Biotechnol, 23, 96–102.

14. Vonk AG, Verdijk R, den Boer H, van der Lee H, Rijs T, Jensen HE. 2020. Histopathological diagnosis using conventional staining techniques, with a key to identification. In: Atlas of Clinical Fungi. de Hoog GS, Guarro J, Gené J, Ahmed S, Al-Hatmi AMS, Figueras MJ, Vitale RG, Eds. CBS Utrecht. https://atlasclinicalfungi.org.

15. Montone KT, Livolsi VA, Lanza DC, Feldman MD, Kennedy DW et al. 2011. Rapid in-situ hybridization for dematiaceous fungi using a broad-spectrum oligonucleotide DNA probe. Diagn Mol Pathol, 20, 180–183.

16. Shinozaki M, Okubo Y, Sasai D, Nakayama H, Murayama SY et al. 2011. Identification of *Fusarium* species in formalin-fixed and paraffin-embedded sections by in situ hybridization using peptide nucleic acid probes. J Clin Microbiol, 49, 808–813.

17. Teertstra WR, Lugones LG, Wösten HAB. 2004. In situ hybridization in filamentous fungi using peptide nucleic acid probes. Fungal Genet Biol, 41, 1099–1103.

18. Montone KT. 2009. Differentiation of *Fusarium* from *Aspergillus* species by colorimetric in situ hybridization in formalin-fixed, paraffin-embedded tissue sections using dual fluorogenic-labeled LNA probes. Am J Clin Pathol, 132, 866–870.

19. Montone KT. 2014. In situ hybridization for fungal ribosomal RNA sequences in paraffin-embedded tissue using biotin-labeled nucleic acid probes. Methods Mol Biol, 1211, 229–235.

20. Zhang Y, Huang C, Song Y, Ma Y, Wan Z et al. 2021. Primary cutaneous aspergillosis in a patient with CARD9 deficiency and *Aspergillus* susceptibility of card9 knockout mice. J Clin Immunol, 41, 427–440.

21. Choi S, Song JS, Kim JY, Cha HH, Yun JH et al. 2019. Diagnostic performance of immunohistochemistry for the aspergillosis and mucormycosis. Mycoses, 62, 1006–1014.

22. Kaufman L, Standard PG, Jalbert M, Kraft DE. 1997. Immunohistologic identification of *Aspergillus* spp. and other hyaline fungi by using polyclonal fluorescent antibodies. J Clin Microbiol, 35, 2206–2209.

23. Fukuzawa M, Inaba H, Hayama M, Sakaguchi N, Sano K et al. 1995. Improved detection of medically important fungi by immunoperoxidase staining with polyclonal antibodies. Virchows Arch, 427, 407–414.

24. Hayden RT, Isotalo PA, Parrett T, Wolk DM, Qian X et al. 2003. In situ hybridization for the differentiation of *Aspergillus*, *Fusarium*, and *Pseudallescheria* species in tissue section. Diag Mol Pathol, 12, 21–26.

25. Jensen HE. 2021. Histopathology in the diagnosis of invasive fungal diseases. Curr Fungal Infect Rep, 15, 23–31.

26. Saito T, Imaizumi M, Kudo K, Hotchi M, Chikaoka S et al. 1999. Disseminated *Fusarium* infection identified by immunohistochemical staining in a patient with a refractory leukemia. J Exp Med, 187, 71–77.

27. Okubo Y, Shinozaki M, Wakayama M, Nakayama H, Sasai D et al. 2013. Applied gene histopathology: Identification of *Fusarium* species in FFPE tissue sections by in situ hybridization. Methods Mol Biol, 968, 141–147.

28. Jackson JA, Kaplan W, Kaufman L, Standard P. 1983. Development of fluorescent-antibody reagents for demonstration of *Pseudallescheria boydii* in tissues. J Clin Microbiol, 18, 668–673.

29. Kimura M, Maenishi O, Ito H, Ohkusu K. 2010. Unique histological characteristics of *Scedosporium* that could aid in its identification: Case report. Pathol Int, 60, 131–136.

30. Sadamoto S, Shinozaki M, Nagi M, Nihonyanagi Y, Ejima K et al. 2021. Histopathological study on the prevalence of trichosporonosis in formalin-fixed and paraffin-embedded tissue autopsy sections by in situ hybridization with peptide nucleic acid probe. Med Mycol, 58, 460–468.

31. Kobayashi M, Kotani S, Fujishita M, Taguchi H, Moriki T et al. 1988. Immunohistochemical identification of *Trichosporon beigelii* in histologic section by immunoperoxidase method. Am J Clin Pathol, 89, 100–105.

32. Alves RC, Ferreira JS, Alves AS, Maia LA, Dutra V et al. 2020. Systemic and gastrohepatic mucormycosis in dogs. J Comp Pathol, 175, 90–94.

33. Verdi CM, Jesus FPK, Kommers G, Ledur PC, Azevedo MI et al. 2018. Embryonated chicken eggs: An experimental model for *Pythium insidiosum* infection. Mycoses, 61, 104–110.

34. Heck LC, Bianchi MV, Pereira PR, Lorenzett MP, de Lorenzo C et al. 2018. Gastric pythiosis in a bactrian camel (*Bactrianus camelus*). J Zoo Wildl Med, 49, 784–787.

35. da Silva TM, Flores MM, Lamego EC, Lorenzetti DM, Ramos CP et al. 2020. Segmental enteritis associated with *Pythium insidiosum* infection in a horse. Pub. 570. Acta Sci Vet, 48, 1–4.

36. Romero A, García J, Balestié S, Malfatto F, Vicentino A et al. 2019. Equine pythiosis in the eastern wetlands of Uruguay. Pesqui Vet Bras, 39, 469–475.

37. de Souto EPF, Maia LÂ, Assis DM, de Miranda Neto EG, Kommers GD et al. 2019. Mastitis by *Pythium insidiosum* in mares. Pub. 387. Acta Sci. Vet, 47, 1–4.

38. Firmino MO, Frade MTS, Alves RC, Maia LA, Olinda RG et al. 2017. Intestinal intussusception secondary to enteritis caused by *Pythium insidiosum* in a bitch. Arq Bras Med Vet Zootec, 69, 623–626.

39. Bianchi MV, Mello LS, de Lorenzo C, Lopes BC, Snel GGM et al. 2018. Lung lesions of slaughtered horses in southern Brazil. Pesqui Vet Bras, 38, 2065–2069.

40. Rossato CK, Fiss L, Sperotto VR, Cardona ROC, Silva RB. 2018. Pythiosis with atypical location in the soft palate in a horse in southern Brazil. Arq Bras Med Vet Zootec, 70, 641–643.

41. Maia LA, Souto EPF, Frade MTS, Pimentel LA, Azevedo EO et al. 2020. Pythiosis in cattle in northeastern Brazil. Pesqui Vet Bras, 40, 340–345.

42. Frade MTS, Diniz PVN, Olinda RG, Maia LA, de Galiza GJN et al. 2017. Pythiosis in dogs in the semiarid region of northeast Brazil. Pesqui Vet Bras, 37, 485–490.

43. Souto EPF, Maia LA, Virgínio JP, Carneiro RS, Kommers GD et al. 2020. Pythiosis in cats in northeastern Brazil. J Mycol Med, 30, 1–5.

44. Schmith R, Lemos VZ, Rondon DA, Moscon LA, Schild AL et al. 2020. Cranioesophageal pythiosis in a horse. Pub. 551. Acta Sci Vet, 48, 1–5.

45. Soares LMC, Schenkel DM, Rosa JMA, Azevedo LS, Tineli TR. 2019. Feline subcutaneous pythiosis. Cienc Rural, 49, 1–4.

46. Alonso R, Pisa D, Fernández-Fernández AM, Rábano A, Carrasco L. 2017. Fungal infection in neural tissue of patients with amyotrophic lateral sclerosis. Neurobiol Dis, 108, 249–260.

47. Pisa D, Alonso R, Carrasco L. 2020. Parkinson's disease: A comprehensive analysis of fungi and bacteria in brain tissue. Int J Biol Sci, 16, 1135–1152.

48. Lim W, Ahmed SA, Fahal AH, Sande W van de. 2018. In situ hybridisation for Madurella mycetomatis in formalin-fixed paraffin-embedded specimens. Erasmus MC. University Medical Center Rotterdam.

49. Alonso R, Pisa D, Fernández-Fernández AM, Carrasco L. 2018. Infection of fungi and bacteria in brain tissue from elderly persons and patients with Alzheimer's disease. Front Aging Neurosci. doi: 10.3389/fnagi.2018.00159.

50. Alves RC, Carneiro RDS, Kommers GD, de Souza AP, de Galiza GJN et al. 2020. Systemic candidosis in dogs associated with canine distemper virus. Pub. 575. Acta Sci Vet, 48, 1–7.

51. Marcilla A, Monteagudo C, Mormeneo S, Sentandreu R. 1999. Monoclonal antibody 3H8: A useful tool in the diagnosis of candidiasis. Microbiology, 145, 695–701.

52. Williams DW, Jones HS, Allison RT, Potts AJC, Lewis MAO. 1998. Immunocytochemical detection of *Candida albicans* in formalin fixed, paraffin embedded material. J Clin Pathol, 51, 857–859.

53. Monteagudo C, Marcilla A, Mormeneo S, Llombart-Bosch A, Sentandreu R. 1995. Specific immunohistochemical identification of *Candida albicans* in paraffin-embedded tissue with a new monoclonal antibody (1B12). Clin Microbiol Infect Dis, 103, 130–135.

54. Witchley JN, Penumetcha PM, Noble SM. 2019. Visualization of *Candida albicans* in the murine gastrointestinal tract using fluorescent in situ hybridization. J Vis Exp, 153. doi:10.3791/60283.

55. Hayden RT, Qian X, Roberts GD, Lloyd RV. 2001. In situ hybridization for the identification of yeastlike

organisms in tissue section. Diagn Mol Pathol, 10, 15–23.

56. Headley SA, Pimentel LA, Michelazzo MZ, Toma HS, Pretto-Giordano LG et al. 2019. Pathologic, histochemical, and immunohistochemical findings in pulmonary and encephalitic cryptococcosis in a goat. J Vet Diagn Invest, 31, 69–73.

57. Myers A, Meason-Smith C, Mansell J, Krockenberger M, Peters-Kennedy J et al. 2017. Atypical cutaneous cryptococcosis in four cats in the USA. Vet Dermatol, 28, 405–411.

58. da Silva EC, Guerra JM, Torres LN, Lacerda AMD, Gomes RG et al. 2017. *Cryptococcus gattii* molecular type VGII infection associated with lung disease in a goat. BMC Vet Res, 13. doi:10.1186/s12917-017-0950-6.

59. Green JH, Harrell WK, Johnson JE, Benson R. 1979. Preparation of reference antisera for laboratory diagnosis of blastomycosis. J Clin Microbiol, 10, 1–7.

60. Fortin JS, Calcutt MJ, Nagy DW, Kuroki K. 2017. Intestinal histoplasmosis in a captive reindeer (*Rangifer tarandus*), Missouri, USA. J Zoo Wildl Med, 48, 925–928.

61. Ku NK, Pullarkat ST, Kim YS, Cheng L, O'Malley D. 2018. Use of CD42b immunohistochemical stain for the detection of *Histoplasma*. Ann Diagn Pathol, 32, 47–50.

62. Pakasa N, Biber A, Nsiangana S, Imposo D, Sumaili E et al. 2018. African histoplasmosis in HIV-negative patients, Kimpese, Democratic Republic of the Congo. Emerg Infect Dis, 24, 2068–2070.

63. Silva ME, Kaplan W. 1965. Specific fluorescin-labeled antiglobulins for the yeast form of *Paracoccidioides brasiliensis*. Am J Trop Med Hyg, 290, 290–294.

64. Arantes TD, Theodoro RC, Teixeira MM, Bagagli E. 2017. Use of fluorescent oligonucleotide probes for differentiation between *Paracoccidioides brasiliensis* and *Paracoccidioides lutzii* in yeast and mycelial phase. Mem Inst Oswaldo Cruz, 112, 140–145.

65. Gonsales FF, Fernandes NCCA, Mansho W, Montenegro H, Guerra JM et al. 2019. Feline *Sporothrix* spp. detection using cell blocks from brushings and fine-needle aspirates: Performance and comparisons with culture and histopathology. Vet Clin Pathol, 48, 143–147.

66. Silva JN, Miranda LHM, Menezes RC, Gremião IDF, Oliveira RVC et al. 2018. Comparison of the sensitivity of three methods for the early diagnosis of sporotrichosis in cats. J Comp Pathol, 160, 72–78.

67. Marques MEA, Coelho KIR, Sotto MN, Bacchi CE. 1992. Comparison between histochemical and immunohistochemical methods for diagnosis of sporotrichosis. J Clin Pathol, 45, 1089–1093.

68. Estrada JA, Stynen D, van Cutsem J, Piérard-Franchimont C, Piérard GE. 1992. Immunohistochemical identification of *Penicillium marneffei* by monoclonal antibody. Int J Dermatol, 31, 410–412.

69. Ning C, Lai J, Wei W, Zhou B, Huang J et al. 2018. Accuracy of rapid diagnosis of *Talaromyces marneffei*: A systematic review and meta-analysis. PLOS ONE, 13. doi:10.1371/journal.pone.0195569.

70. Sakashita T, Kaneko Y, Izzati UZ, Hirai T, Fuke N et al. 2020. Disseminated pneumocystosis in a toy poodle. J Comp Pathol, 175, 85–89.

71. Kobayashi M, Moriki T, Uemura Y, Takehara N, Kubonishi I et al. 1992. Immunohistochemical detection of *Pneumocystis carinii* in transbronchial lung biopsy specimens: Antigen difference between human and rat *Pneumocystis carinii*. Jpn J Clin Oncol, 22, 387–392.

72. Weissenbacher-Lang C, Fuchs-Baumgartinger A, Klang A, Kneissl S, Pirker A et al. 2017. *Pneumocystis carinii* infection with severe pneumomediastinum and lymph node involvement in a whippet mixed-breed dog. J Vet Diagn Invest, 29, 757–762.

73. Haidaris PJ, Wright TW, Gigliotti F, Fallon MA, Whitbeck AA et al. 1993. In situ hybridization analysis of developmental stages of *Pneumocystis carinii* that are transcriptionally active for a major surface glycoprotein gene. Mol Microbiol, 7, 647–656.

74. Kaplan W, Clifford MK. 1964. Production of fluorescent antibody reagents specific for the tissue form of *Coccidioides immitis*. Am Rev Respir Dis, 89, 651–658.

75. Jensen HE, Aalbæk B, Bloch B, Huda A. 1998. Bovine mammary protothecosis due to *Prototheca zopfii*. Med Mycol, 36, 89–95.

76. Kang Y, Zeng Y, Zhang Q. 2017. Detection of cutaneous protothecosis by fluorescence in situ hybridization. Int J Clin Exp Med, 10, 820–825.

6

Glossary of medical mycology

Many people find fungal taxonomy and the terminology used to describe mycoses confusing. Molecular techniques have advanced our understanding of the relationships among fungi and some new terminologies have been introduced.

These recent developments have increased the potential for confusion. Therefore, the following glossary has been included.

Term	Definition
Adiaconidium	Asexual conidium (spore) that enlarges after formation *in vitro* or implantation *in vivo*; adiaconidia do not reproduce *in vivo*
Adventitious sporulation	Fungal differentiated reproductive structures within infected tissue
Anamorph	A somatic or reproductive structure of the asexual cycle. Asexual form of sporulation
Arthroconidium	Asexual conidium (spore) formed by mycelial fragmentation
Ascus	Sac-like structure containing ascospores (sexual reproduction)
Aseptate	Lacking cross-walls/separating membranes
Ascospore	Spores (sexually) formed in sac-like cells (ascus)
Asteroid body	Radially oriented Splendore–Hoeppli material (phenomenon) that sometimes surrounds yeasts and hyphae in tissue
Basidiospore	Sexual spore formed by the union of two nuclei after meiosis
Blastospore/ blastoconidium	Asexual spore formed from a budding process. Produced by blastic conidiogenesis
Bud	Variety of conidium produced by lateral outgrowth (inflation) from a parent cell; buds may be single or multiple
Budding	Asexual reproductive process characteristic of unicellular fungi or conidia in which a lateral outgrowth from the parent cell is pinched off to form a new cell
Capsule	Hyaline (colourless) mucopolysaccharide coat external to the wall of a fungal cell or conidium. Formed from terminal or intercalary hyphae
Chlamydoconidium/ chlamydospore	Thick-walled, rounded, resistant conidium formed by direct differentiation of the mycelium
Coenocytic	Non-septate (used to describe hyphae) with multiple nuclei
Conidiophore	Specialized hypha that produces and bears conidia
Conidium	Asexual propagule formed on, but easily detached from, a hypha, conidiophore, or other parent cells. Asexual fungal spore
Dematiaceous	Naturally pigmented, usually brown or black; also termed phaeoid
Dichotomous	Hyphae forking into two equal branches from the same original stem
Dimorphic	Having two forms; growth as hyphae *in vitro* at 25°C (environmental) and as budding yeasts, muriform cells, or spherules in infected tissues or *in vitro* at 37°C (invasive)
Endospore	Asexual spore formed within a closed structure such as a spherule
Endosporulation	Process of producing endospores, formation of a wall around a fraction of cytoplasm
Eukaryotes	Organisms possessing a true nucleus, such as fungi
Fission	A cell is divided by a septum and two cells are produced
Fruiting body	Imprecise term for conidia-bearing organs produced by fungi

DOI: 10.1201/9781003306177-6

Germ tube	Tube-like process, produced by a germinating conidium, which eventually develops into a hypha
Granule (grain)	Mass of organized mycelia that may be embedded in a cement-like matrix; formed in actinomycosis and in mycetomas caused by fungi and actinomycetes
Hyaline/hyalo	Colourless/transparent
Hypha	Filament that forms the thallus or body of most fungi; tube-like structural units; may contain septa
Hyphomycete	A fungus that produces mycelia/hyphae without discernible dark pigment
Intercalary	The location between hyphal cells
Macroconidium	The larger of two types of conidia produced in the same manner by the same fungus
Microconidium	The smaller of two types of conidia produced in the same manner by the same fungus
Muriform	Having horizontal and vertical septations or cross-walls (brick wall arrangement)
Mycelium	Mass of intertwined and branched hyphae
Mycosis	Disease caused by a fungus
Perfect state	The developmental state of a fungus when sexual reproduction takes place and sexual spores are produced
Phaeoid	Dark, dusky; term applied to fungal cell walls darkened by melanins
Phialide	A conidiogenous cell that successively produces and extrudes conidia from within. Flask-shaped projection from the vesicle
Progeny	The offspring
Propagule	Cell or cellular element serving dispersal
Pseudohyphae	Short hyphal-like filaments produced by successive yeast buds that elongate and fail to separate (not true hyphae)
Septate	Having cross-walls
Septum	Cross-wall of a mycelial filament or conidium
Schizogony	Process of multiplication of yeasts by the splitting and separation of a septum that permits adjacent cells to be set free
Sclerotic	Grown rigid or unresponsive
Spherule	Closed, thick-walled, spherical structure within which asexual endospores are produced by progressive cytoplasmic cleavage
Splendore–Hoeppli material (phenomenon)	Eosinophilic, refractile, homogeneous, and often radially oriented material sometimes found around fungi in tissue sections; represents a localized antigen–antibody reaction in a hypersensitized host. The material is also known as the asteroid body
Sporangium	A closed structure within which asexual spores (sporangiospores) are produced by cytoplasmic cleavage
Spore	Reproductive propagule in fungi
Sterigma	Short or elongated specialized projection of a conidiophore on which conidia develop (see phialide)
Teleomorph	Sexual form of a fungus (sporulation)
Thallus	Vegetative body of a fungus
Vesicle	Swollen end of a conidiophore or sporangiophore
Yeast	Spherical to oval unicellular fungus that reproduces by budding or fission
Zygospore	Thick-walled, resting spore formed during sexual reproduction

7

Aspergillosis

INTRODUCTION

Aspergillosis is caused by species of the genus *Aspergillus* and occurs worldwide. Of the hundreds of *Aspergillus* species, only a few cause most infections: *A. fumigatus, A. flavus, A. niger,* and *A. terreus* (1, 2). *A. fumigatus* is the most frequent cause of infections. The frequency of *A. flavus, A. terreus,* and *A. niger* infections is related to climate (1–4). Occasionally, other species such as *A. oryzae, A. udagawae, A. quadrilineatus, A. pseudoviridinutans, A. tanneri, A. subramanianii, A. fumisynnematus,* and *A. felis* are identified in individual cases, but these rarely affect patients who do not have hereditary defects in host antifungal defence pathways (5, 6). *Aspergillus* spp. are ubiquitous within the environment and may be isolated from the air (outdoors and indoors), soil, decomposing organic matter, food, or water. Moreover, several *Aspergillus* species are used widely in industry. All reproduce asexually and produce chains of conidia from fruiting bodies (2).

EPIDEMIOLOGY

Infections involving *Aspergillus* spp. occur almost exclusively in individuals with underlying health problems, and immunocompromised individuals are particularly at risk. Reasons for an increased susceptibility to infection may include hematopoietic stem cell or solid organ transplants, long-term treatment with corticosteroids or broad-spectrum antibiotics, and neutrophil dysfunction (1, 2). In addition, patients with lung lesions caused by tuberculosis have a higher risk of developing aspergillomas (1, 2). Most frequently, *Aspergillus* fungi enter the respiratory system when spores are inhaled. However, traumatic implantation in the eyes or skin may also cause invasive aspergillosis. Primary cutaneous infections may be associated with intravenous catheters, trauma, burns, occlusive dressings and tapes, or following surgery (7). Although most aspergillosis cases are sporadic and due to patients having underlying health problems, outbreaks of invasive aspergillosis have occurred during construction or renovation work within hospitals or nearby units (1). The mortality rate associated with invasive aspergillosis is between 50% and 100%, depending on underlying health problems, the manifestation of infection, and the delay in obtaining a specific diagnosis (8). However,

in immunocompetent individuals, an early diagnosis may result in successful treatment, even if aspergillosis has spread to multiple organ systems (9).

PATHOLOGY

Several clinical forms of aspergillosis are recognized (1, 10). In the airways and sinuses, these include the following: acute and chronic invasive pulmonary aspergillosis and sinusitis; tracheo-bronchitis and obstructive bronchial aspergillosis; and pulmonary and paranasal sinus aspergilloma formation (Figs. 7.1–7.4). In very rare cases, invasive aspergillosis may also be situated in the epiglottis (11). In practice, any organ may be infected following the hematogenous spread of *Aspergillus* spp. Aspergillosis lesions may occur in the brain, skin, endocardium (mainly on prosthetic valves [8]), bones (osteomyelitis), and the eyes (causing endophthalmitis, which has been linked to several *Aspergillus* spp., but especially *A. flavus* in developing countries [8, 12]) (Figs. 7.5–7.9). Cerebral infections may also develop following invasive *Aspergillus* sinusitis (8), and cerebral aspergillosis abscesses have occurred following surgery (13).

The invasive form of pulmonary aspergillosis typically affects immunocompromised individuals, including transplant recipients, premature babies, and individuals with prolonged neutropenia or acquired immune deficiency syndrome (AIDS) (1, 2). Particular clinical observations may suggest invasive pulmonary aspergillosis, including information from X-rays, computed tomography scans, and molecular haematology tests. However, the gold standard test for invasive aspergillosis, and several other opportunistic fungal infections, is demonstrating the presence of fungal hyphae in biopsies, fine-needle aspirates, or material obtained during necropsies (14) (Figs. 7.10–7.12).

Systemic hematogenous spread may result from hyphal penetration into blood vessels, which may be a complication to infection of the lungs and upper respiratory tract. *Aspergillus* spp. may spread hematogenously to almost any organ including the skin. In rare cases, *Aspergillus* spp. may enter the body through the gastrointestinal tract (15, 16), which can also become infected following hematogenous spread (8). The acute lesions that occur in the lungs, or other organs following hematogenous spread, exhibit necrosis and may affect blood vessels causing subsequent

DOI: 10.1201/9781003306177-7

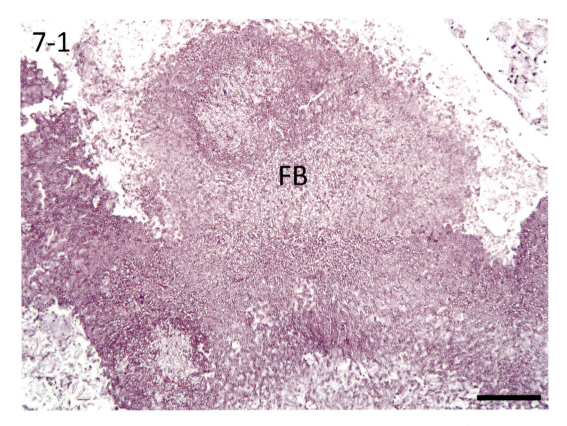

Figure 7.1 Pulmonary fungus ball (FB) due to *A. fumigatus*. The masses of hyphae occupy a pulmonary cavern. HE. Bar = 150 µm.

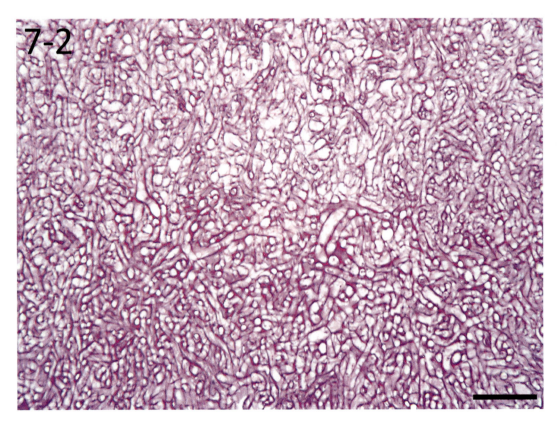

Figure 7.2 Close-up of a fungus ball due to *A. fumigatus*; the hyphae are growing densely and vary considerably in width. HE. Bar = 30 µm.

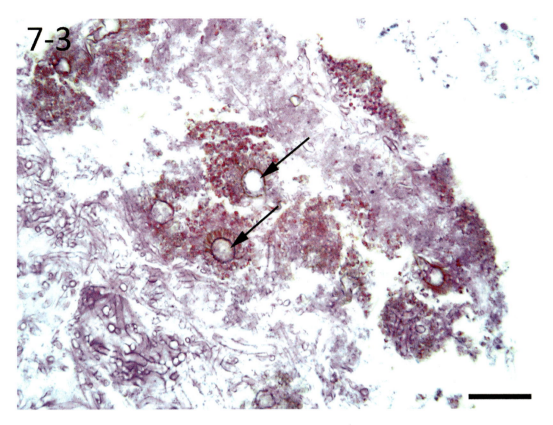

Figure 7.3 Sinus aspergilloma due to growth of *A. fumigatus*. Several fruiting bodies (arrows) are releasing conidia. HE. Bar = 85 µm.

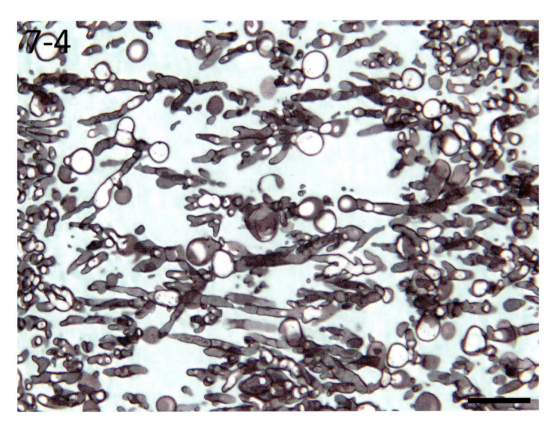

Figure 7.4 The hyphae within a sinus aspergilloma due to *A. fumigatus* are shown. There are multiple dilatations within hyphae and at the termini of hyphae due to antimycotic therapy. GMS. Bar = 30 µm.

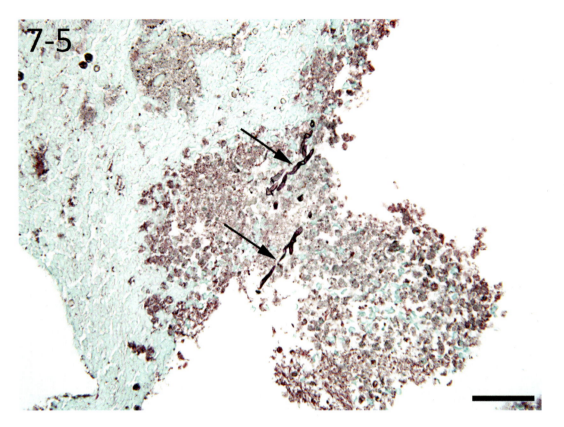

Figure 7.5 Cerebral aspergillosis. A few uncharacteristic *Aspergillus* hyphae (arrows) are shown within this biopsy taken from the brain of a patient with acquired immunodeficiency syndrome (AIDS). GMS. Bar = 100 μm.

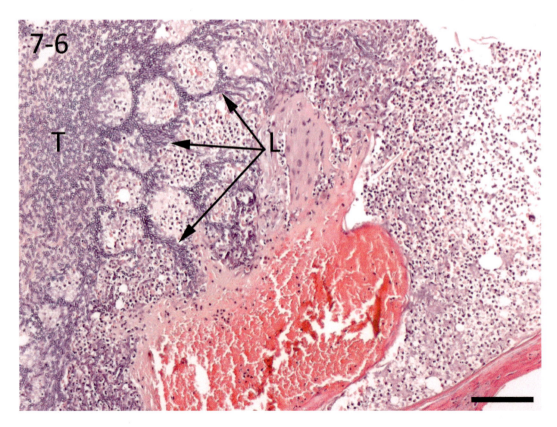

Figure 7.6 Acute, suppurative, haemorrhagic, necrotizing dermal aspergillosis due to *A. fumigatus* following hematogenous spread. Both transversely (T) and longitudinally (L) sectioned hyphae are present. HE. Bar = 150 μm.

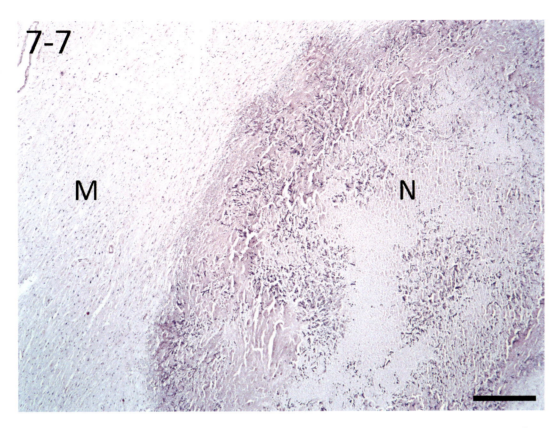

Figure 7.7 Acute, suppurative, and necrotizing myocardial aspergillosis due to *A. flavus*. Next to the area of necrosis (N), normal myocardial tissue (M) is present. HE. Bar = 200 μm.

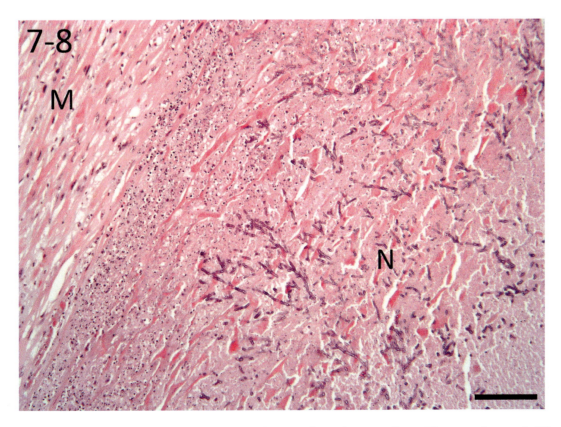

Figure 7.8 Acute, suppurative, and necrotizing myocardial aspergillosis due to *A. flavus*. The area of necrosis (N) containing hyphae is towards the normal myocardial tissue (M), bordered by a zone of infiltrating neutrophils. HE. Bar = 100 μm.

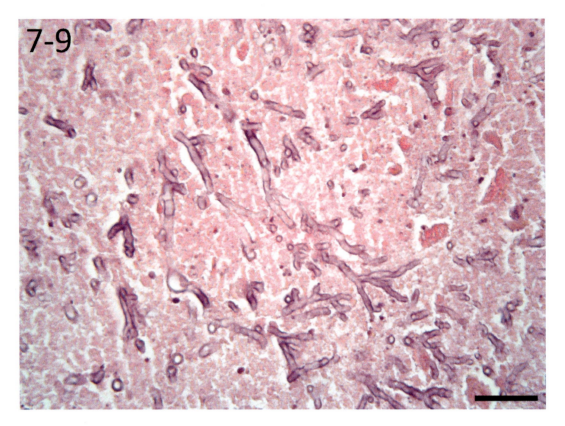

Figure 7.9 Acute and necrotizing myocardial aspergillosis due to *A. flavus*. HE. Bar = 40 μm.

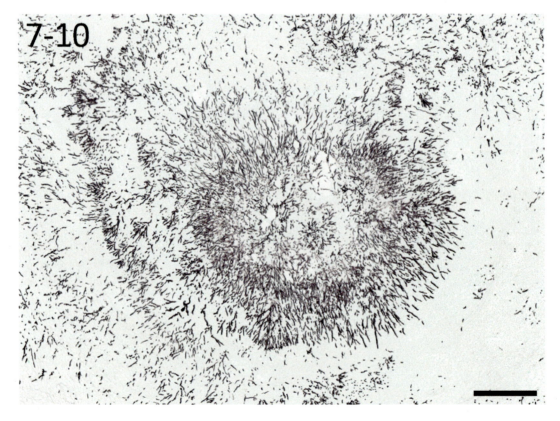

Figure 7.10 Chronic, invasive necrotizing pulmonary aspergillosis due to *A. fumigatus*. The hyphae are growing out from a small blood vessel in a globose-like pattern following hematogenous spread. GMS. Bar = 150 μm.

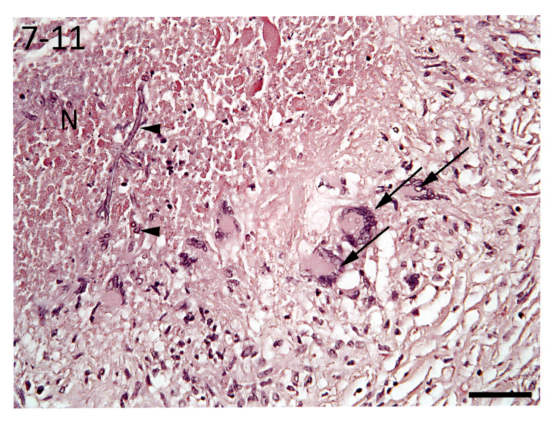

Figure 7.11 Chronic, invasive necrotizing pulmonary aspergillosis due to *A. fumigatus*. Hyphae are present (arrowheads) at the periphery of the necrotic lesion (N). Multinucleate giant cells with hyphae (arrows) are also present. HE. Bar = 60 μm.

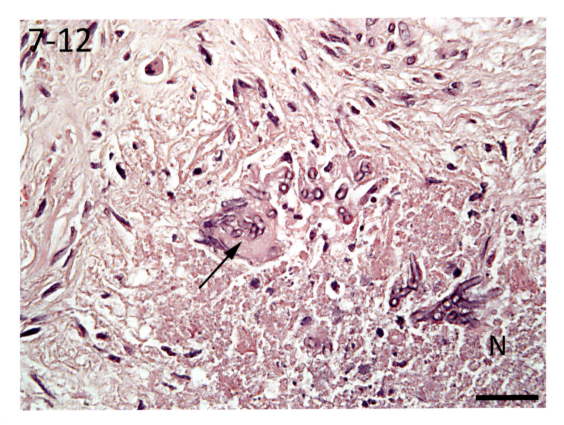

Figure 7.12 Chronic, invasive necrotizing pulmonary aspergillosis due to *A. fumigatus*. Hyphae are present within the necrotic tissue (N) and have been phagocytosed by a multinucleate giant cell (arrow). HE. Bar = 40 μm.

thrombosis. Acute necrosis results from heavy infiltration with neutrophils producing suppurative inflammation (Figs. 7.6 and 7.9). If the host survives the acute infections, the inflammation will develop into lesions containing multifocal coalescing chronic pyogranulomas (17) or non-suppurative granulomatous inflammation that is characterized by heavy infiltration of macrophages, formation of epithelioid cells, and multinuclear giant cells (3, 4, 18) (Figs. 7.11–7.13). Chronic inflammatory lesions are accomplished by the infiltration of lymphocytes and plasma cells. Frequently, hyphal Aspergillus spp. fragments can be identified within multinuclear giant cells (Figs. 7.12 and 7.13). Apart from the frequently occurring hematogenous spread of fungi, Aspergillus elements may also be spread by the lymphatic system to regional lymph nodes, where inflammation occurs, similar to that in other organs. At gross inspection, the chronic granulomatous lesions that occur in lymph nodes are indistinguishable from those caused by tuberculosis.

Pulmonary aspergillomas (i.e., fungus balls) are usually a result of Aspergillus growth within pulmonary cavities established following tuberculosis, pneumoconiosis, sarcoidosis, or bronchiectasis due to non-fungal chronic bronchopneumonia (1, 2). These non-preformed cavities are encapsulated by fibrous walls and can be classified as thin-walled aspergillomas or chronic necrotizing (cavity forming) pulmonary aspergillosis (2). The fungus balls grow as a dense amorphous mass within the cavities but are not usually invasive (Figs. 7.1 and 7.2). However, occasionally the hyphae may invade the cavity wall and surrounding vessels leading to hematogenous spread (Fig. 7.14) (19). Fungus balls are most frequently caused by A. fumigatus, A. flavus, or A. niger, but may occasionally be caused by A. terreus, A. nidulans, or A. oryzae (20). Cavities with fungus balls may contain fruiting bodies (fructification organs), facilitating a species diagnosis (Fig. 7.3).

There are also non-invasive aspergilloma forms of aspergillosis that cause hypersensitivity reactions. In particular, these include allergic bronchopulmonary aspergillosis (ABPA) and sinusoidal aspergillosis (1). In each of these disease complexes, histological examination of sputum from the lungs or mucin from the sinus system can generate a diagnosis due to the presence of abundant dichotomously branching hyphae. The presence of fungal elements together with eosinophilia, high immunoglobulin (Ig) E in serum, and specific IgE and IgG towards Aspergillus spp. are of diagnostic significance (1, 2).

FUNGAL HISTOMORPHOLOGY

In tissues, Aspergillus spp. usually grow as septate hyphae with parallel walls that are 3–6 µm apart. However, hyphae that are up to 12 µm wide have also been reported (2–4). The hyphae, which are frequently transversely septate, branch dichotomously at an angle of 45° (Fig. 7.15). In many tissues, the hyphae grow in all directions; however, in soft tissues, such as lung tissue, hyphae often exhibit globous growth (Fig. 7.10). This characteristic feature of hyphal growth, with the fungal process resembling "globose balls," may also occur when the fungus has been spread to the small blood vessels within solid organs. Here, cross-sections of multiple hyphae may resemble yeast cells (Figs. 7.16 and 7.17) (10). In rare cases of invasive aspergillosis, asteroid body formation (Splendore–Hoeppli phenomenon) may be present, as it may in several other non-aspergillosis mycoses (Fig. 7.18) (10, 21). In such cases, immunohistochemical staining techniques may be used to identify the fungus (Fig. 7.19). Birefringent calcium oxalate crystals, which can be detected by polarized light, may occur in or around infected tissue, especially in A. niger infections (Fig. 7.20) (10, 22). Fungal balls caused by A. nidulans may also exhibit birefringence. In these cases, the fungal balls resemble Maltese crosses (22).

Fruiting bodies do not develop in solid tissue but may develop from fungal mycelia when the oxygen tension is high (e.g., in the lungs, sinuses, or lung cavities). The fruiting bodies resemble vesicles, and layers of phialides produce spores (10). The presence of fructification organs may allow the fungal species to be determined (Fig. 7.3). A. terreus is the only Aspergillus species that produces aleurioconidia on the hyphae when it grows in solid tissues, facilitating its identification (2).

Notably, antifungal therapy may alter the hyphal morphology of Aspergillus, especially in necrotic tissue, usually resulting in much broader and irregular hyphae that stain weakly (Fig. 7.4) (2, 3).

DIFFERENTIAL DIAGNOSIS

Stating a specific diagnosis of aspergillosis based only on hyphal morphology is challenging. In tissues, Aspergillus spp. hyphal morphology is difficult to distinguish from that of Scedosporium spp., Fusarium spp., or Pseudallescheria spp., which all share the same morphological characteristics (7, 10, 23). Moreover, in histopathological sections, Aspergillus spp. have also been confused with hyphae-forming infections due to Candida albicans and several Mucorales genera that cause mucormycosis (10, 23). As described above, if antimycotic treatment has been given, the hyphae may be broader and less regular. Therefore, aspergillosis infections may be misdiagnosed as mucormycosis, whereas mucormycosis is less likely to be misdiagnosed as aspergillosis (24, 25). Although the elements of Candida tend to be thinner than those of Aspergillus spp., these may be swollen due to the surrounding necrotic tissue and/or changes caused by antimycotic drugs. Specific identification of Aspergillus spp. can be obtained by both immunohistochemistry (10, 16, 21, 26–28) and in situ hybridization (29–31). Because double and triple infections with Aspergillus spp. can occur (3, 25, 26, 32), specific diagnoses in such cases may require in situ diagnostic techniques such as immunohistochemistry (Figs. 7.17, 7.19, and 7.21) or in situ hybridization (Fig. 7.22). Notably, additional infections with opportunistic pathogenic fungi may occur, and the growth of these fungi and/ or the presence of their DNA/RNA in tissue samples does

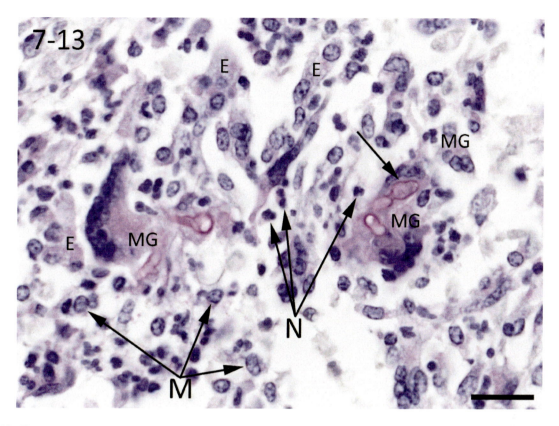

Figure 7.13 Chronic, invasive necrotizing pulmonary aspergillosis due to *A. fumigatus*. The pyogranulomatous inflammation exhibits an influx of neutrophils (N), macrophages (M), and the formation of epithelioid cells (E) and multinucleate giant cells (MG). Hyphae have been phagocytosed by a multinucleate giant cell (arrow). PAS. Bar = 35 μm.

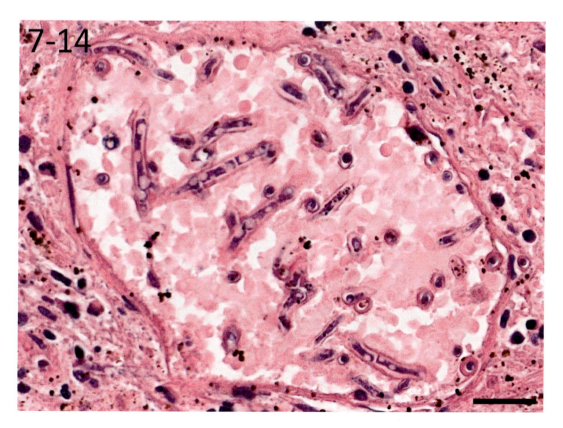

Figure 7.14 Acute, pulmonary thrombosing vasculitis due to invasion of *Aspergillus* hyphae, which contain vacuoles. HE. Bar = 25 μm.

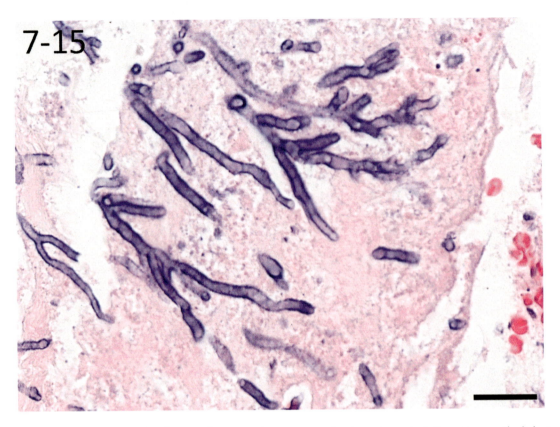

Figure 7.15 Abundant, septate, and uniform A. *fumigatus* hyphae growing in a characteristic pattern with dichotomous branching. HE. Bar = 25 µm.

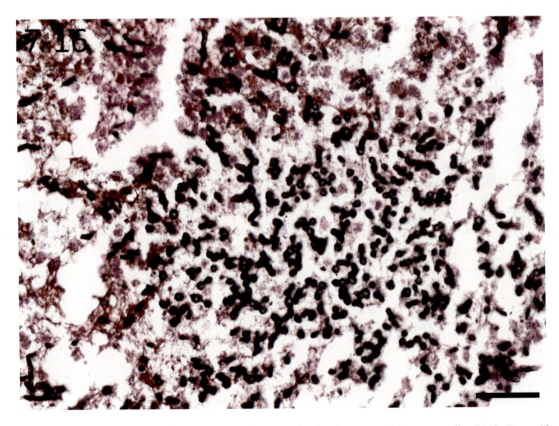

Figure 7.16 Acute, renal aspergillosis. Cross-sections of *Aspergillus* hyphae resemble yeast cells. GMS. Bar = 60 µm.

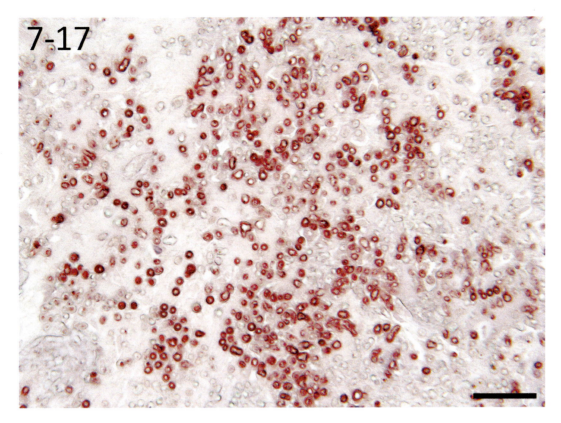

Figure 7.17 Acute, renal aspergillosis. Immunohistochemical identification of cross-sectioned *Aspergillus* hyphae. IHC. Bar = 40 μm.

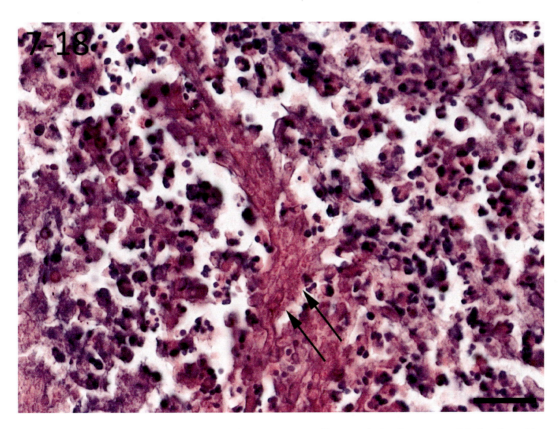

Figure 7.18 Chronic, suppurative, and necrotizing pulmonary aspergillosis with the formation of Splendore–Hoeppli material on the surface of hyphae (arrows). HE. Bar = 50 μm.

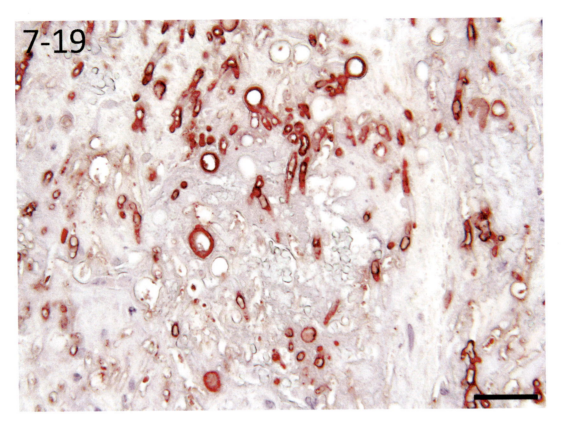

Figure 7.19 Chronic, suppurative, and necrotizing pulmonary aspergillosis. The hyphae are easily identified by specific primary monoclonal antibodies using immunohistochemical techniques. IHC. Bar = 50 μm.

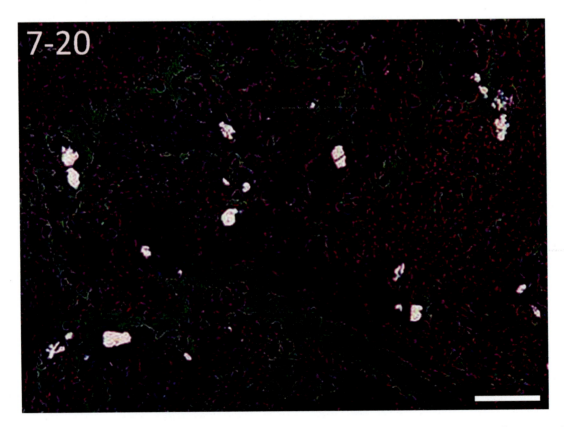

Figure 7.20 Acute, cerebral aspergillosis due to infection with *A. niger*. Within the necrotic tissue, birefringent calcium oxalate crystals are present. HE with polarized light. Bar = 75 μm.

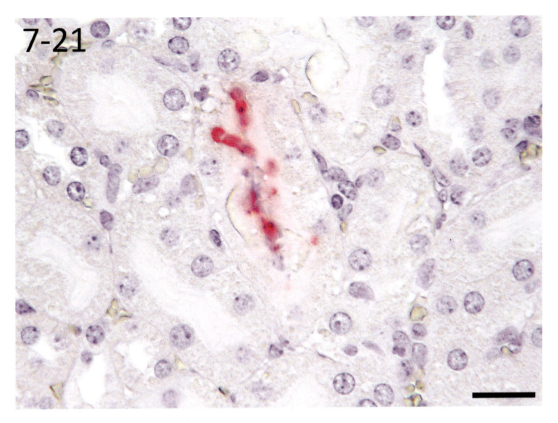

Figure 7.21 Acute, renal aspergillosis. The *Aspergillus* hyphae are identified by an *Aspergillus*-specific monoclonal antibody using immunohistochemical staining. IHC. Bar = 25 μm.

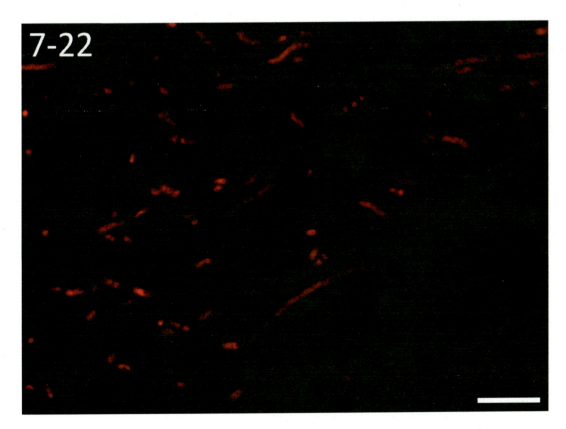

Figure 7.22 Acute, pulmonary aspergillosis. Hyphae of *A. fumigatus* are identified by *in situ* hybridization with a specific probe. ISH. Bar = 40 μm.

not prove that these are invasive, because they may be present as saprophytes without eliciting lesions or symptoms. Fructification organs within the tissue may be used to identify species, but released spores and hyphal cross-sections may be confused with the small yeast-like cells of several fungal species (10).

REFERENCES

1. Richardson MD, Warnock, DW. 2003. Aspergillois. In: Fungal Infection Diagnosis and Management. 3rd ed. Blackwell Publishing. pp 156–184.
2. Guarner J, Brandt, ME. 2011. Histopathologic diagnosis of fungal infections in the 21st century. Clin Microbiol Rev, 24, 247–280.
3. Jensen HE, Chandler FW. 2007. Histopathological diagnoses of mycoses. In: Topley and Wilson's Microbiology & Microbial Infections. Medical Mycology. 10th ed. Merz WG, Hay RJ, Eds. Hodder Arnold. pp 121–143.
4. Jensen HE. 2021. Histopathology in the diagnosis of invasive fungal diseases. Curr Fungal Infect Rep, 15, 23–31.
5. Seyedmousavi S, Lionakis MS, Parta M, Peterson SW, Kwon-Chung KJ. 2018. Emerging Aspergillus species almost exclusively associated with primary immunodeficiencies. Open Forum Infect Dis, 5. doi: 10.1093/ofid/ofy213.
6. Barrs VR, van Doorn TM, Houbraken J, Kidd SE, Martin P et al. 2013. Aspergillus felis sp. nov., an emerging agent of invasive aspergillosis in humans, cats, and dogs. PLOS ONE, 8. doi: org/10.1371.
7. Saghrouni F, Gheith S, Yaacoub A, Ammous O, Ben Abdeljelil J et al. 2011. Primary cutaneous aspergillosis due to Aspergillus flavus in a neutropenic patient. J Med Mycol, 21, 285–288.
8. Chakrabarti A, Chatterjee SS, Das A, Shivaprakash MR. 2011. Invasive aspergillosis in developing countries. J Med Mycol, 49, Suppl 1, S35–S47
9. Phuttharak W, Hesselink JR, Wixom C. 2005. MR features of cerebral aspergillosis in an immunocompetent patient: Correlation with histology and elemental analysis. Am J Neuroradiol, 26, 835–838.
10. Kradin RL, Mark EJ. 2008. The pathology of pulmonary disorders due to Aspergillus spp. Arch Pathol Lab Med, 132, 606–614.
11. Ohashi T, Mizuta K, Kuze B, Aoki M, Ito Y. 2015. Invasive epiglottic aspergillosis: A case report and literature review. Auris Nasus Larynx, 42, 501–504.
12. Jain V, Dabir S, Shome D, Dadu T, Natarajan S. 2009. Aspergillus iris granuloma: A case report with review of literature. Surv Ophthalmol, 54, 286–291.
13. Bao ZS, You G, Li WB, Jiang T. 2014. A single Aspergillus fumigatus intracranial abscess in an immunocompetent patient with parietal lobe tumorectomy. World J Surg Oncol, 12, 181–185.
14. Naaraayan A, Kavian R, Lederman J, Basak P, Jesmajian S. 2015. Invasive pulmonary aspergillosis – case report and review of literature. J Community Hosp Intern Med Perspect, 5, 3–6.
15. Fuqua TH, Sittitavornwong S, Knoll M, Said-Al-Naief N. 2010. Primary invasive oral aspergillosis: An updated literature review. J Oral Maxillofac Surg, 68, 2557–2563.
16. Gjeorgjievski M, Amin MB, Cappell MS. 2015. Characteristic clinical features of Aspergillus appendicitis: Case report and literature review. World J Gastroenterol, 21, 12713–12721.
17. do Carmo PMS, Portela RA, de Oliveira-Filho JC, Dantas AFM, Simões SVD et al. 2014. Nasal and cutaneous aspergillosis in a goat. J Comp Pathol, 150, 4–7.
18. Mayahi M, Esmaeilzadeh S, Kiani R. 2008. Aspergillus fumigatus infection in a green parrot. Comp Clin Pathol, 17, 279–281.
19. Gupta K, Das A, Joshi K, Singh N, Aggarwal R et al. 2010. Aspergillus endocarditis in a known case of allergic bronchopulmonary aspergillosis: An autopsy report. Cardiovasc Pathol, 19, 137–139.
20. Zander DS. 2011. Allergic bronchopulmonary aspergillosis: A report of a case and an update. Pathol Case Rev, 16, 224–229.
21. Ahmed SA, Abbas MA, Jouvion G, Al-Hatmi AMS, de Hoog GS et al. 2015. Seventeen years of subcutaneous infection by Aspergillus flavus; eumycetoma confirmed by immunohistochemistry. Mycoses, 58, 728–734.
22. Leite-Filho RV, Fredo G, Lupion CG, Spanamberg A, Carvalho G et al. 2016. Chronic invasive pulmonary aspergillosis in two cats with diabetes mellitus. J Comp Pathol, 155, 141–144.
23. Shah AA, Hazen KC. 2013. Diagnostic accuracy of histopathologic and cytopathologic examination of Aspergillus species. Am J Clin Pathol, 139, 55–61.
24. Kung VL, Chernock RD, Burnham, CAD. 2018. Diagnostic accuracy of fungal identification in histopathology and cytology specimens. Eur J Clin Microbiol Infect Dis, 37, 157–165.
25. Jensen HE, Salonen J, Ekfors, TO. 1997. The use of immunohistochemistry to improve sensitivity and specificity in the diagnosis of systemic mycoses in patients with haematological malignancies. J Pathol, 181, 100–105.
26. Abdo W, Kawachi T, Sakai H, Fukushi H, Kano R et al. 2012. Disseminated mycosis in a killer whale (Orcinus orca). J Vet Diagn Invest, 24, 211–218.
27. Challa S, Uppin SG, Uppin MS, Pamidimukkala U, Vemu L. 2015. Diagnosis of filamentous fungi on tissue sections by immunohistochemistry using anti-Aspergillus antibody. Med Mycol, 53, 470–476.
28. Jung J, Park YS, Sung H, Song JS, Lee SO et al. 2015. Using immunohistochemistry to assess the accuracy of histomorphologic diagnosis of aspergillosis and mucormycosis. Clin Infect Dis, 61, 1664–1670.

29. Hayden RT, Isotalo PA, Parrett T, Wolk DM, Qian X et al. 2003. In situ hybridization for the differentiation of *Aspergillus*, *Fusarium*, and *Pseudallescheria* species in tissue section. Diagn Mol Pathol, 12, 21–26.

30. Kobayashi M, Sonobe H, Ikezoe T, Hakoda E, Ohtsuki Y et al. 1999. In situ detection of *Aspergillus* 18S ribosomal RNA in invasive pulmonary aspergillosis. Intern Med, 38, 563–569.

31. Montone KT. 2009. Differentiation of *Fusarium* from *Aspergillus* species by colorimetric in situ hybridization in formalin-fixed, paraffin-embedded tissue sections using dual fluorogenic-labeled LNA probes. Am J Clin Pathol, 132, 866–870.

32. Jensen HE, Schønheyder HC, Hotchi M, Kaufmanet L. 1996. Diagnosis of systemic mycoses by specific immunohistochemical tests. APMIS, 104, 241–258.

8

Fusariosis

INTRODUCTION

Several *Fusarium* species may cause fusariosis; however, *F. solani*, *F. oxysporum*, and *F. moniliforme* are the most frequently identified pathogens (1, 2). Fusariosis predominantly affects individuals with impaired immunological function; for example, patients with neutropenia who are undergoing stem cell transplantation (3–6). The *Fusarium* fungi are ubiquitous in soil and water, and fusariosis occurs worldwide (2, 7).

EPIDEMIOLOGY

Fusarium spp. cause both superficial and invasive disseminated infections. Invasive keratitis, which may lead to endophthalmitis (Figs. 8.1–8.6), affects individuals who wear contact lenses, but invasive lesions of the skin and underlying tissues following burns and wounds have also been reported (1, 5–7). Systemic hematogenous spread involving several organ systems is particularly common in immunosuppressed patients (Figs. 8.7–8.12) (2, 4, 8). During dissemination, *Fusarium* spp. exhibit a propensity for causing secondary skin lesions (Figs. 8.13–8.18) (1, 3, 5, 9–11). Apart from infections, *Fusarium* spp. also cause mycotoxicosis in humans and animals (1, 7).

PATHOLOGY

As for all mycoses, the characteristics of lesions depend on the immune status of patients. However, angioinvasion, necrosis, and the influx of neutrophils typically occur in acute lesions (Figs. 8.1, 8.4, and 8.14) (1, 6, 12). Necrosis is typically present in chronic lesions, together with infiltration by macrophages, epithelioid cells, and multinucleate giant cells (Figs. 8.7, 8.8, and 8.10) (13, 14). Several laboratory animal models have been developed to study different aspects of fusariosis, including pathogenesis and strategies for therapy (15, 16). Fusariosis lesions also occur in domestic animals, especially dogs (3, 17), as well as in wild animals (18, 19).

FUNGAL HISTOMORPHOLOGY

Fusarium hyphae are comparable to those of *Aspergillus* and those of other pathogens that cause hyalohyphomycoses in tissues: they are hyaline, septate, and exhibit frequent branching dichotomously or at right angles (Figs. 8.12, 8.13, 8.15–8.17) (12, 20, 21). The outline of these parallel hyphae is highlighted best with periodic acid-Schiff and Grocott's methenamine stains (Figs. 8.10–8.12, 8.15–8.17) (1, 20, 21). *Fusarium* hyphae are 3–8 μm wide, may contain local vesicles, and often exhibit constrictions that are associated with the formation of septa (Figs. 8.6, 8.11, and 8.17; see the chapter on aspergillosis). *Aspergillus* hyphae may also exhibit these characteristics, but to a lesser extent. In particular, the terminal vesicles often resemble those of *Aspergillus* hyphae when antimycotic therapy has been initiated. As with aspergillosis, *in situ* sporulation may occur in fusariosis lesions (7).

DIFFERENTIAL DIAGNOSIS

Because it is almost impossible to differentiate *Fusarium* spp., *Aspergillus* spp., and other pathogens that cause hyalohyphomycoses in tissues, specific *in situ* identification techniques such as immunohistochemistry (13, 22) and *in situ* hybridization (23–25) are needed to obtain a reliable diagnosis (Fig. 8.18). In addition, specific polymerase chain reaction techniques may also be applied to tissue specimens. However, the possibility of contamination with other pathogens, including other hyalohyphomycotic pathogens, must be excluded when using these techniques.

DOI: 10.1201/9781003306177-8

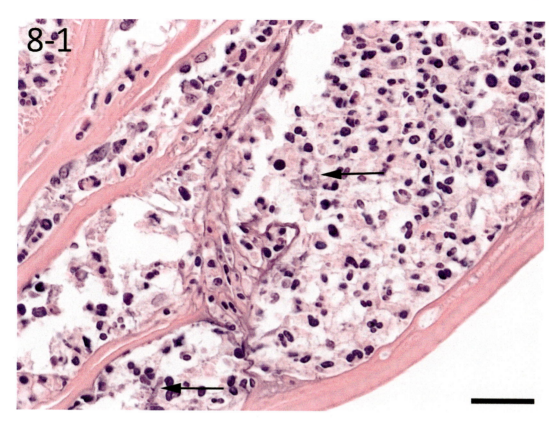

Figure 8.1 Invasive keratitis caused by *F. solani*. Acute suppurative keratitis is present due to the invasion of *Fusarium* hyphae (arrows). HE. Bar = 50 μm.

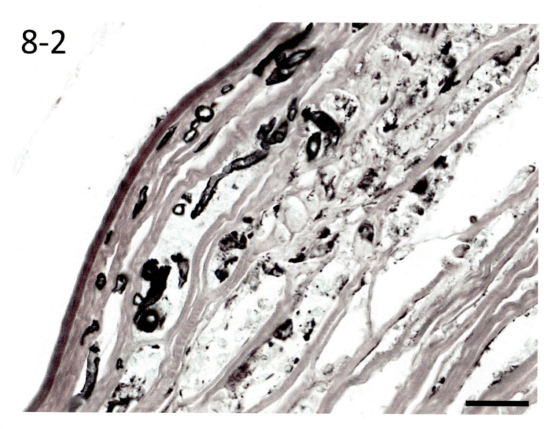

Figure 8.2 Invasive keratitis caused by *F. solani*. Within the suppurative keratitis, the invasion of *Fusarium* hyphae is optimally visualized by Grocott's methenamine silver stain. Same case as in Fig. 8.1. GMS. Bar = 50 μm.

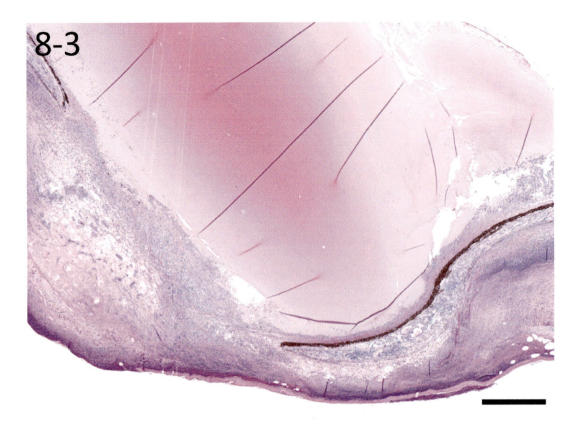

Figure 8.3 Panophthalmitis caused by *F. solani*. Necrotizing and suppurative inflammation is present in all layers of the eye. HE. Bar = 250 μm.

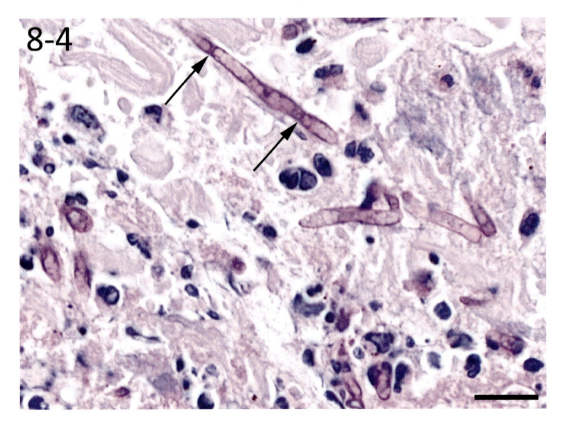

Figure 8.4 Panophthalmitis caused by *F. solani*. *Fusarium* hyphae that exhibit narrowing at septation sites (arrows) are present within necrotic debris, together with hyphae that vary in shape. Same case as in Fig. 8.3. HE. Bar = 50 μm.

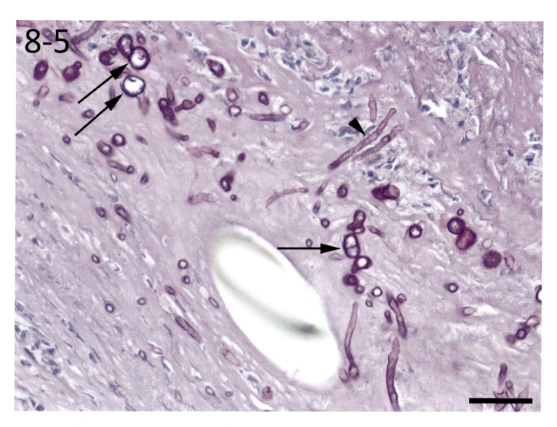

Figure 8.5 Panophthalmitis caused by *F. solani*. Both vesicles (arrows) and narrowing at a septation site (arrowhead) are visible in the *Fusarium* hyphae. Same case as in Fig. 8.3. PAS. Bar = 60 μm.

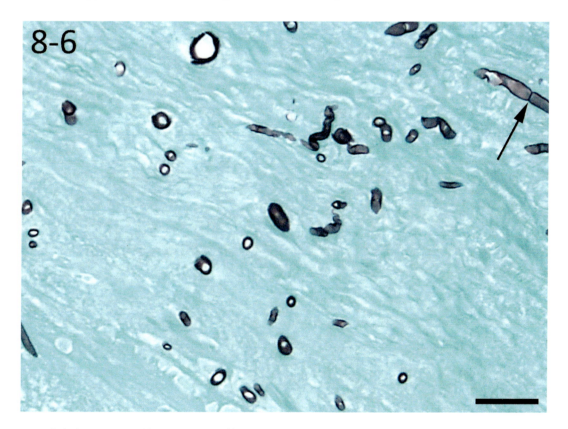

Figure 8.6 Panophthalmitis caused by *F. solani*. Different shaped *Fusarium* elements are present within the necrotic lesions. Narrowing at a septation site is shown (arrow), as is the formation of dilatations/vesicles. Same case as in Fig. 8.3. GMS. Bar = 50 μm.

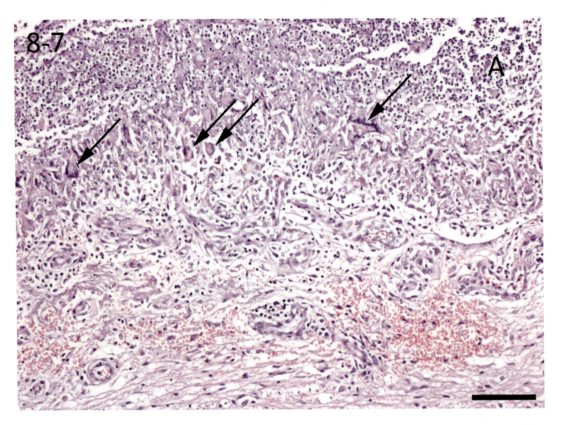

Figure 8.7 Chronic cerebral fusariosis following systemic hematogenous spread. A rim of granulomatous inflammation with multinucleate giant cells (arrows) surrounds an abscess (A). HE. Bar = 120 μm.

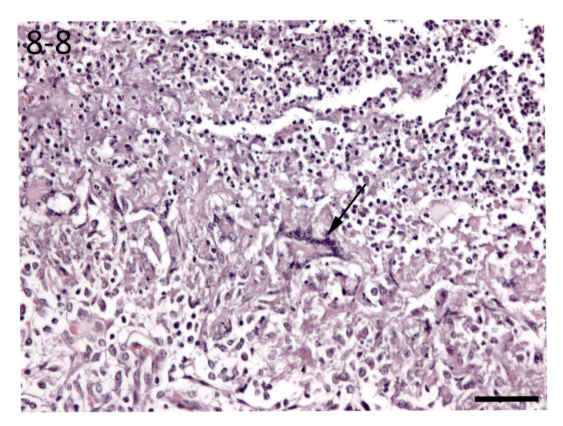

Figure 8.8 Chronic cerebral fusariosis following systemic hematogenous spread. Macrophages and a multinucleate giant cell (arrow) containing a hyphal fragment near the suppurative inflammation are magnified. Same case as in Fig. 8.7. HE. Bar = 60 μm.

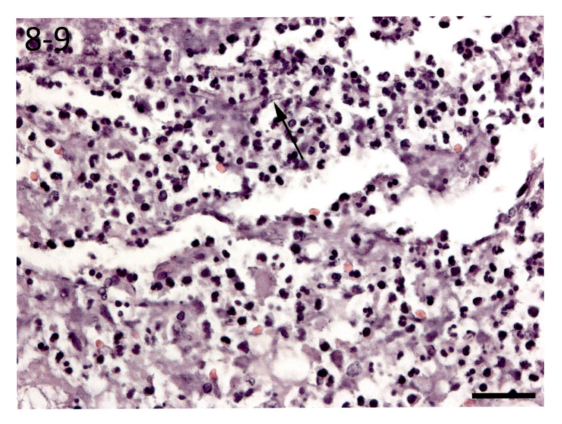

Figure 8.9 Chronic cerebral fusariosis following systemic hematogenous spread. The *Fusarium* hyphae are only faintly stained (arrow) by haematoxylin and eosin within the suppurative abscess. Same case as in Fig. 8.7. HE. Bar = 40 μm.

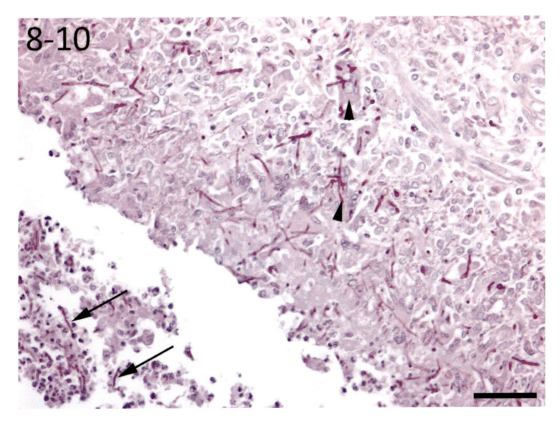

Figure 8.10 Chronic cerebral fusariosis following systemic hematogenous spread. Periodic acid-Schiff staining shows the *Fusarium* hyphae within the suppurative abscess (arrows) and the surrounding multinucleate giant cells (arrowheads). PAS. Bar = 60 μm.

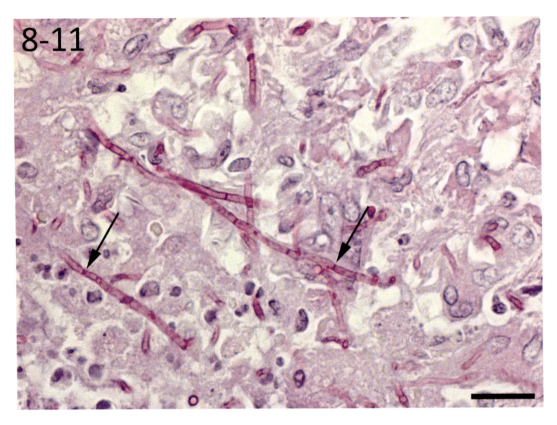

Figure 8.11 Chronic cerebral fusariosis following systemic hematogenous spread. Frequent septation is present within the uniform outline of the *Fusarium* hyphae, and narrowing is visible in some places (arrows). PAS. Bar = 30 μm.

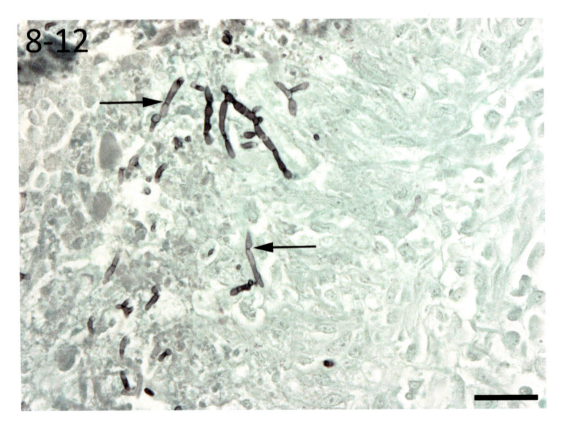

Figure 8.12 Chronic cerebral fusariosis following systemic hematogenous spread. Narrowing is visible at septation sites (arrows) within the uniform outline of the *Fusarium* hyphae. GMS. Bar = 40 μm.

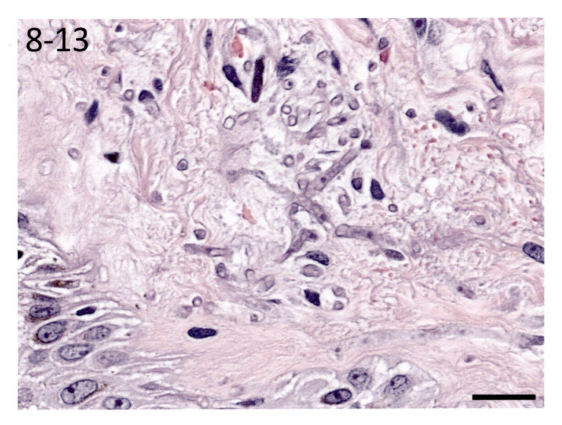

Figure 8.13 Dermal fusariosis following the systemic hematogenous spread of *F. solani*. Many *Fusarium* hyphae are present within the dermis. HE. Bar = 50 µm.

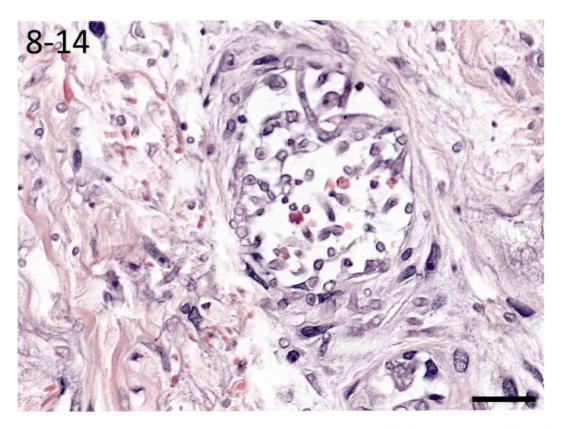

Figure 8.14 Dermal fusariosis following the systemic spread of *F. solani*. *Fusarium* hyphae are present within a dermal vessel following hematogenous spread. HE. Bar = 50 µm.

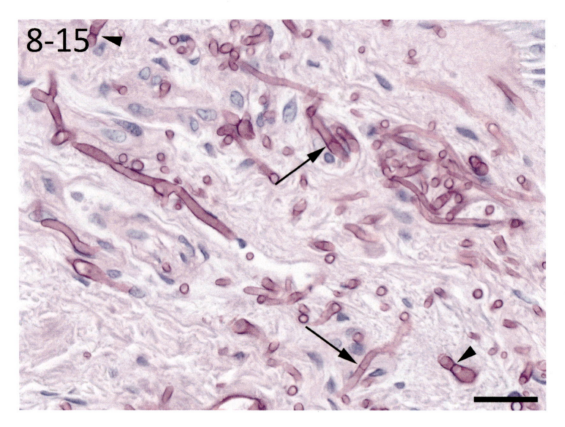

Figure 8.15 Dermal fusariosis following the systemic spread of *F. solani*. Uniform hyphae with septa (arrows) are present within the dermis, following hematogenous spread. In some hyphae, narrowing is present at septation points (arrowheads). PAS. Bar = 40 μm.

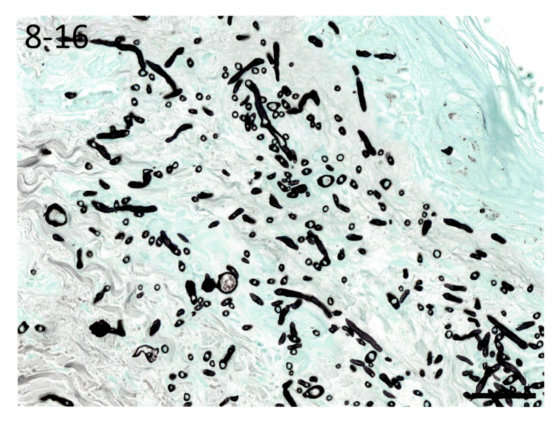

Figure 8.16 Dermal fusariosis following the systemic hematogenous spread of *F. solani*. Vesicles are clearly visible within several *Fusarium* hyphae. GMS. Bar = 80 μm.

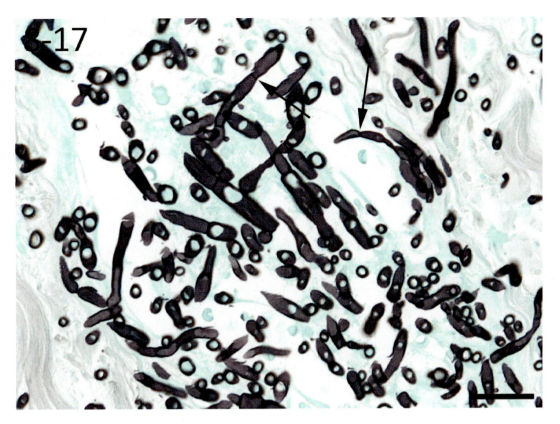

Figure 8.17 Dermal fusariosis following the systemic hematogenous spread of *F. solani*. Vesicles are present within longitudinally cut hyphae, and some hyphae exhibit narrowing where the septa form (arrows). GMS. Bar = 40 μm.

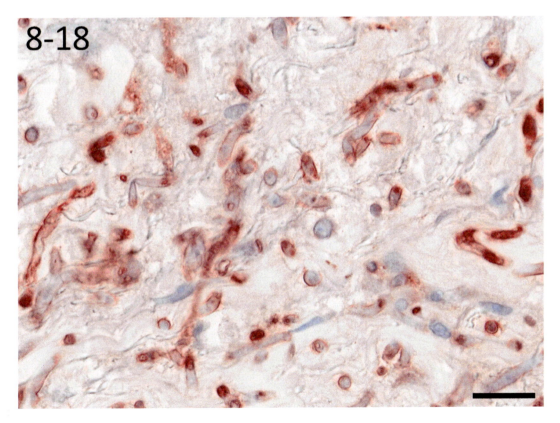

Figure 8.18 Dermal fusariosis following the systemic hematogenous spread of *F. solani*. *Fusarium* hyphae are identified by immunohistochemistry using genus-specific monoclonal antibodies. IHC. Bar = 50 μm.

REFERENCES

1. Hospenthal DR. 2015. Hyalohyphomycosis: Infection due to hyaline moulds: In: Diagnosis and Treatment of Fungal Infections. Hospenthal DR, Rinaldi MG, Eds. Springer. pp 141–149.

2. Del Alcazar E, Jaka A, Camino N, Gancho G, Tuneu A. 2015. Fever and skin lesions in an immunocompromised patient. Clin Exp Dermatol, 40, 219–221.

3. Avelino-Silva VI, Ramos JF, Leal FE, Testagrossa L, Novis YS. 2014. Disseminated *Fusarium* infection in autologous stem cell transplant recipient. Braz J Infect Dis, 19, 90–93.

4. Busemann C, Krüger W, Schwesinger G, Kallinich B, Schröder G et al. 2009. Myocardial and aortal involvement in a case of disseminated infection with *Fusarium solani* after allogeneic stem cell transplantation: Report of a case. Mycoses, 52, 372–376.

5. Gardner JM, Nelson MM, Heffernan MP. 2005. Chronic cutaneous fusariosis. Arch Dermatol, 141, 794–795.

6. Romano C, Caposciutti P, Ghilardi A, Miracco C, Fimiani M. 2010. A case of primary localized cutaneous infection due to *Fusarium oxysporum*. Mycopathologia, 170, 39–46.

7. Guarner J, Brandt, ME. 2011. Histopathologic diagnosis of fungal infections in the 21st century. Clin Microbiol Rev, 24, 247–280.

8. Sandberg Y, van Groningen MCC, Ammatuna E. 2015. Disseminated fusariosis. Int J Infect Dis, 30, 154–155.

9. Cooke NS, Feighery C, Armstrong DKB, Walsh M, Dempsey S. 2009. Cutaneous *Fusarium solani* infection in childhood acute lymphoblastic leukaemia. Clin Exp Dermatol, 34, 117–119.

10. Mohanty NK, Sahu S. 2014. *Fusarium solani* infection in a kidney transplant recipient. Indian J Nephrol, 24, 312–314.

11. Nakai K, Yoneda K, Imataki O, Kida J, Uemura M et al. 2014. Transepidermal growth in disseminated *Fusarium* infection. J Dermatol, 41, 770–771.

12. Schuetz AN, Walsh TJ. 2015. Importance of fungal histopathology in immunocompromised pediatric patients. Am J Clin Pathol, 144, 185–187.

13. Evans J, Levesque D, De Lahunta A, Jensen HE. 2004. Intracranial fusariosis: A novel cause of fungal meningoencephalitis in a dog. Vet Pathol, 41, 510–514.

14. Sugahara G, Kiuchi A, Usui R, Usui R, Mineshige T et al. 2014. Granulomatous pododermatitis in the digits caused by *Fusarium proliferatum* in a cat. J Vet Med Sci, 76, 435–438.

15. Schäfer K, Di Pietro A, Gow NAR, MacCallum D. 2014. Murine model for *Fusarium oxysporum* invasive fusariosis reveals organ-specific structures for dissemination and long-term persistence. PLOS ONE, 9, 1–9.

16. Abou Shousha M, Santos ARC, Oechsler RA, Iovieno A, Maestre-Mesa J et al. 2013. A novel rat contact lens model for *Fusarium* keratitis. Mol Vis, 19, 2596–2605.

17. Day MJ, Holt PE. 1994. Unilateral fungal pyelonephritis in a dog. Vet Pathol, 31, 250–252.

18. Salter CE, O'Donnell K, Sutton DA, Marancik DP, Knowles S et al. 2012. Dermatitis and systemic mycosis in lined seahorses *Hippocampus erectus* associated with a marine-adapted *Fusarium solani* species complex pathogen. Dis Aquat Organ, 101, 23–31.

19. Williams SR, Sims MA, Roth-Johnson L, Wickes B. 2012. Surgical removal of an abscess associated with *Fusarium solani* from a Kemp's ridley sea turtle (*Lepidochelys kempii*). J Zoo Wildl Med, 43, 402–406.

20. Jensen HE. 2021. Histopathology in the diagnosis of invasive fungal diseases. Curr Fungal Infect Rep, 15, 23–31.

21. Jensen HE, Chandler FW. 2007. Histopathological diagnoses of mycoses. In: Topley and Wilson's Microbiology & Microbial Infections. Medical Mycology. 10th ed. Merz WG, Hay RJ, Eds. Hodder Arnold. pp 121–143.

22. Jensen HE, Aalbæk B, Jungersen G, Hartvig T, Moser C et al. 2011. Immunohistochemical diagnosis of fusariosis with monoclonal antibodies. Mycoses, 54, 54–55.

23. Hayden RT, Isotalo PA, Parrett T, Wolk DM, Qian X et al. 2003. In situ hybridization for the differentiation of *Aspergillus*, *Fusarium*, and *Pseudallescheria* species in tissue section. Diagn Mol Pathol, 12, 21–26.

24. Montone KT. 2009. Differentiation of *Fusarium* from *Aspergillus* species by colorimetric in situ hybridization in formalin-fixed, paraffin-embedded tissue sections using dual fluorogenic-labeled LNA probes. Am J Clin Pathol, 132, 866–870.

25. Shinozaki M, Okubo Y, Sasai D, Nakayama H, Murayama SY et al. 2011. Identification of *Fusarium* species in formalin-fixed and paraffin-embedded sections by in situ hybridization using peptide nucleic acid probes. J Clin Microbiol, 49, 808–813.

Scedosporiosis and lomentosporiosis

INTRODUCTION

The nomenclature of the genus *Scedosporium/Pseudallescheria* has undergone numerous changes over the last decade, and the formerly named *Scedosporium prolificans* was found to be unrelated to *Scedosporium* and has, therefore, been reclassified as *Lomentospora prolificans* (1). The pathogens that cause scedosporiosis and lomentosporiosis are increasingly recognized as causing mycoses under different circumstances (e.g., trauma, cystic fibrosis, solid organ transplantation, and neutropenia), and they are resistant to many antifungal agents (2–6). The majority of these infections are caused by *S. apiospermum* (which is the asexual state of *P. boydii*), *S. boydii*, *S. aurantiacum*, and *L. prolificans* with some geographical differences in the distribution pattern (1–3). The fungi are ubiquitous in soil and water (7).

EPIDEMIOLOGY

Infections are generally acquired by inhalation of conidia (8). *Scedosporium*, but not *Lomentospora*, has been linked to allergic bronchopulmonary mycoses and the formation of pulmonary fungal balls (Figs. 9.1–9.5) (1, 9). Both genera may cause localized infections of the skin, including local invasive infections and eumycetomas (10, 11); hematogenous spread (12–15) may result in the muscles, joints, and eyes becoming infected, but disseminated infections also occur frequently (1, 7, 16, 17). Solid organ transplant recipients, patients with human immunodeficiency virus or leukaemia, and individuals who have nearly drowned in polluted water are particularly at risk of disseminated infections (1, 9, 10, 18–22). Scedosporiosis and lomentosporiosis have also been diagnosed in several animal species where the pathological and fungal morphology is similar to that in humans (23–29). Moreover, a number of experimental models have been described (30–32).

PATHOLOGY

In acute localized and disseminated lesions in various organs, haemorrhagic necrosis will be present. The fungal elements are found within the necrotic tissue and typically within thrombosed vessels (Figs. 9.6–9.8) (2, 33). The inflammatory reaction in acute lesions is predominantly neutrophilic (34). Approximately one-third of infections are disseminated, and cerebral (e.g., abscesses, meningitis, and ventriculitis) (1, 35) and cardiovascular involvement is common (3). Chronic lesions, such as those that occur in the central nervous system, are characterized by a granulomatous inflammatory reaction involving multinucleated giant cells (36, 37). In addition, mixed inflammatory reactions may occur with the formation of pyogranulomas and the presence of the Splendore–Hoeppli phenomenon on the fungal elements (38).

FUNGAL HISTOMORPHOLOGY

Hyphae of *Scedosporium* and *Lomentospora* are thin-walled, hyaline (although hyphae of *Lomentospora* may appear melanized), septate, and show haphazard branching. Dichotomous branches appear at right angles and in lomentosporiosis, there may be bridges between parallel hyphae (i.e., a letter H pattern) (Figs. 9.5 and 9.8) (33). The hyphae are 2–5 μm wide (34, 39), and conidia may be formed within solid organ lesions (33). The fungal elements of scedosporiosis and lomentosporiosis are best visualized by periodic acid-Schiff and Grocott's methenamine silver stains (Figs. 9.5 and 9.8) (39).

DIFFERENTIAL DIAGNOSIS

When conidia are not formed, it may be impossible to differentiate histologically between *Scedosporium/Lomentospora* infections and aspergillosis, fusariosis, or the other pathogens that cause hyalohyphomycoses (7, 40–46). Specific monoclonal antibodies can be used in immunohistochemical staining techniques to differentiate between *Scedosporium/Lomentospora* and other septate fungi (1). Moreover, specific *in situ* hybridization techniques have been developed to differentiate between the pathogens that cause scedosporiosis/lomentosoriosis, aspergillosis, and fusariosis (47).

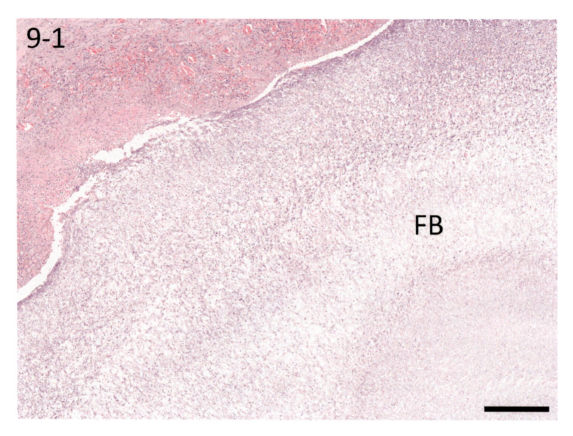

Figure 9.1 Fungus ball (FB) formation in a lung cavity due to *S. apiospermum*. HE. Bar = 200 μm.

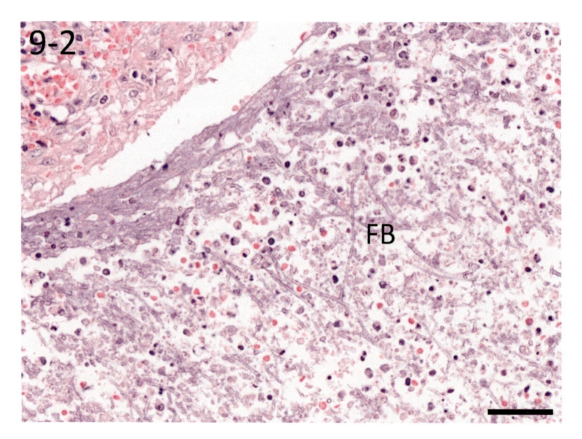

Figure 9.2 Fungus ball (FB) formation due to *S. apiospermum*. Under high magnification, it is evident that the *Scedosporium* hyphae are not invading the peripheral tissue bordering the cavity. Same case as in Fig. 9.1. HE. Bar = 75 μm.

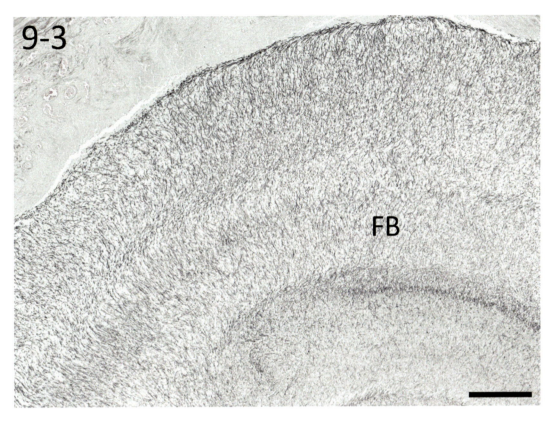

Figure 9.3 Fungus ball (FB) formation due to *S. apiospermum*. The outline of the radiating hyphae of *Scedosporium* is visible in the pulmonary cavity. Same case as in Fig. 9.1. GMS. Bar = 200 μm.

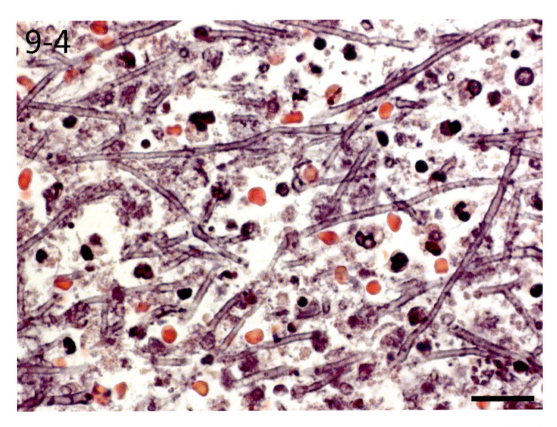

Figure 9.4 Fungus ball formation due to *S. apiospermum*. Within the fungus ball, the hyphal structures of *Scedosporium* are predominantly infiltrated with neutrophils. HE. Bar = 35 μm.

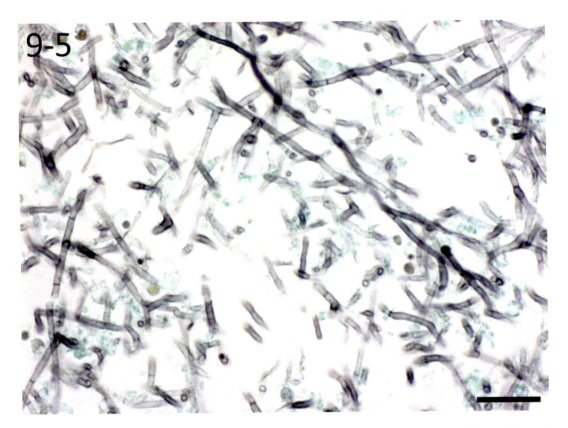

Figure 9.5 Fungus ball formation due to *S. apiospermum*. The hyphae of *S. apiospermum* are uniform, thin-walled, and frequently septate. GMS. Bar = 35 μm.

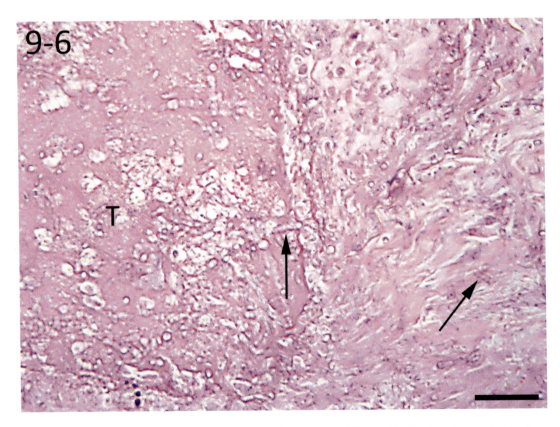

Figure 9.6 Acute, necrotizing, and thrombosing pneumonia due to *L. prolificans*. The hyphae (arrows), which are growing out from a thrombosed vessel (T), are only weakly stained due to the pronounced necrosis. PAS. Bar = 40 μm.

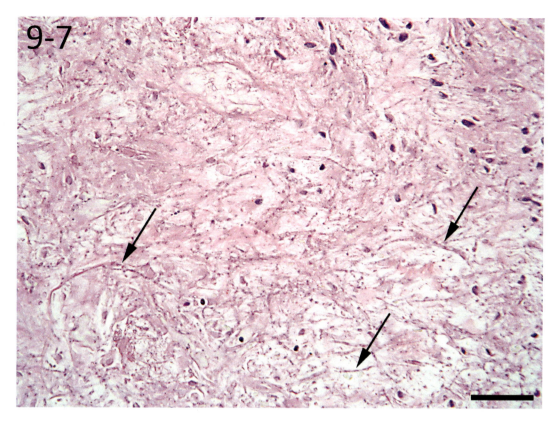

Figure 9.7 Acute, necrotizing, and thrombosing pneumonia due to *L. prolificans*. Hyphae (arrows) are only weakly stained within the tissue by the periodic acid-Schiff stain due to the pronounced necrosis. PAS. Bar = 75 μm.

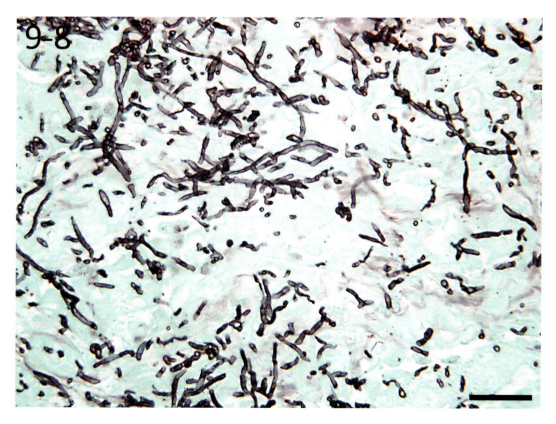

Figure 9.8 Acute, necrotizing, and thrombosing pneumonia due to *L. prolificans*. Multiple, rather uniform, septate hyphae with different branching patterns are present within the necrotic lung tissue. GMS. Bar = 50 μm.

REFERENCES

1. Ramirez-Garcia A, Pellon A, Rementeria A, Buldain I, Barreto-Bergter E et al. 2018. Scedosporium and Lomentospora: An updated overview of underrated opportunists. Med Myco, 58, 102–125.

2. Sharon CAC, Halliday CL, Hoenigl M, Cornely OA, Meyer W. 2021. Scedosporium and Lomentospora infections: Contemporary microbiological tools for the diagnosis of invasive disease. J Fungi, 7, 1–18.

3. Bronnimann D, Garcia-Hermoso D, Dromer F, Lanternier F. 2021. Scedosporiosis/lomentosporiosis observational study (SOS): Clinical significance of Scedosporium species identification. Med Mycol, 59, 486–497.

4. Lackner M, De Hoog GS, Verweij PF, Mohammad JN, Curfs-Breuker I et al. 2012. Spices-specific anti-fungal susceptibility patterns of Scedosporium and Pseudallescheria species. Antimicrob Agents Chemother, 56, 2635–2642.

5. Fietz T, Knauf W, Schwartz S, Thiel E. 2003. Intramedullary abscess in a patient with disseminated Scedosporium apiospermum infection. Br J Haematol, 120, 724.

6. Jabado N, Casanova JL, Haddad E, Dulieu F, Fournet JC et al. 1998. Invasive pulmonary infection due to Scedosporium apiospermum in two children with chronic granulomatous disease. Clin Infect Dis, 27, 1437–1441.

7. Cortez KJ, Roilides E, Quiroz-Telles F, Meletiadis J, Antachopoulos C et al. 2008. Infections caused by Scedosporium spp. Clin. Microbiol. Rev, 21, 157–197.

8. Capilla J, Yustes C, Mayayo E, Fernández B, Ortoneda M et al. 2003. Efficacy of albaconazole (UR-9825) in treatment of disseminated Scedosporium prolificans infection in rabbits. Antimicrob Agents Chemother, 47, 1948–1951.

9. Guarner J, Brandt ME. 2011. Histopathologic diagnosis of fungal infections in the 21st century. Clin Microbiol Rev, 24, 247–280.

10. Allen PB, Koka R, Kleinberg ME, Baer MR. 2013. Scedosporium apiospermum soft tissue infection as the initial presentation of acute myeloid leukemia: A case report. J. Clin Oncol, 31, 98–100.

11. Bower CPR, Oxley JD, Campbell CK, Archer CB. 1999. Cutaneous Scedosporium apiospermum infection in an immunocompromised patient. J Clin Pathol, 52, 846–848.

12. Cardoso JC, Serra D, Cardoso R, Reis JP, Tellechea Ó et al. 2009. Cutaneous Pseudallescheria boydii infection in a renal transplant patient: A case report. Dermatol Online J, 15. PMID: 19951626.

13. Boyce Z, Collins N. 2015. Scedosporium apiospermum: An unreported cause of fungal sporotrichoid-like lymphocutaneous infection in Australia and review of the literature. Australas J Dermatol, 56, 39–42.

14. Harrison MK, Hiatt KH, Smoller BR, Cheung WL. 2012. A case of cutaneous Scedosporium infection in an immunocompromised patient. J Cutan Pathol, 39, 458–460.

15. Kusne S, Ariyanayagam-Baksh S, Strollo DC, Abernethy J. 2000. Invasive Scedosporium apiospermum infection in a heart transplant recipient presenting with multiple skin nodules and a pulmonary consolidation. Transpl Infect Dis, 2, 194–196.

16. Fernandez-Flores A, Lopez-Medrano R, Fuster-Foz C. 2016. Histopathological clues in the diagnosis of fungal infection by Scedosporium in a case of endophthalmitis starting as conjunctivitis. J Cutan Pathol, 43, 461–467.

17. Lin D, Qurat-Ul-Ain K, Lai S, Musher DM, Hamill R. 2013. Cerebral Scedosporium apiospermum infection presenting with intestinal manifestations. Infection, 41, 723–726.

18. Nonaka D, Yfantis H, Southall P, Sun CC. 2002. Pseudallescheriasis as an aggressive opportunistic infection in a bone marrow transplant recipient. Arch Pathol Lab Med, 126, 207–209.

19. Ortmann C, Wüllenweber J, Brinkmann B, Fracasso T. 2010. Fatal mycotic aneurysm caused by Pseudallescheria boydii after near drowning. Int J Legal Med, 124, 243–247.

20. Smith AG, Crain M, Dejongh C, Thomas GM, Vigorito R. 1995. Systemic pseudallescheriasis in a patient with acute myelocytic leukemia. Mycopathologia, 90, 85–89.

21. Beier F, Kittan N, Holzmann T, Schardt K, Andreesen R et al. 2010. Successful treatment of Scedosporium apiospermum soft tissue abscess with caspofungin and voriconazole in a severely immunocompromised patient with acute myeloid leukemia. Transpl Infect Dis, 12, 538–542.

22. Makino K, Fukushima S, Maruo K, Egawa K, Nishimoto K et al. 2009. Cutaneous hyalohyphomycosis by Scedosporium apiospermum in an immunocompromised patient. Mycoses, 54, 259–261.

23. Baszler T, Chandler FW, Bertoy RW, Smith CW, Whiteley HE. 1988. Disseminated pseudallescheriasis in a dog. Vet Pathol, 25, 95–97.

24. Elad D, Perl S, Yamin G, Blum S, David D. 2010. Disseminated pseudallescheriosis in a dog. Med Mycol, 48, 635–638.

25. Elad D. 2011. Infections caused by fungi of the Scedosporium/Pseudallescheria complex in veterinary species. Vet J, 187, 33–41.

26. Singh K, Boileau MJ, Streeter RN, Welsh RD, Meier WA et al. 2007. Granulomatous and eosinophilic rhinitis in a cow caused by Pseudallescheria boydii species complex (anamorph Scedosporium apiospermum). Vet Pathol, 44, 917–920.

27. Berzina I, Trumble NS, Novicki T, Sharkey LC. 2011. Subconjunctival mycetoma caused by Scedosporium apiospermum infection in a horse. Vet Clin Pathol, 40, 84–88.

28. McCowan C, Bibby S, Scott PC. 2014. Mycotic keratitis due to *Scedosporium apiospermum* in layer pullets. Vet Ophthalmol, 17, 63–66.

29. Haynes SM, Hodge PJ, Tyrrell D, Abraham LA. 2012. Disseminated *Scedosporium prolificans* infection in a German Shepherd dog. Aust Vet J, 90, 1–2.

30. Levievre B, Legras P, Godon C, Franconi F, Saint-André JP et al. 2013. Experimental models of disseminated scedosporiosis with cerebral involvement. J Pharmacol Exp Ther, 345, 198–205.

31. Xisto MIDS, Liporagi-Lopes LC, Munoz JE, Bittencourt VCB, Santos GMP et al. 2016. Peptidorhamnomannan negatively modulates the immune response in a scedosporiosis murine model. Med Mycol, 54, 846–855.

32. Elizondo-Zertuche M, Montoya AM, Robledo-Leal E, Garza-Veloz I, Sánchez-Núñez AL et al. 2017. Comparative pathogenicity of *Lomentospora prolificans* (*Scedosporium prolificans*) isolates from Mexican patients. Mycopathologia, 182, 681–689.

33. Kimura M, Maenishi O, Ito H, Ohkusu K. 2010. Unique histological characteristics of *Scedosporium* that could aid in its identification. Pathol Int, 60, 131–136.

34. Albernaz V, Huston B, Castillo M, Mukherji S, Bouldin TW. 1996. *Pseudallescheria boydii* infection of the brain: Imaging with pathologic confirmation. Am J Neuroradiol, 17, 589–592.

35. Vamseedhar A, Athaniker VS, Yelikar BR. 2008. Isolated frontal sinusitis due to *Pseudallescheria boydii*. Indian J Pathol Microbiol, 51, 435–436.

36. Busaba NY, Poulin M. 1997. Invasive *Pseudallescheria boydii* fungal infection of the temporal bone. Otolaryngol Head Neck Surg,117, 91–94.

37. Ginter G, Petutschnig B, Pierer G, Soyer HP, Reischle S et al. 1999. Case report. Atypical cutaneous pseudallescheriosis refractory to antifungal agents. Mycoses, 42, 507–511.

38. Wangchinda W, Chongtrakool P, Tanboon J, Jitmuang A. 2018. *Lomentospora prolificans* vertebral osteomyelitis with spinal epidural abscess in an immunocompetent woman: Case report and literature review. Med Mycol Case Rep, 21, 26–29.

39. Jensen HE, Chandler FW. 2007. Histopathological diagnoses of mycoses. In: Topley and Wilson' Microbiology & Microbial Infections. Medical Mycology. 10th ed. Merz WG, Hay RJ, Eds. Hodder Arnold. pp 121–143.

40. Campagnaro EL, Woodside KJ, Early MG, Gugliuzza KK, Colome-Grimmer MI et al. 2002. Disseminated *Pseudallescheria boydii* (*Scedosporium apiospermum*) infection in a renal transplant patient. Transpl Infect Dis, 4, 207–211.

41. Khurshid A, Barnett VT, Sekosan M, Ginzburg AS, Önal E. 1999. Disseminated *Pseudallescheria boydii* infection in a nonimmunocompromised host. Chest 116, 572–574.

42. Lam SM, Lau ACW, Ma MW, Yam LYC. 2008. *Pseudallescheria boydii* or *Aspergillus fumigatus* in a lady with an unresolving lung infiltrate, and a literature review. Respirology, 13, 478–480.

43. Raj R, Frost AE. 2002. *Scedosporium apiospermum* fungemia in a lung transplant recipient. Chest, 121, 1714–1716

44. Shinohara MM, George E. 2009. *Scedosporium apiospermum*: An emerging opportunistic pathogen that must be distinguished from *Aspergillus* and other hyalohyphomycetes. J Cutan Pathol, 36, 39–41.

45. Takeuchi M, Yoshida C, Ota Y, Fujiwara Y. 2011. Deep skin infection of *Scedosporium apiospermum* in a patient with refractory idiopathic thrombocytopenic purpura. Internal Med, 50, 1339–1343.

46. Rabodonirina M, Paulus S, Thevenet F, Loire R, Gueho E et al. 1994. Disseminated *Scedosporium prolificans* (*S. inflation*) infection after single-lung transplantation. Clin Infect Dis, 19, 138–142.

47. Hayden RT, Isotalo PA, Parrett T, Wolk DM, Qian X et al. 2003. In situ hybridization for the differentiation of *Aspergillus*, *Fusarium*, and *Pseudallescheria* species in tissue section. Diagn Mol Pathol, 12, 21–26.

10

Mucormycosis

INTRODUCTION

Mucormycosis, which occurs worldwide, is the term used to describe infections caused by fungi of the order Mucorales. The most frequently identified animal and human pathogenic genera of mucormycosis are *Rhizopus* spp., *Mucor* spp., and *Lichtheimia* spp., followed by *Rhizomucor* spp., *Cunninghamella* spp., *Apophysomyces* spp., and *Saksenaea* spp. (1). The genera of Mucorales are ubiquitous in the environment and are found in soil, decomposing matter, air (outdoors and indoors), and in food (2). Invasive mucormycosis is a rapidly progressing and often fatal fungal infection which is difficult to diagnose (1). In particular, the most common reason for an incorrect morphological diagnosis is the misidentification of genera within Mucorales as *Aspergillus* spp. (3, 4). Such misdiagnosis of mucormycosis as aspergillosis may have serious adverse consequences because invasive mucormycosis and aspergillosis are treated with different classes of antifungal agents (4). Identifying the infective pathogen rapidly and accurately is crucial for effective treatment.

EPIDEMIOLOGY

Most cases of mucormycosis are sporadic and occur in individuals with underlying diseases (1). Apart from immunocompromised patients, uncontrolled diabetes mellitus (which can cause acidosis) and treatment with corticosteroids are risk factors for the development of mucormycosis (5–7). Patients receiving cancer chemotherapy and immunosuppressive treatment for stem cell or solid organ transplantation are also at risk of developing mucormycosis (6, 8). The mortality rate from mucormycosis is often more than 50% and may be over 80% if the brain is affected or hematogenous spread occurs (1, 7). Infections most frequently result from inhalation of spores. Therefore, for aspergillosis, the respiratory system is the most important site of initial infection (1, 6, 9–12). Also similar to aspergillosis, mucormycosis is often established within the sinuses and the lungs (1, 6, 13). Infections due to genera of Mucorales may also result from trauma or ingesting food contaminated with fungal elements (5, 14, 15).

PATHOLOGY

Although mucormycotic lesions may be present in almost any organ system, their propensity for localization has led to the recognition of the following major clinical forms: rhinocerebral, pulmonary, gastrointestinal (especially in infants), cutaneous, and disseminated mucormycosis (5, 8–10, 14–16). Infections are often aggressive and develop rapidly because the disease is highly angiotrophic. Thrombosis, infarct formation, and hematogenous spread to other organs (disseminated mucormycosis) may occur (Figs. 10.1 and 10.2), as with many other mycoses including aspergillosis (1, 5, 6).

In rhinocerebral infections, where the gross lesions typically develop into dark gangrenous masses, hyphae invade tissue in the face and eventually reach the brain (1, 6, 7). Lung lesions either develop as necrotizing bronchopneumonias or are disseminated by hematogenous spread from other primary infection sites (Fig. 10.3) (10–12, 17). However, in both cases, the lesions are predominantly necrotic and often accompanied by haemorrhage (10). Pulmonary necrosis may lead to the development of cavities (11, 12). Necrotizing lesions are the most obvious sign of mucormycosis in the gastrointestinal tract and primary skin infections. The skin may become infected after a burn or other trauma, but surgical dressings or frequent injections (e.g., of insulin) may also lead to infections (5, 14).

Mucormycosis lesions are not specific, but share common features regardless of the tissue infected or the genus involved. In acute infections, infarction due to angioinvasion of arteries and venules and thrombosis accompanied by haemorrhage and coagulation necrosis are typical initial manifestations. These processes are followed by neutrophilic infiltration in non-neutropenic hosts (Fig. 10.4) (1, 5). However, in some acute infections, there is almost no inflammatory reaction in the lungs (Figs. 10.5 and 10.6) (8). In chronic lesions, the inflammatory reaction is associated with an influx of macrophages and the formation of epithelioid cells and multinucleate giant cells. Therefore, when neutrophils are also present, multifocal pyogranulomas form (Figs. 10.7 and 10.8) (1, 18, 19). This pattern of inflammatory reaction development is common among

DOI: 10.1201/9781003306177-10

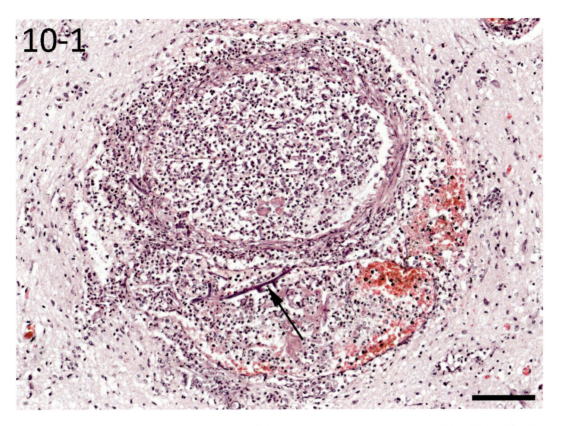

Figure 10.1 Chronic, necrotizing, pyogranulomatous, and thrombosing mucormycotic vasculitis with hyphae formation (arrow) is present within the cerebrum following hematogenous spread. HE. Bar = 150 μm.

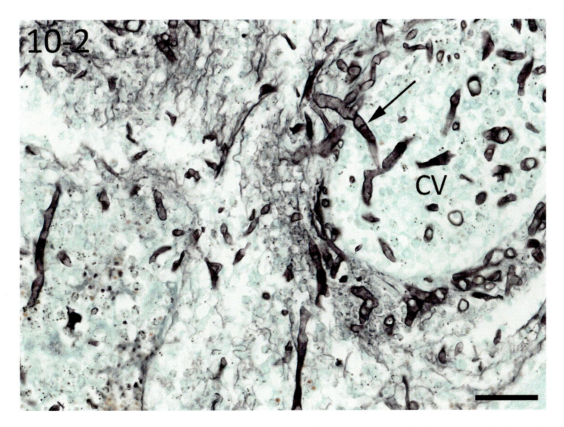

Figure 10.2 A magnified view of the specimen shown in Fig. 10.1. The mucormycotic hyphae are visible in and around the cerebral vessel (CV). In one hypha, a septum is present (arrow). GMS. Bar = 50 μm.

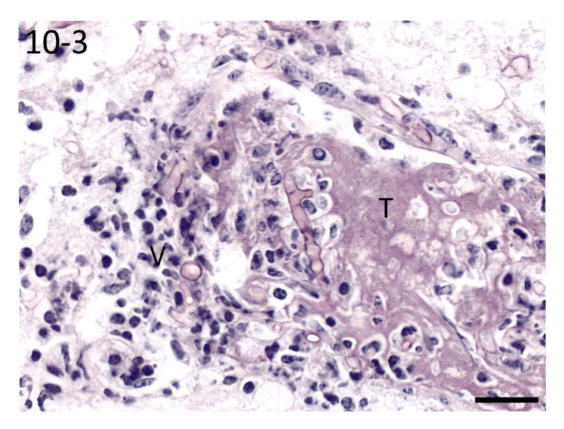

Figure 10.3 Acute, necrotizing, suppurative, and thrombosing pulmonary mucormycosis. The hyphae are penetrating the vessel wall, causing thrombosis (T) and vasculitis (V). PAS. Bar = 50 μm.

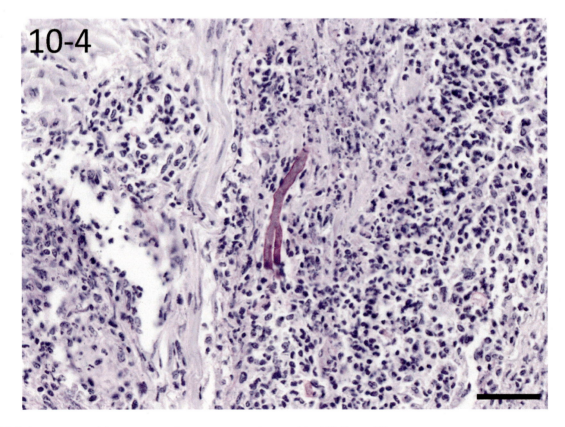

Figure 10.4 Acute, necrotizing, suppurative mucormycotic myositis. HE. Bar = 70 μm.

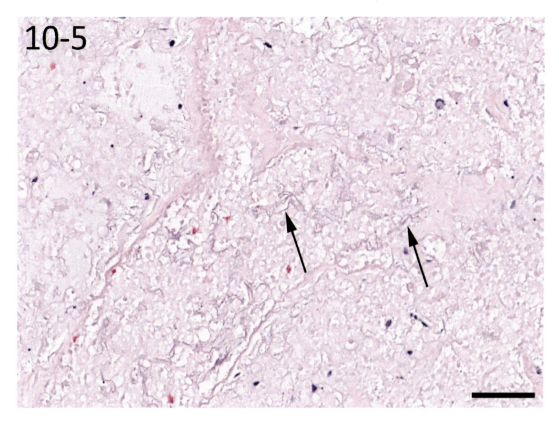

Figure 10.5 Acute, necrotizing pulmonary mucormycosis. The growth of hyphae (faintly stained (arrows) by haematoxylin and eosin) is not accompanied by an inflammatory reaction. HE. Bar = 70 μm.

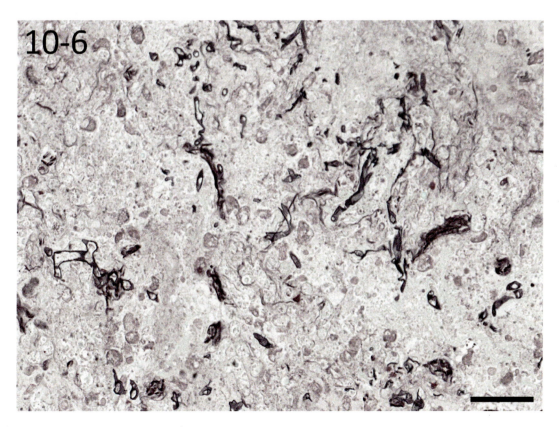

Figure 10.6 Acute, necrotizing pulmonary mucormycosis. The growth of hyphae (strongly stained by Grocott's methenamine silver) is not accompanied by an inflammatory reaction. Same case as in Fig. 10.5. GMS. Bar = 70 μm.

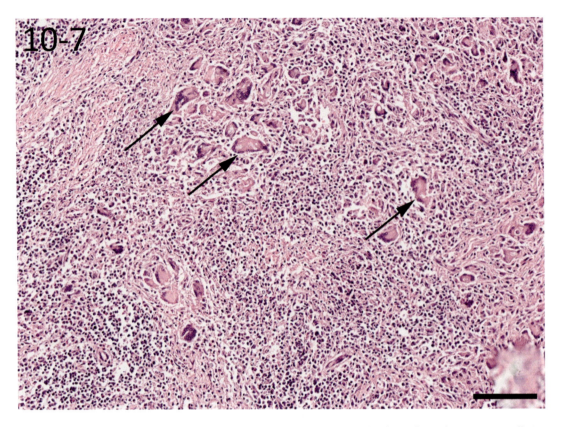

Figure 10.7 Chronic, pyogranulomatous mucormycotic lymphadenitis with multiple multinucleate giant cells (arrows) present. HE. Bar = 150 μm.

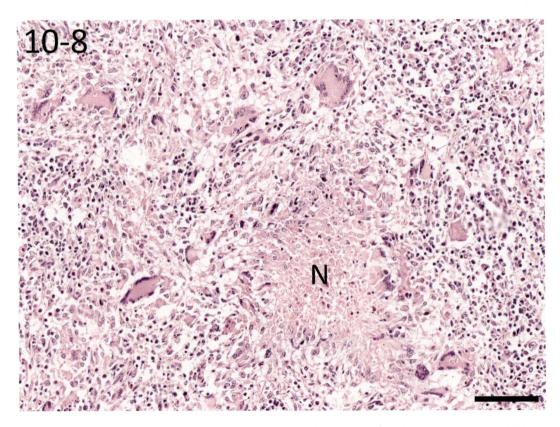

Figure 10.8 Chronic, necrotizing, pyogranulomatous mucormycotic lymphadenitis. The necrotic center (N) is surrounded by multinucleate giant cells. HE. Bar = 100 μm.

mycoses, including aspergillosis. Multinucleate giant cells may phagocytose hyphae (Figs. 10.9 and 10.10). In other chronic cases, the hyphae may be covered by asteroid bodies (i.e., the Splendore-Hoeppli phenomenon), which are eosinophilic (in haematoxylin and eosin-stained sections) and surround the pathogen (Fig. 10.11) (1). Chronic lesions may also be infiltrated with lymphocytes and plasma cells and encapsulated by fibrotic tissue. In addition, angiolymphatic invasion may occur, with fungal spread to local lymph nodes, where chronic, pyogranulomas or granulomatous necrotizing lesions are established (5, 20, 21).

FUNGAL HISTOMORPHOLOGY

The hyphae of Mucorales fungi are generally non-pigmented and broad, with a width of 6–25 µm (Figs. 10.2–10.6). The hyphal walls are typically not linear, and the width of an individual hypha often changes considerably along its length. The thickness of the walls of the Mucorales fungi also varies considerably. Hyphal septation is rarely present and the hyphae branch haphazardly, sometimes at right angles (Fig. 10.3) (3, 15, 17, 20, 22, 23). The variations in hyphal width and wall thickness, as well as the twists and folds in shape, have led to the hyphae being described as "hollow trees," especially when stained with Grocott's methenamine silver (Figs. 10.2–10.6) (24, 25). The hyphae are readily stained by haematoxylin and eosin (Fig. 10.5), periodic acid-Schiff stain, and Gridley's stain, and prolonged exposure to silver nitrate in Grocott's methenamine silver stains the hyphae black (Figs. 10.2, 10.6, and 10.10) (1, 12, 24–26). In tissues, hyphae often penetrate blood vessels, where thrombosis occurs (Figs. 10.1–10.3) (1, 24, 25). Intra- and peri-neuronal invasion is an important histological feature of rhinocerebral mucormycosis and indicates an advanced level of invasion (27). Mucormycosis hyphae penetrate a variety of tissues and may grow along corneal (28) and nerve (18, 19, 27) fibres. Cross-sections of hyphae growing in tissues exposed to air may mimic large yeast-forming fungi (e.g., spherules of *Coccidioides immitis*) (3, 17).

As described for *Aspergillus*, members of the Mucorales may occasionally produce fructification bodies, especially in the upper respiratory system where oxygen is plentiful (Fig. 10.12). As with aspergillosis, these elements may be used to identify pathogens to the genus level (24, 29).

DIFFERENTIAL DIAGNOSIS

Using histomorphology to make a mucormycosis diagnosis is not straightforward, and Mucorales fungi may be misidentified as *Aspergillus* spp. In tissues, *Aspergillus* spp. are morphologically similar to *Fusarium* spp. and *Scedosporium* spp. Therefore, mucormycosis fungi are sometimes mistaken for these too (1, 6, 24, 25, 29) (Fig. 10.4). Furthermore, the pseudohyphae and true hyphae of *Candida albicans* have been confused with those of mucormycosis genera (24, 25, 30). In lesions, Mucorales hyphae are similar to those of the Entomophthorales, which cause entomophthoromycosis. However, Entomophthorales hyphae tend to be narrower and have thinner walls. Moreover, infiltration with eosinophils is more common in Entomophthorales lesions and the Splendore-Hoeppli phenomenon is more frequently observed around hyphae in entomophthoromycosis cases than in mucormycosis cases (6). Mucorales hyphae have few septa but they have folds that resemble septa. As described above, hyphal cross-sections may be misidentified as large yeast cells.

The immunohistochemical application of commercially available monoclonal antibodies (1, 8, 30–32) and polymerase chain reaction-based techniques to either fresh or formalin-fixed paraffin-embedded tissue (Fig. 10.13) (1, 4, 32–38) have been used to identify mucormycosis pathogens, although variation in sensitivity has been reported. In addition, several specific DNA/RNA *in situ* hybridization probes are available for differentiating mucormycosis pathogens (some to the genus level) from other filamentous fungi that cause infections, including those that cause aspergillosis and yeast infections (13, 39, 40).

Mortierella wolfii, a saprophytic fungus of the family Mortierellaceae, has a worldwide distribution. *M. wolfii* is an important cause of animal infections and is only rarely causing human infections. However, in lesions the hyphae of *M. wolfii* are similar to those of the Mucorales fungi (41, 42).

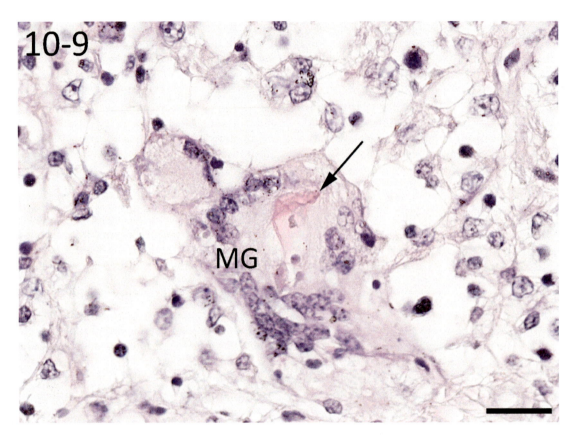

Figure 10.9 A mucormycotic hyphal fragment is visible (arrow) within the multinucleate giant cell (MG). PAS. Bar = 50 μm.

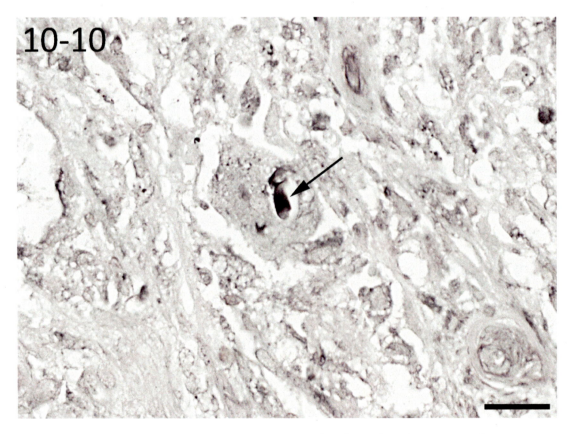

Figure 10.10 A mucormycotic hyphal fragment is present (arrow) within the multinucleate giant cell. GMS. Bar = 50 μm.

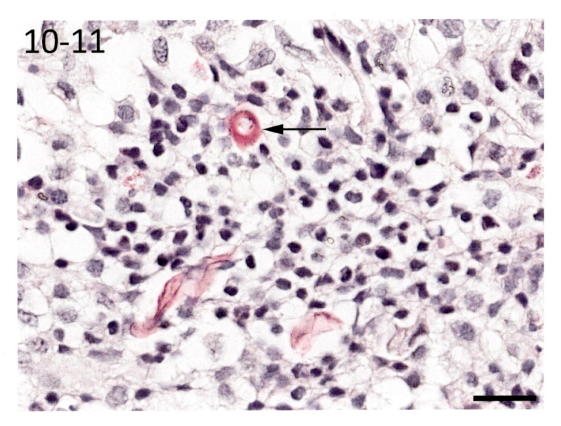

Figure 10.11 Chronic, pyogranulomatous mucormycotic pneumonia. Splendore-Hoeppli material has formed (arrow) around the cross-sectioned hyphae. HE. Bar = 40 μm.

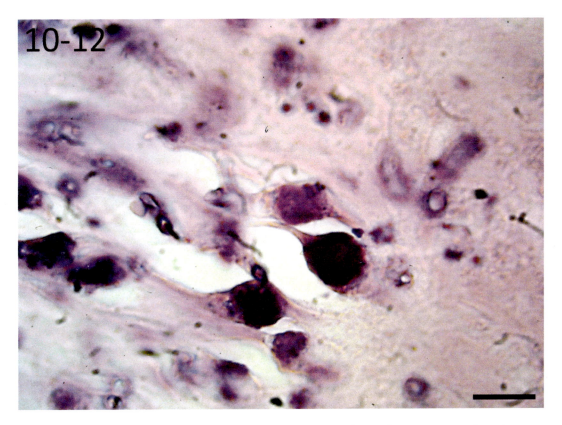

Figure 10.12 In the upper respiratory tract, the oxygen tension may be sufficient for sporangia to form in mucormycosis lesions. In the present case of acute necrotizing mucormycotic sinusitis, sporangia have formed. HE. Bar = 40 μm.

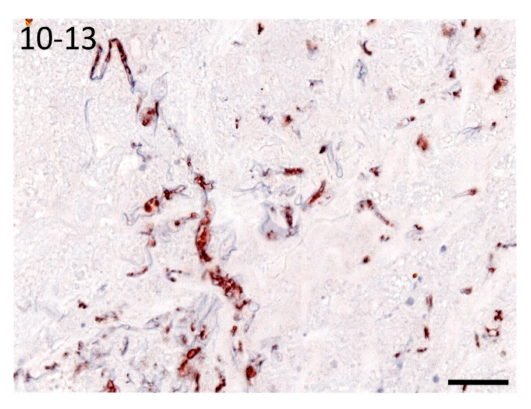

Figure 10.13 Acute, necrotizing pulmonary mucormycosis. A Mucorales-specific monoclonal antibody reacts strongly with the hyphae. IHC. Bar = 70 μm.

REFERENCES

1. Cornely OA, Alastruey-Izquierdo A, Arenz D, Chen, SCA, Dannaoui E et al. 2019. Global guideline for the diagnosis and management of mucormycosis: An initiative of the European Confederation of Medical Mycology in cooperation with the Mycoses Study Group Education and Research Consortium. Lancet Infect Dis, 19, 405–421.

2. Hoffmann K, Pawłowska J, Walther G, Wrzosek M, de Hoog GS et al. 2013. The family structure of the Mucorales: A synoptic revision based on comprehensive multigene-genealogies. Persoonia, 30, 57–76.

3. Kung VL, Chernock RD, Burnham, CAD. 2018. Diagnostic accuracy of fungal identification in histopathology and cytology specimens. Eur J Clin Microbiol Infect Dis, 37, 157–165.

4. Springer J, Lackner M, Ensinger C, Risslegger B, Morton CO et al. 2016. Clinical evaluation of a Mucorales-specific real-time PCR assay in tissue and serum samples. J Med Microbiol, 65, 1414–1421.

5. Arnáiz-García ME, Alonso-Peña D, González-Vela MDC, García-Palomo JD, Sanz-Giménez-Rico JR et al. 2009. Cutaneous mucormycosis: Report of five cases and review of the literature. J Plast Reconstr Aesthet Surg, 62, 434–441.

6. Guarner J, Brandt, ME. 2011. Histopathologic diagnosis of fungal infections in the 21st century. Clin Microbiol Rev, 24, 247–280.

7. Prakash H, Ghosh AK, Rudramurthy SM, Singh P, Xess I et al. 2019. A prospective multicenter study on mucormycosis in India: Epidemiology, diagnosis, and treatment. Med Mycol, 57, 395–402.

8. Mayayo E, Klock C, Goldani L. 2011. Thyroid involvement in disseminated zygomycosis by Cunninghamella bertholletiae: 2 cases and literature review. Int J Surg Pathol, 19, 75–79.

9. Pyrgos V, Shoham S, Walsh TJ. 2008. Pulmonary zygomycosis. Semin Respir Crit Care Med, 29, 111–120.

10. Ben-Ami R, Luna M, Lewis RE, Walsh TJ, Kontoyiannis DP. 2009. A clinicopathological study of pulmonary mucormycosis in cancer patients: Extensive angioinvasion but limited inflammatory response. J Infect, 59, 134–138.

11. Chakrabarti A, Marak RSK, Shivaprakash MR, Gupta S, Garg R et al. 2010. Cavitary pulmonary zygomycosis caused by Rhizopus homothallicus. J Clin Microbiol, 48, 1965–1969.

12. Challa S, Uppin SG, Uppin MS, Paul RT, Prayaga AK et al. 2011. Pulmonary zygomycosis: A clinicopathological study. Lung India, 28, 25–29.

13. Hirayama Y, Yajima N, Kaimori M, Akagi T, Kubo K et al. 2013. Disseminated infection and pulmonary embolization of Cunninghamella bertholletiae complicated with hemophagocytic lymphohistiocytosis. Intern Med, 52, 2275–2279.

14. Flagothier C, Arrese JE, Quatresooz P, Piérard G. 2006. Cutaneous mucormycosis. J Med Mycol, 16, 77–81.

15. Gelman A, Valdes-Rodriguez R, Bhattacharyya S, Yosipovitch G. 2015. A case of primary cutaneous mucormycosis caused by minor trauma. Dermatol Online J, 21, 12–14.

16. McDermott NE, Barrett J, Hipp J, Merino MJ, Richard LCC et al. 2010. Successful treatment of periodontal mucormycosis: Report of a case and literature review. Oral Surg Oral Med Oral Pathol Oral Radiol Endod, 109, 64–69.

17. Kimura M, Ito H. 2009. Vesicular thick-walled swollen hyphae in pulmonary zygomycosis. Case Report. Pathol Int, 59, 175–178.

18. Goel A, Kini U, Shetty S. 2010. Role of histopathology as an aid to prognosis in rhino-orbito-cerebral zygomycosis. Indian J Pathol Microbiol, 53, 253–257.

19. Frater JL, Hall GS, Procop, GW. 2001. Histologic features of zygomycosis: Emphasis on perineural invasion and fungal morphology. Arch Pathol Lab Med, 125, 375–378.

20. Barnett JEF, Davison NJ, Susan M, Riley P, Cooper T et al. 2011. Systemic mucormycosis in a hooded seal (*Cystophora cristata*). J Zoo Wildl Med, 42, 338–341.

21. Ortega J, Uzal FA, Walker R, Kinde H, Diab SS et al. 2010. Zygomycotic lymphadenitis in slaughtered feedlot cattle. Vet Pathol, 47, 108–115.

22. Kulkarni RV, Thakur SS. 2015. Invasive gastric mucormycosis—a case report. Indian J Surg, 77, 87–89.

23. Li H, Hwang SK, Zhou C, Du J, Zhang J. 2013. Gangrenous cutaneous mucormycosis caused by *Rhizopus oryzae*: A case report and review of primary cutaneous mucormycosis in China over past 20 years. Mycopathologia, 176, 123–128.

24. Jensen HE, Chandler FW. 2007. Histopathological diagnoses of mycoses. In: Topley and Wilson's Microbiology & Microbial Infections. Medical Mycology. 10th ed. Merz WG, Hay RJ, Eds. Hodder Arnold. pp 121–143.

25. Jensen HE. 2021. Histopathology in the diagnosis of invasive fungal diseases. Curr Fungal Infect Rep, 15, 23–31.

26. Cunha SCS, Aguero C, Damico CB, Corgozinho KB, Souza HJM et al. 2011. Duodenal perforation caused by *Rhizomucor* species in a cat. J Feline Med Surg, 13, 205–207.

27. Sravani T, Uppin SG, Uppin MS, Sundaram C. 2014. Rhinocerebral mucormycosis: Pathology revisited with emphasis on perineural spread. Neurol India, 62, 383–386.

28. Feizi S, Jafarinasab MR, Kanavi MR. 2012. A zygomycetes-contaminated corneal graft harvested from a donor with signs of orbital trauma. Cornea, 31, 84–86.

29. Suzuta F, Kimura K, Urakawa R, Kusuda Y, Tanaka S et al. 2015. Variations in the morphology of *Rhizomucor pusillus* in granulomatous lesions of a Magellanic penguin (*Spheniscus magellanicus*). J Vet Med Sci, 77, 1029–1031.

30. Jensen HE, Salonen J, Ekfors TO.1997. The use of immunohistochemistry to improve sensitivity and specificity in the diagnosis of systemic mycoses in patients with haematological malignancies. J Pathol, 181, 100–105.

31. Jung J, Park YS, Sung H, Song JS, Lee SO et al. 2015. Using immunohistochemistry to assess the accuracy of histomorphologic diagnosis of aspergillosis and mucormycosis. Clin Infect Dis, 61, 1664–1670.

32. Abdo W, Kakizoe Y, Ryono M, Dover SR, Fukushi H et al. 2012. Pulmonary zygomycosis with *Cunninghamella bertholletiae* in a killer whale (*Orcinus orca*). J Comp Pathol, 147, 94–99.

33. Salehi E, Hedayati MT, Zoll J, Rafati H, Ghasemi M et al. 2016. Discrimination of aspergillosis, mucormycosis, fusariosis, and scedosporiosis in formalin-fixed paraffin-embedded tissue specimens by use of multiple real-time quantitative PCR assays. J Clin Microbiol, 54, 2798–2803.

34. Drogari-Apiranthitou M, Panayiotides I, Galani I, Konstantoudakis S, Arvanitidis G et al. 2016. Diagnostic value of a semi-nested PCR for the diagnosis of mucormycosis and aspergillosis from paraffin-embedded tissue: A single center experience. Pathol Res Pract, 212, 393–339.

35. Dhaliwal HS, Singh A, Sinha SK, Nampoothiri, RV, Goyal A et al. 2015. Diagnosed only if considered: Isolated renal mucormycosis. Lancet, 385, 2322.

36. Bernal-Martínez L, Buitrago MJ, Castelli MV, Rodriguez-Tudela JL, Cuenca-Estrella M. 2012. Development of a single tube multiplex real-time PCR to detect the most clinically relevant Mucormycetes species. Clin Microbiol Infect, 19, 1–7.

37. Zaman K, Rudramurthy SM, Das A, Panda N, Honnavar P et al. 2017. Molecular diagnosis of rhino-orbito-cerebral mucormycosis from fresh tissue samples. J Med Microbiol, 66, 1124–1129.

38. Springer J, Goldenberger D, Schmidt F, Weisser M, Wehrle-Wieland E et al. 2016. Development and application of two independent real-time PCR assays to detect clinically relevant Mucorales species. J Med Microbiol, 65, 227–234.

39. Hayden RT, Qian X, Procop GW, Roberts GD, Lloyd RV. 2002. In situ hybridization for the identification of filamentous fungi in tissue section. Diagn Mol Pathol 11, 119–126.

40. Louie C, Schwartz LE, Litzky LA, Nachamkin I, Montone KT. 2011. Disseminated fungal infections at autopsy: Multiple fungal species identified by in situ hybridization. Pathol Case Rev, 16, 260–265.

41. Therese KL, Lakshmipathy M, Lakshmipathy D. 2020. First report of Mortierella wolfii causing fungal keratitis from a tertiary eye hospital in India. Indian J Ophthalmol, 68, 2272–2274.

42. Munday JS, Laven RA, Orbell GMB, Pandey SK. 2006. Meningoencephalitis in an adult cow due to Mortierella wolfii. J Vet Diagn Invest, 18, 619–622.

11

Entomophthoromycosis

INTRODUCTION

Entomophthoromycosis is due to infection with pathogens of the genera *Basidiobolus* or *Conidiobolus*, causing basidiobolomycosis or conidiobolomycosis, respectively (1–3). The clinically most important species within these two genera are *B. ranarum* and *C. coronatus*. However, infections with other species, such as *C. incongruus* and *C. lamprauges*, have also been reported (3, 4).

Previously, the term zygomycosis was used to describe two different clinicopathological diseases: mucormycosis due to infection by members of the order Mucorales and entomophthoromycosis caused by members of the order Entomophthorales (1, 3). Infection by *Basidiobolus* or *Conidiobolus* predominantly occurs in tropical areas of South America, Africa, and Asia (3, 5).

EPIDEMIOLOGY

Members of the Entomophthorales are found within arthropod carcasses, and they are pathogens of some insects. In the environment, they occur in tropical rain forests, soil, and rotten vegetation and they may be present within the gastrointestinal tracts of insectivorous animals (3).

Both pathogenic genera (*Basidiobolus* and *Conidiobolus*) of the Entomophthorales cause primary infections in the skin and subcutaneous tissue. However, whereas basidiobolomycosis primarily occurs on the body extremities and the trunk, conidiobolomycosis typically occurs in the sinuses, orbital regions, and the skin on the head (2, 3). Dermal infections result from trauma, including insect bites (6). Infection of the upper respiratory system, and in particular the sinuses, results from the inhalation of spores, which may lie dormant within the sinuses (3). In animals, especially sheep, conidiobolomycosis causes head infections, including outbreaks of both rhinocerebral and rhinopharyngeal conidiobolomycosis that have occurred in particular regions of Brazil (7–9). Despite the typical pattern of infection sites, both basidiobolomycosis and conidiobolomycosis have also been diagnosed in the gastrointestinal tracts of both humans and animals, probably following ingestion of soil, animal faeces, or contaminated food (5, 6, 10, 11). In rare cases, the systemic spread may also occur (3).

PATHOLOGY

Basidiobolomycosis and conidiobolomycosis cause similar and characteristic tissue reactions. In acute lesions, necrosis and haemorrhage are accompanied by eosinophilic exudation, which may result in eosinophilic abscesses (3, 5, 6, 10). Hemosiderin-loaded macrophages will be present due to haemorrhage. Neutrophils will also be present, together with the eosinophils. In chronic lesions, multiple pyogranulomas are formed, with abundant infiltration of eosinophils, macrophages, epithelioid cells, multinucleate giant cells, lymphocytes, and plasma cells (Figs. 11.1–11.4) (2, 3, 6).

Typically, angioinvasion does not occur in infections that solely affect the skin and subcutaneous tissues (2, 3). Lymphangiectasia causes lymphoedema, resulting in facial elephantiasis when infections occur in the head of humans or animals such as sheep (7–9, 12). Entomophthoromycosis has been experimentally introduced into several animal species including gerbils, and the same infective elements that occur in spontaneous cases have been detected (4).

Angioinvasion occurs in systemically spread *Conidiobolus* infections, but in most of these cases, the Splendore-Hoeppli phenomenon is absent (3, 10). Therefore, the formation of the Splendore-Hoeppli material may be due to an effective host immune response that hampers invasion of surrounding tissues and blood vessels, preventing the dissemination of the infection (3).

FUNGAL HISTOMORPHOLOGY

Within tissues, the fungal morphology of *Basidiobolus* spp. and *Conidiobolus* spp. is identical (3). The hyphae exhibit frequent septation with an irregular pattern. They are thin walled, with a mean width of approximately 8 μm. However, among lesions, variation in mean width from 6 to 12 μm has been reported (3), and widths of up to 25 μm (9) and 30 μm (8) have been observed (Figs. 11.5 and 11.6). The hyphae, which are not stained by haematoxylin and eosin, are well stained by both periodic acid-Schiff and Grocott's methenamine silver stains and clearly exhibit septation (Figs. 11.7 and 11.8) (6, 10, 13). Characteristic and pronounced Splendore-Hoeppli phenomena are clearly visible around the hyphae. This material, which is eosinophilic and proteinaceous,

DOI: 10.1201/9781003306177-11

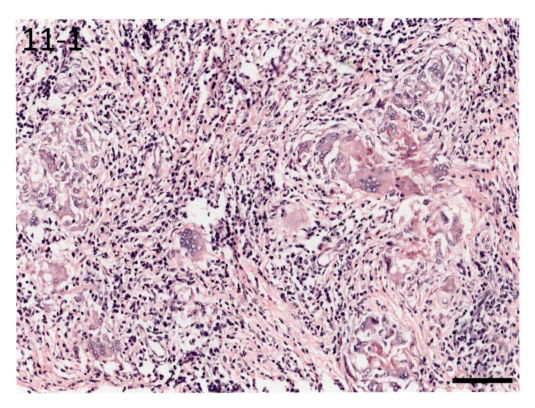

Figure 11.1 Chronic, subcutaneous pyogranulomatous entomophthoromycosis due to *B. ranarum*. Multiple multinucleate giant cells are present together with neutrophils and eosinophils. The processes are interspersed with fibrous tissue. HE. Bar = 60 μm.

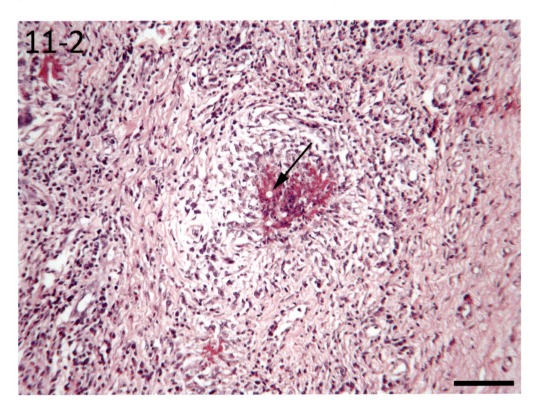

Figure 11.2 Chronic, subcutaneous pyogranulomatous entomophthoromycosis due to *B. ranarum*. Within a pyogranuloma, a hyphal cross-section (arrow) is surrounded by eosinophilic material (Splendore-Hoeppli phenomenon), which is surrounded by macrophages and epithelioid cells arranged in a palisade pattern. HE. Bar = 75 μm.

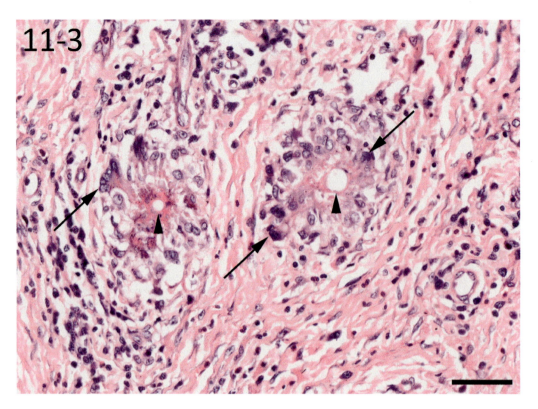

Figure 11.3 Chronic, subcutaneous pyogranulomatous entomophthoromycosis due to *B. ranarum*. A magnified pyogranuloma. Multinucleate giant cells (arrows) are present, together with macrophages and epithelioid cells. Arrowheads: cross-sections of hyphae. HE. Bar = 30 μm.

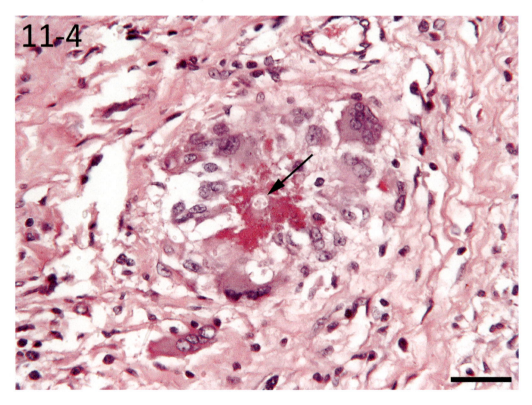

Figure 11.4 Chronic, subcutaneous pyogranulomatous entomophthoromycosis due to *B. ranarum*. A magnified central cross-section of *B. ranarum* (arrow) is surrounded by an eosinophilic mass (Splendore-Hoeppli phenomenon), which is surrounded by multinucleate giant cells and eosinophils. HE. Bar = 20 μm.

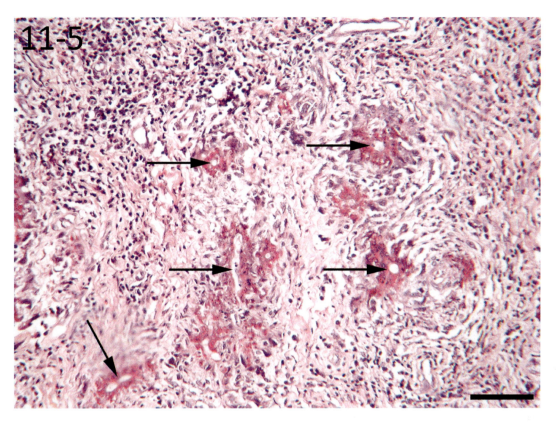

Figure 11.5 Chronic, submucosal nasal pyogranulomatous entomophthoromycosis due to *C. coronatus*. The outline of the non-stained hyphae (arrows) is surrounded by Splendore-Hoeppli material. HE. Bar = 75 μm.

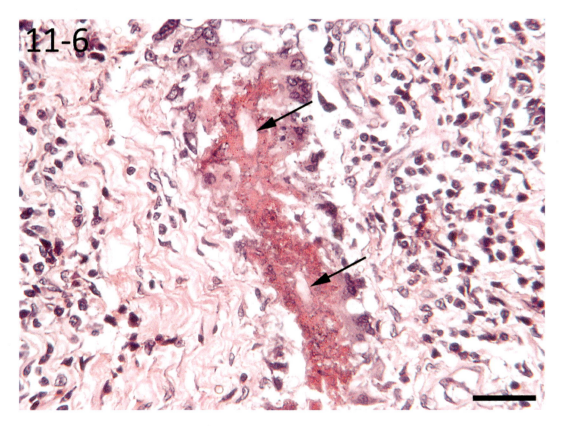

Figure 11.6 Chronic, submucosal nasal pyogranulomatous entomophthoromycosis due to *C. coronatus*. Magnified non-stained hyphae (arrows) are surrounded by Splendore-Hoeppli material, which is surrounded by multinucleate giant cells and epithelioid cells. HE. Bar = 20 μm.

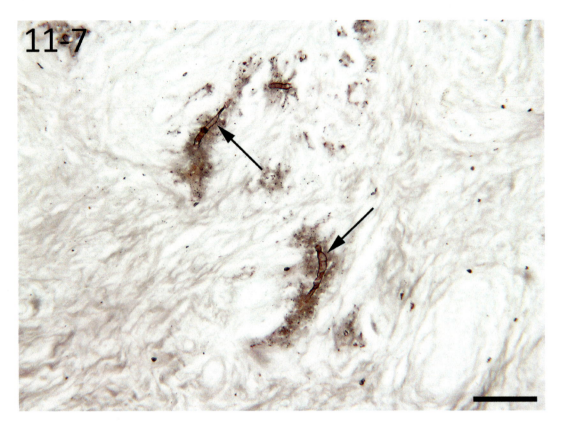

Figure 11.7 Chronic, submucosal nasal pyogranulomatous entomophthoromycosis due to *C. coronatus*. The hyphae (arrows) and the surrounding Splendore-Hoeppli material are stained brown/black with Grocott's methenamine silver stain. GMS. Bar = 75 μm.

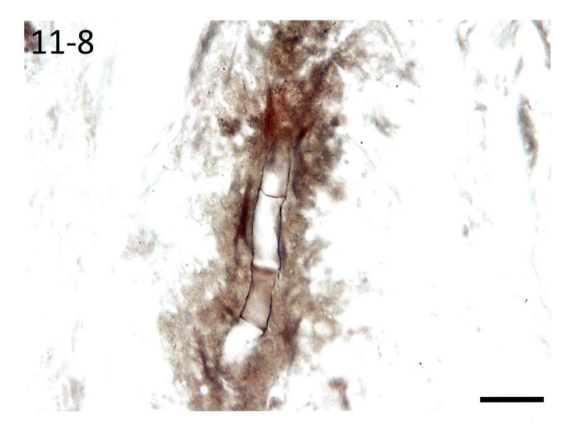

Figure 11.8 Chronic, submucosal nasal pyogranulomatous entomophthoromycosis due to *C. coronatus*. Hyphal septation is clearly shown by Grocott's methenamine silver stain. GMS. Bar = 15 μm.

is faintly stained by Grocott's methenamine silver stain (Figs. 11.7 and 11.8) (6). The hyphae are often found together with material reminiscent of the Splendore-Hoeppli phenomenon within Langhans-type and/or foreign-body-type multinucleate giant cells (Figs. 11.1 and 11.4) (6).

DIFFERENTIAL DIAGNOSIS

Although the Splendore-Hoeppli phenomenon may be observed in several mycoses (e.g., sporotrichosis, coccidioidomycosis, blastomycosis, mucormycosis, aspergillosis, pythiosis, and paracoccidioidomycosis), in cases of entomophthoromycosis it is very prominent around the hyphae (2, 3, 6). Mucormycosis and pythiosis often generate pyogranulomatous lesions, and the hyphae present in these mycoses are similar to those observed in entomophthoromycosis (11). However, in contrast to entomophthoromycosis, the hyphae in both mucormycosis and pythiosis, although broad with irregularly branched, exhibit sparse septation. The Splendore-Hoeppli material consists of antigen–antibody complexes, tissue debris, and fibrin, and it is often manifest in entomophthoromycosis cases. It may also occur, to a lesser extent, in chronic cases of both mucormycosis and pythiosis (11, 13). However, mucormycosis and pythiosis lesions are not heavily infiltrated with eosinophils, if infiltrated by these cells at all. Interestingly, Splendore-Hoeppli material also forms in some bacterial infections (e.g., around *Staphylococcus aureus* colonies in botryomycosis), around several migrating parasites (e.g., schistosomiasis and helminths), and may cover inert foreign bodies (3, 13).

REFERENCES

1. Kwon-Chung KJ. 2012. Taxonomy of fungi causing mucormycosis and entomophthoramycosis (zygomycosis) and nomenclature of the disease: Molecular mycologic perspectives. Clin Infect Dis, 54, 8–15.
2. Guarner J, Brandt, ME. 2011. Histopathologic diagnosis of fungal infections in the 21st century. Clin Microbiol Rev, 24, 247–280.
3. Choon SE, Kang J, Neafie RC, Ragsdale B, Klassen-Fischer M et al. 2012. Conidiobolomycosis in a young Malaysian woman showing chronic localized fibrosing leukocytoclastic vasculitis: A case report and meta-analysis focusing on clinicopathologic and therapeutic correlations with outcome. Am J Dermatopathol, 34, 511–522.
4. de Godoy I, de Campos CG, Pescador CA, Galceran JVA, Cândido SL et al. 2017. Experimental infection in gerbils by *Conidiobolus lamprauges*. Microb Pathog, 105, 251–254.
5. Saadah OI, Farouq MF, Daajani NA, Kamal JS, Ghanem AT. 2012. Gastrointestinal basidiobolomycosis in a child; an unusual fungal infection mimicking fistulising Crohn's disease. J Crohn's Colitis, 6, 368–372.
6. Nemenqani D, Yaqoob N, Khoja H, Al Saif O, Amra NK et al. 2009. Gastrointestinal basidiobolomycosis: An unusual fungal infection mimicking colon cancer. Arch Pathol Lab Med, 133, 1938–1942.
7. Câmara ACL, Soto-Blanco B, Batista JS, Vale AM, Feijó FMC et al. 2011. Rhinocerebral and rhinopharyngeal conidiobolomycosis in sheep. Ciênc Rural, 41, 862–868.
8. Silva SMMDS, Castro RS, Costa FAL, Vasconcelos AC, Batista MCS et al. 2007. Conidiobolomycosis in sheep in Brazil. Vet Pathol, 44, 314–319.
9. Mendonça FS, Albuquerque RF, Evêncio-Neto J, Dória RGS, de Camargo LM et al. 2012. Conidiobolomycosis in sheep in the state of Pernambuco. Rev Bras Med Vet, 34, 241–246.
10. van den Berk GEL, Noorduyn LA, van Ketel RJ, van Leeuwen J, Bemelman WA et al. 2006. A fatal pseudo-tumour: Disseminated basidiobolomycosis. BMC Infect Dis, 6, 140–144.
11. Okada K, Amano S, Kawamura Y, Kagawa Y. 2015. Gastrointestinal basidiobolomycosis in a dog. J Vet Med Sci, 77, 1311–1313.
12. Azadeh B, McCarthy DO, Dalton A, Campbell F. 2004. Gastrointestinal zygomycosis: Two case reports. Histopathology, 44, 298–300.
13. Hussein MR. 2010. Mucocutaneous Splendore-Hoeppli phenomenon. J. Cutan Pathol, 56, 3–23.

12

Pythiosis

INTRODUCTION

Species of the genus *Pythium* are found worldwide in soil but especially in aquatic environments and are important plant pathogens (1). One of these species, *P. insidiosum*, is the cause of pythiosis in animals and humans (1–10). This organism is an oomycete, which implies that it is more an algae-like organism than a fungus. Uncontrolled pythiosis in both animals and humans is life-threatening (4, 6–8, 10, 11). From a histomorphological viewpoint, it may be difficult to distinguish pythiosis from entomophthoromycosis. However, pythiosis and mucormycosis may also be confused with one another.

EPIDEMIOLOGY

Pythiosis mainly occurs in tropical and subtropical regions of Asia, Australia, New Zealand, South and Central America, and in the Gulf coast states of the United States. However, it also occurs in the central United States (6, 12–14). Infections occur in several animal species (e.g., horses, donkeys, dogs, cattle, and goats, as well as domestic and exotic cats) and in humans (6, 7, 9–11, 15–17). The gastrointestinal tract of dogs (14, 18), the nasal cavities of horses, and subcutaneous tissues in all animals and humans are particularly susceptible to infections (10, 11, 16, 19, 20). Subcutaneous infections occur in humans, and sometimes the eyes and vasculature are affected (3, 4, 19). In animals, pythiosis is not considered an opportunistic infection, because it is not predominantly associated with immunodeficiency or underlying disease. However, a survey from Thailand showed that most patients with cutaneous/subcutaneous, vascular, and disseminated pythiosis had underlying thalassemia-hemoglobinopathy syndrome (3). Infections are often linked to contact with stagnant water, and small skin injuries increase the risk of subcutaneous and eye infections, whereas contaminated drinking water causes gastrointestinal infections (21).

PATHOLOGY

The pathological reaction that occurs in animals and humans with pythiosis is similar and typically consists of well-defined eosinophilic coagulative to liquefactive necrosis involving fibrin and neutrophils (Figs. 12.1 and 12.2).

Lesions are surrounded by macrophages, epithelioid cells, and Langhans-type and/or foreign-body-type multinucleate giant cells (Figs. 12.3 and 12.4) (2, 10, 11, 22). In chronic cases, extensive fibrosis occurs and plasma cells will be present (Figs. 12.5 and 12.6) (23). Some lesions are heavily infiltrated with eosinophils (Fig. 12.2) (2, 9–11). Local angioinvasion regularly occurs in infections of both animals and humans (10, 11). In humans, this will often lead to thrombosis and infarct formation, resulting in gangrenous necrosis that requires amputation (3, 4). In pythiosis lesions, hyphae are found within necrotic areas and may be engulfed by multinucleate giant cells (Fig. 12.4) (24).

FUNGAL HISTOMORPHOLOGY

The fungal hyphae of pythiosis are not stained by hematoxylin and eosin and only weakly stained by periodic acid-Schiff stain, if at all. Therefore, any hyphae (there may be few within lesions) are best visualized by applying Grocott's methenamine silver stain (Figs. 12.7 and 12.8) (5, 6, 10, 11, 14). The outline of hyphae may be visualized by negative staining with hematoxylin and eosin (Figs. 12.2 and 12.4), and the width of these hyphae reportedly varies in different studies: 5–8 μm (18), 7–10 μm (5), 5–7 μm (14), 2–8 μm (16), 3–7 μm (20), 4.8–7.2 μm; the mean width of hyphae was 6.34 μm (25). The hyphae are rarely septate and they may exhibit irregular branching, including at right angles (Figs. 12.7 and 12.8). The hyphal walls generally run parallel, are relatively thick, and sometimes exhibit globose dilatations (24) (Fig. 12.8). In several cases of pythiosis, the hyphae were surrounded by eosinophilic Splendore-Hoeppli material (Figs. 12.2 and 12.5) (10, 18).

DIFFERENTIAL DIAGNOSIS

In lesions, the hyphae of *P. insidiosum* are morphologically similar to those of species within the orders Mucorales and Entomophthorales (*Basidiobolus* spp. and *Conidiobolus* spp.) (12, 13, 19, 20). Compared to hyphae of genera within the Mucorales, *P. insidiosum* hyphae tend to be more uniform and have parallel walls. Moreover, in mucormycosis cases, eosinophils are not usually abundant and the Splendore-Hoeppli phenomenon rarely forms around hyphae. It is much more difficult to differentiate pythiosis and entomophthoromycosis

DOI: 10.1201/9781003306177-12

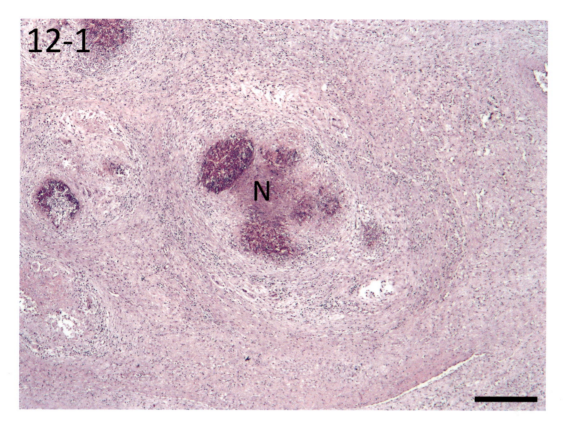

Figure 12.1 Chronic, subcutaneous eosinophilic coagulative necrosis (N) due to *P. insidiosum*. The lesion is encapsulated by fibrous tissue. HE. Bar = 150 μm.

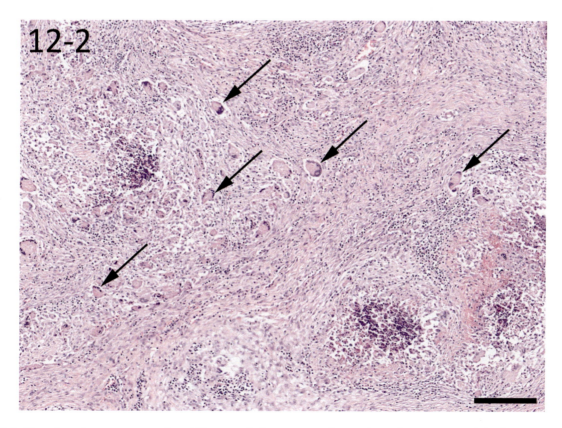

Figure 12.2 Chronic, subcutaneous eosinophilic coagulative necrosis due to *P. insidiosum*. Around the lesions, several multinucleate giant cells (arrows) are present. HE. Bar = 100 μm.

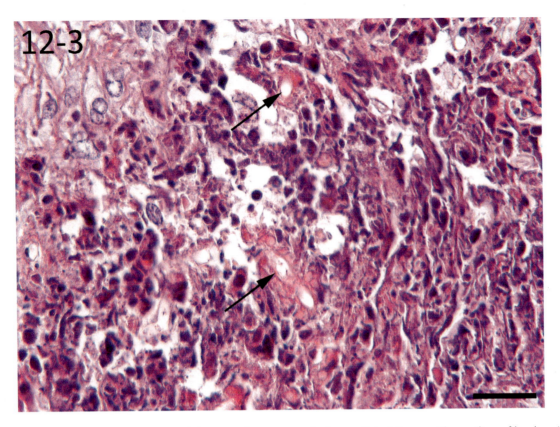

Figure 12.3 Chronic, subcutaneous eosinophilic coagulative necrosis due to *P. insidiosum*. The outline of hyphae (arrows), surrounded by Splendore-Hoeppli material, is visible within the necrotic lesion, together with the infiltration of macrophages. HE. Bar = 60 μm.

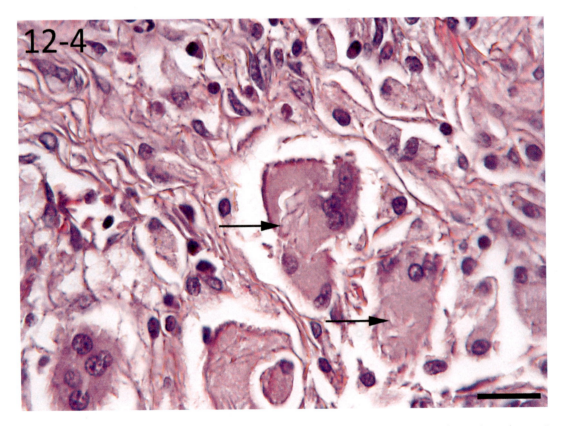

Figure 12.4 Chronic, subcutaneous eosinophilic coagulative necrosis due to *P. insidiosum*. The multinucleate giant cells contain fragments of hyphae (arrows). HE. Bar = 25 μm.

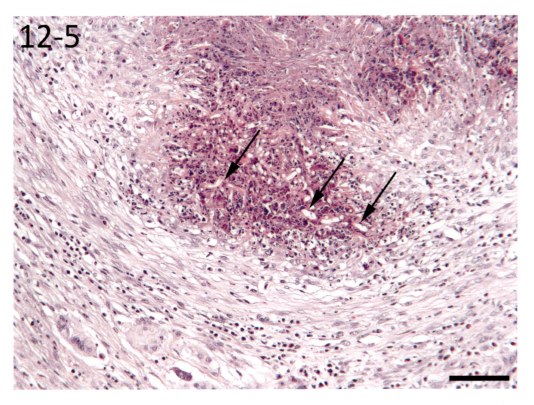

Figure 12.5 Chronic, subcutaneous eosinophilic coagulative necrosis due to *P. insidiosum*. Chronic lesions of pythiosis with hyphae (arrows) surrounded by Splendore-Hoeppli material are encapsulated by fibrosis and interspersed with macrophages, macrophage-derived cells, lymphocytes, and plasma cells. HE. Bar = 60 µm.

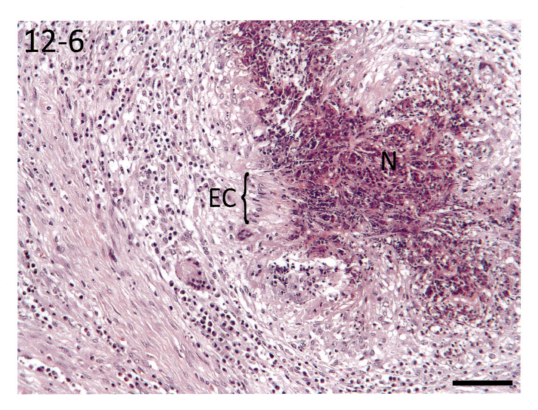

Figure 12.6 Chronic, subcutaneous eosinophilic coagulative necrosis due to *P. insidiosum*. Hematoxylin and eosin staining shows the outline of hyphae, which are surrounded by Splendore-Hoeppli material, within the necrotic area (N). There are also epithelioid cells (EC) around the necrotic area. HE. Bar = 60 µm.

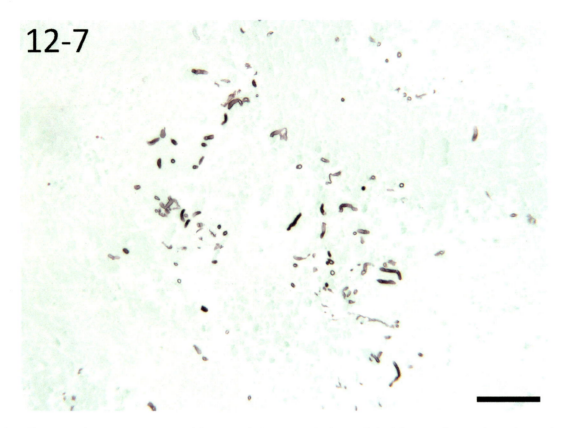

Figure 12.7 Chronic, subcutaneous eosinophilic coagulative necrosis due to *P. insidiosum*. Grocott's methenamine silver stain shows the hyphae of *P. insidiosum* within the necrotic lesions. GMS. Bar = 80 μm.

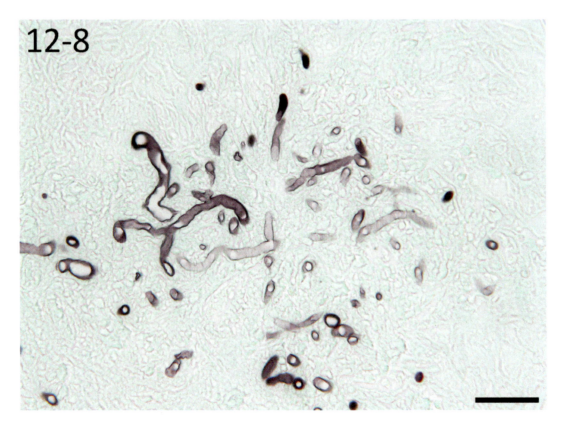

Figure 12.8 Chronic, subcutaneous eosinophilic coagulative necrosis due to *P. insidiosum*. The irregular pattern of branching is clearly visible in Grocott's methenamine silver-stained sections. GMS. Bar = 25 μm.

lesions because the latter also exhibit an influx of eosinophils and hyphae are also surrounded by Splendore-Hoeppli material (see chapter on Entomophthoromycosis). Therefore, to make an accurate diagnosis of pythiosis *in situ*, a specific and sensitive immunohistochemical protocol (e.g., based on a rabbit anti-ELI025 antibody) is required (5, 10, 16, 17, 26).

REFERENCES

1. Mendoza L, Hernandez F, Ajello L. 1993. Life cycle of the human and animal Oomycete pathogen *Pythium insidiosum*. J Clin Microbiol, 31, 2967–2973.

2. Triscott JA, Weedon D, Cabana E. 1993. Human subcutaneous pythiosis. J Cutan Pathol, 20, 267–271.

3. Krajaejun T, Sathapatayavongs B, Pracharktam R, Nitiyanant P, Leelachaikul P et al. 2006. Clinical and epidemiological analyses of human pythiosis in Thailand. Clin Infect Dis, 43, 569–576.

4. Chitasombat, MN, Larbcharoensub N, Chindamporn A, Krajaejun T. 2018. Clinicopathological features and outcomes of pythiosis. Inter J Infect Dis, 71, 33–41.

5. Bernardo FD, Conhizak C, Ambrosini F, de Jesus FPK, Santurio JM et al. 2015. Pythiosis in sheep from Paraná, Southern Brazil. Pesqui Vet Bras, 35, 513–517.

6. Berryessa NA, Marks SL, Pesavento PA, Krasnansky T, Yoshimoto SK et al. 2008. Gastrointestinal pythiosis in 10 dogs from California. J Vet Intern Med, 22, 1065–1069.

7. Buergelt C, Powe J, White T. 2006. Abdominal pythiosis in a Bengal tiger (*Panthera tigris tigris*). J Zoo Wildl Med, 37, 186–189.

8. Camus AC, Grooters AM, Aquilar RF. 2004. Granulomatous pneumonia caused by *Pythium insidiosum* in a central American jaguar, *Panthera onca*. J Vet Diagn Invest, 16, 567–571.

9. Do Carmo PMS, Portela RA, Silva TR, Oliveira-Filho JC, Riet-Correa F. 2015. Cutaneous pythiosis in a goat. J Comp Pathol, 152, 103–105.

10. Martins TB, Kommers GD, Trost ME, Inkelmann MA, Fighera RA et al. 2012. A comparative study of the histopathology and immunohistochemistry of pythiosis in horses, dogs and cattle. J Comp Pathol, 146, 122–131.

11. Kirzhner M, Arnold SR, Lyle C, Mendoza LL, Fleming JC. 2015. *Pythium insidiosum*: A rare necrotizing orbital and facial infection. J Pediatr Infect Dis Soc, 4, 10–13.

12. Connolly SL, Frank C, Thompson CA, Van Alstine WG, Gelb H et al. 2012. Dual infection with *Pythium insidiosum* and *Blastomyces dermatitidis* in a dog. Vet Clin Pathol, 41, 419–423.

13. Dykstra MJ, Sharp NJH, Olivry T, Hillier A, Murphy KM et al. 1999. A description of cutaneous-subcutaneous pythiosis in fifteen dogs. Med Mycol, 37, 427–433.

14. Helman RG, Oliver J. 1999. Pythiosis of the digestive tract in dogs from Oklahoma. J Am Anim Hosp Assoc, 35, 111–114.

15. Rakich PM, Grooters AM, Tang KN. 2005. Gastrointestinal pythiosis in two cats. J Vet Diagn Invest, 17, 262–269.

16. Souto EPF, Maia LA, Olinda RG, Galiza GJN, Kommers GD et al. 2016. Pythiosis in the nasal cavity of horses. J Comp Pathol, 155, 126–129.

17. Ubiali DG, Cruz RAS, De Paula DAJ, Silva MC, Mendonça FS et al. 2013. Pathology of nasal infection caused by *Conidiobolus lamprauges* and *Pythium insidiosum* in sheep. J Comp Pathol, 149, 137–145.

18. Fischer JR, Pace LW, Turk JR, Kreeger JM, Miller MA et al. 1994. Gastrointestinal pythiosis in Missouri dogs: Eleven cases. J Vet Diagn Invest, 6, 380–382.

19. Tanhehco TY, Stacy RC, Mendoza L, Durand ML, Jakobiec FA et al. 2011. *Pythium insidiosum* keratitis in Israel. Eye Contact Lens, 37, 96–98.

20. Morton LD, Morton DG, Baker GJ, Gelberg HB. 1991. Chronic eosinophilic enteritis attributed to *Pythium* sp. in a horse. Vet Pathol, 28, 542–544.

21. Neto RT, Bosco SMG, Amorim RL, Brandao CV, Fabris VE et al. 2010. Cutaneous pythiosis in a dog from Brazil. Vet Dermatol, 21, 202–204.

22. LeBlanc CJ, Echandi RL, Moore RR, Souza C, Grooters AM. 2008. Hypercalcemia associated with gastric pythiosis in a dog. Vet Clin Pathol, 37, 115–120.

23. Pereira DIB, Schild AL, Motta MA, Fighera RA, Sallis ESV et al. 2010. Cutaneous and gastrointestinal pythiosis in a dog in Brazil. Vet Res Commun, 34, 301–306.

24. Pessoa CRM, Riet-Correa F, Pimentel LA, Garino F, Dantas AFM et al. 2012. Pythiosis of the digestive tract in sheep. J Vet Diagn Invest, 24, 1133–1136.

25. Howerth EW, Brown CC, Crowder C. 1989. Subcutaneous pythiosis in a dog. J Vet Diagn Invest, 1, 81–83.

26. Inkomlue R, Larbcharoensub N, Karnsombut P, Lerksuthirat T, Aroonroch R et al. 2016. Development of an anti-elicitin antibody-based immunohistochemical assay for diagnosis of pythiosis. J Clin Microbiol, 54, 43–48.

13

Hyalohyphomycosis, minor

INTRODUCTION

Fungal infections caused by hyaline (non-coloured) and septate hyphae are termed hyalohyphomycoses. Separate chapters have focused on the most frequently (major forms) occurring hyalohyphomycoses (e.g., aspergillosis, fusariosis, scedosporiosis/lomentosporiosis, trichosporonosis, mucormycosis, entomophthoromycosis, and pythiosis). Therefore, in the present chapter, the focus is on the rare and minor causes of hyalohyphomycoses. These include species of *Paecilomyces*, *Purpureocillium*, *Acremonium*, *Gliomastix*, *Sarocladium*, *Scopulariopsis/Microascus* (teleomorphs), *Penicillium*, *Trichoderma*, *Beauveria*, *Schizophyllum*, *Phaeoacremonium*, *Saprochaete*, *Rasamsonia*, and *Geotrichum candidum* (1–3).

EPIDEMIOLOGY

Similar to those responsible for the major forms of hyalohyphomycosis, the fungal agents responsible for the rare hyalohyphomycoses occur ubiquitously in the environment. Some of these organisms are commensal and may be present in the gastrointestinal tract, on the skin, and mucosa and are found worldwide, although they may be more common in particular geographic locations (1–5). Generally, pathogens that cause rare hyalohyphomycoses predominantly produce mucocutaneous infections, but they may also produce systemic infections that have a high mortality rate (1, 2, 4, 6–8). As with aspergillosis, fusariosis, and mucormycosis, the rare forms of hyalohyphomycosis are generally opportunistic and are usually associated with different forms of immunosuppression and/or underlying diseases, premature birth, organ transplantation, diabetes, or dialysis (1, 4, 5, 9–15).

PATHOLOGY

As with the major forms of hyalohyphomycosis (e.g., aspergillosis, fusariosis, scedosporiosis/lomentosporiosis, trichosporonosis, mucormycosis, entomophthoromycosis, and pythiosis), acute lesions caused by the rare forms of hyalohyphomycosis are necrotic and suppurative, whereas chronic lesions may exhibit granulomatous or pyogranulomatous inflammation containing macrophages, multinucleate giant cells, and epithelioid cells (Figs. 13.1–13.6) (5, 11, 16–18). Chronic infections caused by the rare forms of hyalohyphomycosis are typically associated with fibrosis and abscesses (14, 15).

FUNGAL HISTOMORPHOLOGY

The pathogens that cause rare hyalohyphomycosis cannot be distinguished from one another in tissue sections. Furthermore, these pathogens cannot be distinguished from those that cause aspergillosis, fusariosis, and scedosporiosis/lomentosporiosis solely based on histomorphology (3, 19, 20). Moreover, the pathogens that cause hyalohyphomycoses are common throughout the environment. Therefore, histopathological identification of invasive non-pigmented (hyaline) septate hyphae with branches is mandatory for stating that a lesion is due to mycosis rather than colonization or contamination (3). In addition to exhibiting the dichotomous branching and septate hyphae that are typical of *Aspergillus* and *Scedosporium*, some pathogens that cause rare hyalohyphomycoses (e.g., *Scopulariopsis* spp. and *Microascus* spp.) also produce pseudohyphae-like structures due to vesicular swellings of the hyphae (Figs. 13.3, 13.7–13.11) (1, 7, 8). All pathogens that cause hyalohyphomycoses are well stained by periodic acid-Schiff and Grocott's methenamine silver stains. These stains should be applied to confirm whether lesions contain hyphal elements. As with all invasive mycosis lesions, it is important to show fungal invasion when the infection is due to *Schizophyllum* and other basidiomycetes, which may occasionally exhibit spicules on hyphae from lung and sinus samples (1). Similarly, in lesions caused by *Purpureocillium* spp., invading septate hyaline hyphae may produce conidiospores (arthroconidia) within granulomas (1). Invasive infections due to *Trichoderma* spp. are predominantly caused by *T. longibrachiatum*, which forms hyaline branching septate hyphae in tissues (Figs. 13.8 and 13.9) (11, 21). Lesions due to *Saprochaete* spp. infections, whether local or disseminated, contain thin septate hyphae with narrow-angle branching and yeast cells (1). It is of outmost importance to verify the presence of parallel-walled septate hyphae that are 3–5 µm wide combined with the invasion of lung, heart, or brain tissue to diagnose infections caused by *Rasamsonia* spp. (1, 22). The same applies to infections with *Penicillium* and non-*marneffei*

DOI: 10.1201/9781003306177-13

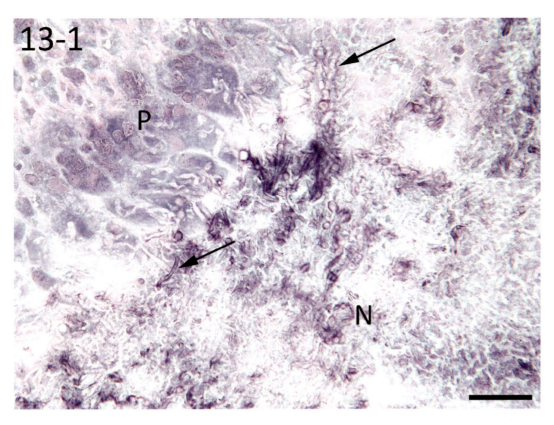

Figure 13.1 Chronic, necrotizing myelitis due to systemic *M. cirrosus* infection. Hyaline hyphae (arrows) are visible within necrotic tissue (N), which is bordered by macrophages and epithelioid cells (P). HE. Bar = 45 μm.

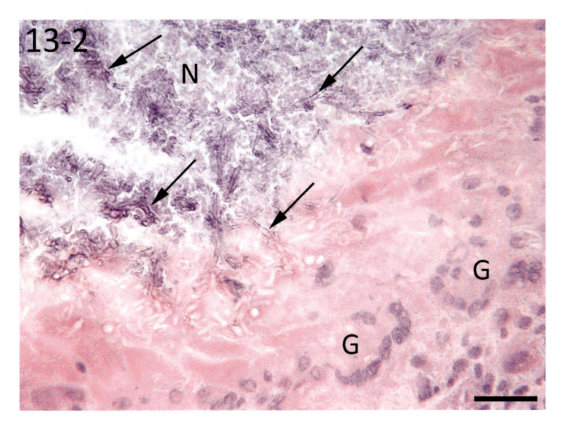

Figure 13.2 Chronic, necrotizing myelitis due to systemic *M. cirrosus* infection. Multinucleate giant cells (G) have formed around the necrotic area (N), which contains hyphal elements (arrows). HE. Bar = 45 μm.

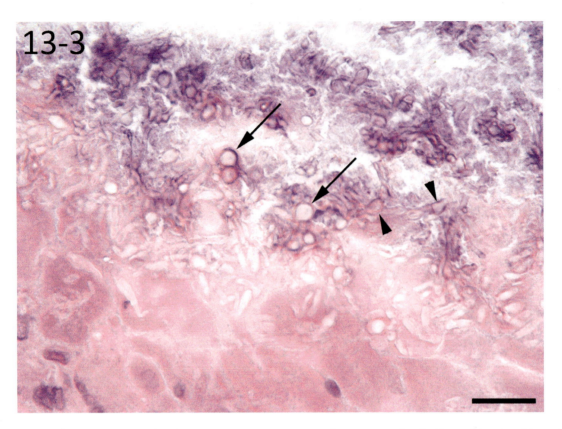

Figure 13.3 Chronic, necrotizing myelitis due to systemic *M. cirrosus* infection. Vesicles (bulbous dilatations) have formed at hyphal termini (arrows) and along the hyphae (arrowheads). HE. Bar = 45 μm.

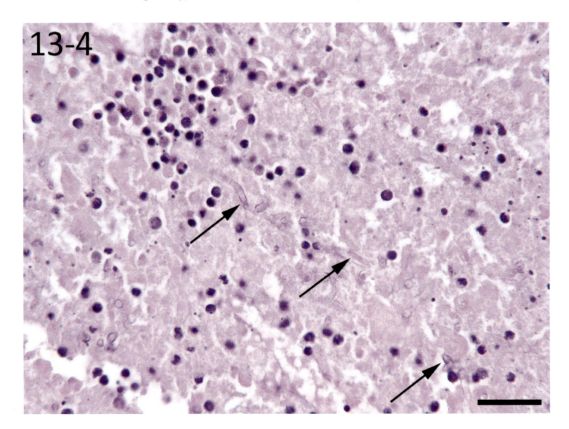

Figure 13.4 Acute, systemic trichodermatosis due to *T. longibrachiatum*. In the acute lesions, the reaction is characterized by necrosis and infiltration by neutrophils. In haematoxylin and eosin-stained sections, the hyphae are only faintly stained (arrows). HE. Bar = 60 μm.

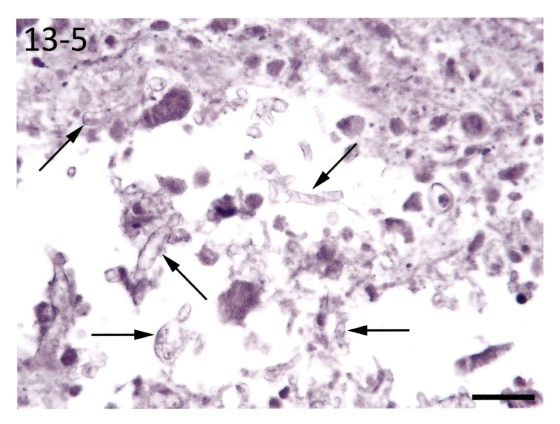

Figure 13.5 Acute, systemic trichodermatosis due to *T. longibrachiatum.* In the acute necrotizing lesion, multiple hyphal elements (arrows) with considerable variations in morphology are present. HE. Bar = 30 μm.

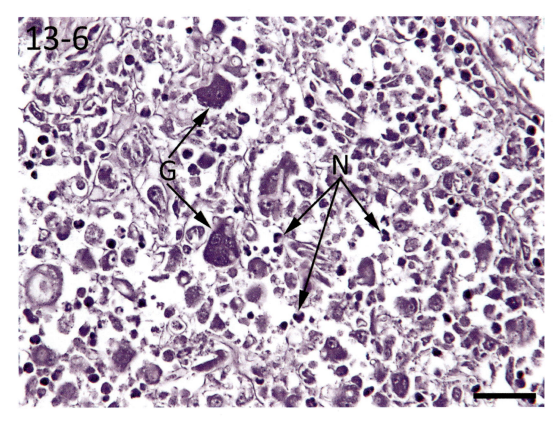

Figure 13.6 Chronic, systemic trichodermatosis due to *T. longibrachiatum.* Chronic lesions are typically pyogranulomatous with infiltration of macrophages and epithelioid cells and the formation of multinucleate giant cells (G) interspersed with neutrophils (N). HE. Bar = 60 μm.

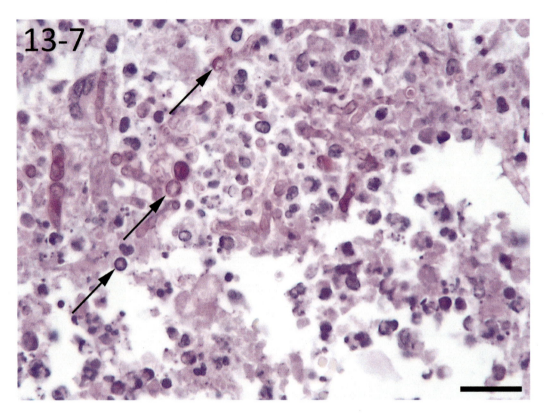

Figure 13.7 Chronic, systemic trichodermatosis due to *T. longibrachiatum*. Periodic acid-Schiff staining shows the fungal structures of *Trichoderma*, and some of the cross-sectioned hyphae and bulbous dilatations resemble yeast cells (arrows). PAS. Bar = 30 µm.

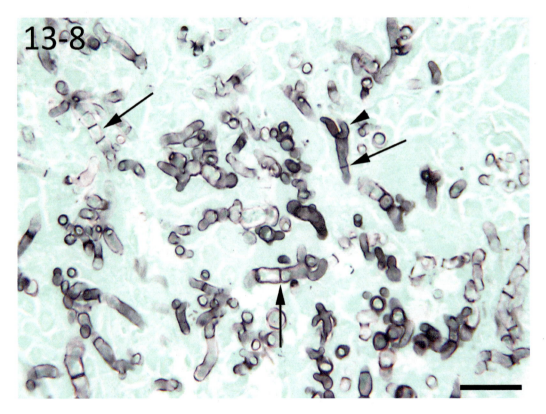

Figure 13.8 Systemic trichodermatosis due to *T. longibrachiatum*. Grocott's methenamine silver staining shows the fungal structures of *Trichoderma*, and the similarities to the major hyalohyphomycoses pathogens are striking due to the dichotomous branching of hyphae (arrowhead) and numerous septate hyphae (arrows). GMS. Bar = 30 µm.

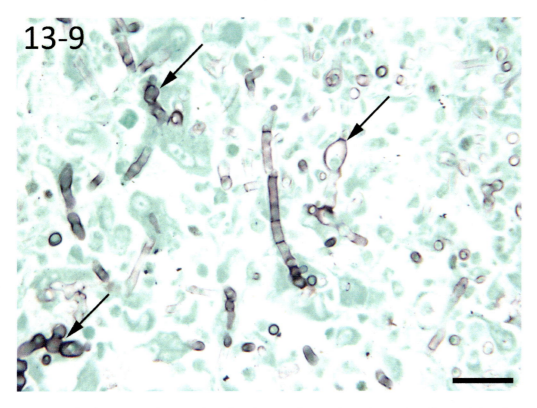

Figure 13.9 Systemic trichodermatosis due to *T. longibrachiatum*. Grocott's methenamine silver staining shows the fungal structures of *Trichoderma*, and the similarities to the major hyalohyphomycoses pathogens are striking due to the frequent septations of hyphae. Dilatations along hyphae (arrows) are also visible in other lesions, such as those caused by aspergillosis. GMS. Bar = 30 μm.

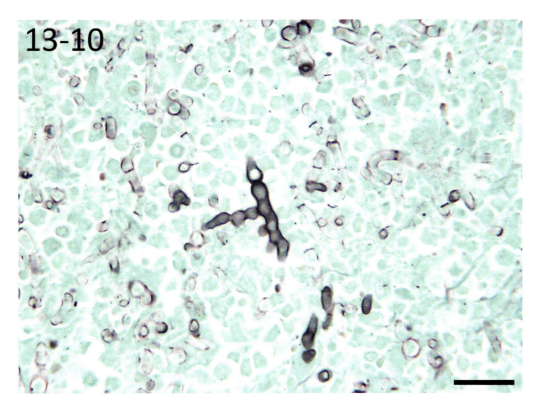

Figure 13.10 Systemic trichodermatosis due to *T. longibrachiatum*. The multiple vesicular dilatations along the hyphae of *Trichoderma* resemble pseudohyphae. GMS. Bar = 30 μm.

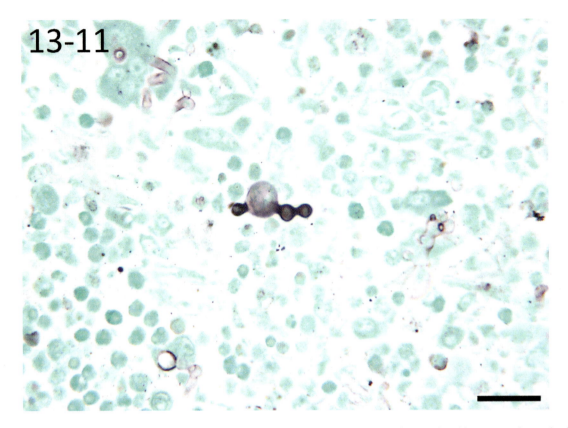

Figure 13.11 Systemic trichodermatosis due to *T. longibrachiatum*. The presence of vesicular dilatations along the hyphae of *Trichoderma* may be pronounced. GMS. Bar = 30 μm.

Talaromyces spp. because these pathogens are usually associated with superficial colonization or infections, but they may be disseminated. Infections with *Paecilomyces* spp. may be caused by several species, but *P. formosus* and *P. variotii* are most likely to cause invasive infections in humans (9). Frequently, *Scopulariopsis* spp./*Microascus* spp. hyphae also have vesicular/bulbous swellings at hyphal termini, or sometimes along the hyphae (7, 8). In geotrichosis infections that are caused by *G. candidum*, the lesions contain infrequently and irregularly branched septate filamentous hyphae (Figs. 13.12 and 13.13), which may vary considerably in size and shape. Arthroconidia and pseudohyphae may also be present (13, 17, 18).

DIFFERENTIAL DIAGNOSIS

To diagnose the rare hyalohyphomycoses, pathology must be demonstrated together with the presence of characteristic invasive hyaline hyphae in lesions. Ideally, this is accomplished by observing a characteristic inflammatory reaction and identifying the pathogen responsible in culture or by polymerase chain reaction. Specific antibodies for immunohistochemical techniques and specific probes for *in situ* hybridization are only commercially available for the organisms that cause the most frequently occurring hyalohyphomycoses (e.g., aspergillosis, fusariosis, and scedosporiosis/lomentosporiosis; see previous chapters). These may be used to exclude the corresponding organisms unless they cross-react with the pathogens that cause rare hyalohyphomycoses. In cases of geotrichosis, yeast cells have also been observed, together with the hyphal/pseudohyphal growth. Therefore, the dual infection may occur, for example, with *G. candidum* and *Candida albicans* (13, 17). However, these genera should not be distinguished on histomorphological criteria alone (17), but also using immunoelectrophoretic and immunohistochemical criteria (23). The gold standard for diagnosing all opportunistic fungal infections, including the rare hyalohyphomycoses, remains a histological demonstration of the pathogen in invasive growth and the repeated isolation of the pathogen from pure growth culture or molecular identification (24).

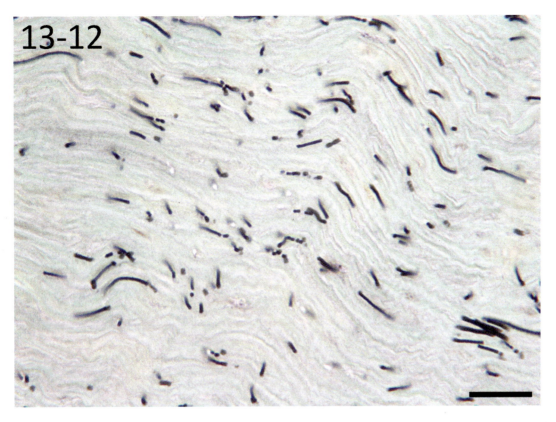

Figure 13.12 Invasive dermal geotrichosis. *G. candidum* hyphae are elongated and exhibit infrequent and irregular branching within the tissue. GMS. Bar = 75 μm.

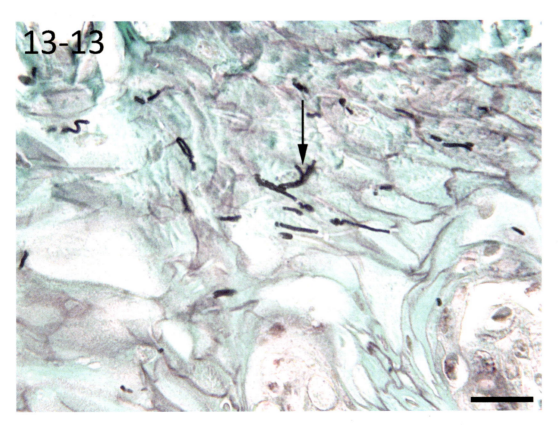

Figure 13.13 Invasive dermal geotrichosis. Within the tissue, the hyphae of *G. candidum* show considerable variation in size and shape, and the infrequent branching often occurs at an acute angle (arrow). GMS. Bar = 60 μm.

REFERENCES

1. Hoenigl M, Salmanton-García J, Walsh TJ, Nucci M, Neoh CF et al. 2021. Global guideline for the diagnosis and management of rare mould infections: An initiative of the European Confederation of Medical Mycology in cooperation with the International Society for Human and Animal Mycology and the American Society for Microbiology. Lancet Infect Dis. doi: 10.1016/S1473-3099(20)30784-2.

2. Hospenthal DR. 2015. Hyalohyphomycosis: Infection due to hyaline moulds. In: Diagnosis and Treatment of Fungal Infections. 2nd ed. Hospenthal DR, Rinaldi MG, Eds. Springer. pp 141–157.

3. Guarner J, Brandt ME. 2011. Histopathologic diagnosis of fungal infections in the 21st century. Clin Microbiol Rev, 24, 247–280.

4. Kuboi T, Okazaki K, Inotani M, Sugino M, Sadamura T et al. 2016. A case of cutaneous Paecilomyces formosus infection in an extremely premature infant. J Infect Chemother, 22, 339–341.

5. Sfakianakis A, Krasagakis K, Stefanidou M, Maraki S, Koutsopoulos A et al. 2007. Invasive cutaneous infection with Geotrichum candidum – sequential treatment with amphotericin B and voriconazole. Med Mycol, 45, 81–84.

6. Tascini C, Cardinali G, Barletta V, Paolo AD, Leonildi A et al. 2016. First case of Trichoderma longibrachiatum CIED (Cardiac Implantable Electronic Device)-associated endocarditis in a non-immunocompromised host: Biofilm removal and diagnostic problems in the light of the current literature. Mycopathologia, 181, 297–303.

7. Miossec C, Morio F, Lepoivre T et al. 2011. Fatal invasive infection with fungemia due to Microascus cirrosus after heart and lung transplantation in a patient with cystic fibrosis. J Clin Microbiol, 49, 2743–2747.

8. Taton O, Bernier B, Etienne I et al. 2017. Necrotizing microascus tracheobronchitis in a bilateral lung transplant recipient. Transpl Infect Dis, 20. doi: 10.1111/tid.12806.

9. Houbraken J, Verweij PE, Rijs AJMM, Borman AM, Samson RA. 2010. Identification of Paecilomyces variotii in clinical samples and settings. J Clin Microbiol, 48, 2754–2761.

10. Batarseh RY, Shehata M, Becker MD, Sigdel S, He P, Shweihat YR. 2020. Paecilomyces in an immune competent host. Case report. IDCases. doi: 10.1016/j.idcr.2020.e00885.

11. Richter S, Cormican MG, Pfaller MA, Lee CK, Gingrich R et al. 1999. Fatal disseminated Trichoderma longibrachiatum infection in an adult bone marrow transplant patient: Species identification and review of the literature. J Clin Microbiol, 37, 1154–1160.

12. Akagi T, Kawamura C, Terasawa N, Yamaguchi K, Kubo K. 2017. Suspected pulmonary infection with Trichoderma longibrachiatum after allogeneic stem cell transplantation. Intern Med, 56, 215–219.

13. Kassamali H, Anaissie E, Ro J, Rolston K, Kantarjian H et al. 1987. Disseminated Geotrichum candidum infection. J Clin Microbiol, 25, 1782–1783.

14. Myint T, Dykhuizen MJ, McDonald CH, Ribes JA. 2015. Post operative fungal endopthalmitis due to Geotrichum candidum. Med Mycol Case Rep, 10, 4–6.

15. Keene S, Sarao MS, McDonald PJ, Veltman J. 2019. Cutaneous geotrichosis due to Geotrichum candidum in a burn patient. Access Microbiol, 1, 1–6.

16. Heshmatnia J, Marjani M, Mahdaviani SA, Adimi P, Pourabdollah M et al. 2017. Paecilomyces formosus infection in an adult patient with undiagnosed chronic granulomatous disease. J Clin Immunol, 37, 342–346.

17. Jagirdar J, Geller SA, Bottone EJ. 1981. Geotrichum candidum as a tissue invasive human pathogen. Human Pathol, 12, 668–671.

18. Reppas GP, Snoeck TD. 1999. Cutaneous geotrichosis in a dog. Aust Vet J, 77, 567–569.

19. Jensen HE, Chandler FW. 2007. Histopathological diagnoses of mycoses. In: Topley and Wilson's Microbiology & Microbial Infections. Medical Mycology. 10th ed. Merz WG, Hay RJ, Eds. Hodder Arnold. pp 121–143.

20. Jensen HE. 2021. Histopathology in the diagnosis of invasive fungal diseases. Curr Fungal Infect Rep, 15, 23–31.

21. Chouaki T, Lavarde V, Lachaud L, Raccurt CP, Hennequin C. 2002. Invasive infections due to Trichoderma species: Report of 2 cases, findings of in vitro susceptibility testing, and review of the literature. Clin Infect Dis, 35, 1360–1367.

22. Doyon JB, Sutton DA, Theodore P, Dhillon G, Jones KD et al. 2013. Rasamsonia argillacea pulmonary and aortic graft infection in an immune-competent patient. J Clin Microbiol, 51, 719–722.

23. Jensen HE, Hau J, Aalbæk B, Schønheyder H. 1990. Indirect immunofluorescence staining and crossed immunoelectrophoresis for differentiation of Candida albicans and Geotrichum candidum. Mycoses, 33, 519–526.

24. Pal M, Sejra S, Sejra A, Tesfaye S. 2013. Geotrichosis: An opportunistic mycosis of humans and animals. Int J Livest Res, 3, 38–44.

14

Phaeohyphomycosis

INTRODUCTION

Phaeohyphomycosis, which occurs worldwide, may be caused by a number of dematiaceous fungi; in particular, *Exophiala* (*E. jeanselmei*), *Alternaria* (*A. alternata*), and *Cladophialophora* (*C. bantiana*) should be mentioned (1–8). The different pathogens tend to infect different tissues and are found in different geographic locations. Within the tissue, the structure of the fungal elements in phaeohyphomycosis differs from that in chromoblastomycosis. In chromoblastomycosis, sclerotic bodies are present (see the chapter on chromoblastomycosis), whereas in phaeohyphomycosis, the fungal elements are present as yeast-like cells, pseudohyphae, and true hyphae (9). In addition, eumycetomas may be caused by dematiaceous fungi; however, in these mycoses, granules are formed in the centre of the lesions (see the chapter on mycetomas).

EPIDEMIOLOGY

Infections occur following trauma or inhalation of the causal fungi, which are found in soil and on plants and are distributed widely in the environment (1–4, 7, 10–13). The infections take different forms and are often grouped as superficial and subcutaneous infections, allergic diseases, pneumonia, brain abscesses, and disseminated infections (1, 12). Phaeohyphomycosis is an opportunistic infection, and lesions in the subcutaneous tissues and other locations may be associated with immunodeficiency or underlying diseases (13–16). However, in individuals who are not immunocompromised, trauma may initiate infections (5, 9, 11). As in chromoblastomycosis, subcutaneous lesions often develop over several months or years (9). Phaeohyphomycosis has also been diagnosed in animals, such as cats (6, 8, 17), horses (18, 19), and alpacas (20).

PATHOLOGY

Invasion of tissues will often result in non-specific inflammatory reactions. These may vary from the formation of abscesses, typically in brain infections (Fig. 14.1) (2), to pyogranulomatous inflammations (Fig. 14.2), which also occur in other mycoses lesions, especially subcutaneous and

submucosal lesions (3, 4, 7, 10, 11). These mixed inflammatory reactions are often characterized by an influx of neutrophils (Fig. 14.1). The neutrophils are surrounded by, or interspersed with, macrophages and macrophage-derived cells such as epithelioid cells and multinucleate giant cells (Fig. 14.2), together with lymphocytes and plasma cells (1, 9). In some cases, eosinophils are also present and liquefactive necrosis occurs (9, 21). Both yeast cells and hyphal fragments may be engulfed by macrophages and multinucleate giant cells (Fig. 14.2) (3, 4, 12).

FUNGAL HISTOMORPHOLOGY

In lesions, the pathogens occur as dematiaceous, yeast-like cells that produce pseudohyphae and true hyphae. The hyphae, which are often septate, may be short, elongated, regular, distorted, swollen, or any combination of these forms (9). These hyphae are visualized best in Grocott's methenamine silver-stained sections (Figs. 14.3 and 14.4).

The yeast cells and hyphae frequently have diameters of 2–6 μm (1). However, when swollen elements are present, diameters may reach 10–20 μm (18) or even 25 μm (Figs. 14.5 and 14.6) (9). The brown fungal elements are visualized best in haematoxylin and eosin-stained sections because the brown colour is masked by periodic acid-Schiff and Grocott's methenamine silver stains. Sections stained with Grocott's methenamine silver may need to be examined to confirm the presence of the disease if lesions contain few fungal elements (Figs. 14.7 and 14.8). Fontana-Masson stain can be used to highlight melanin within the fungal elements (9). It is not possible to state a diagnosis, even at the genus level, based on the histomorphological characteristics observed in slides.

DIFFERENTIAL DIAGNOSIS

Phaeohyphomycosis must be distinguished from other mycoses caused by dematiaceous fungi, such as chromoblastomycosis and black grain eumycetomas. As summarized in the chapters that describe these diseases, the diagnostic sclerotic bodies present in chromoblastomycosis lesions are not present in phaeohyphomycosis lesions. Furthermore, black granules are present in eumycetoma lesions, but not

DOI: 10.1201/9781003306177-14

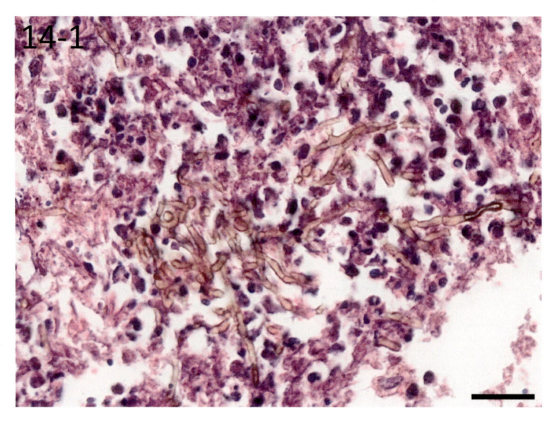

Figure 14.1 Chronic, cerebral, apostematous phaeohyphomycosis with brown hyphae and pseudohyphae. Many neutrophils are visible and are interspersed with fungal elements. HE. Bar = 30 μm.

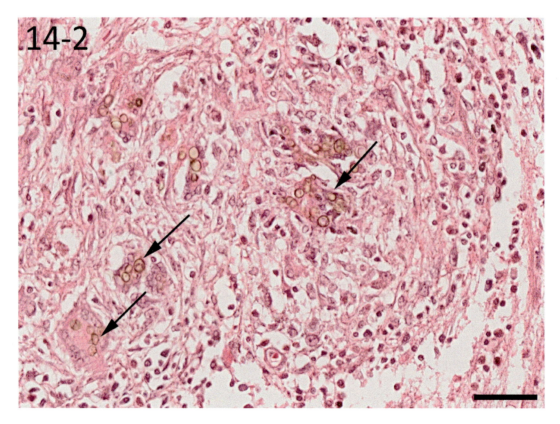

Figure 14.2 Chronic, cerebral, granulomatous phaeohyphomycosis. In the granuloma, brown fungal elements have been engulfed by multinucleate giant cells (arrows). HE. Bar = 60 μm.

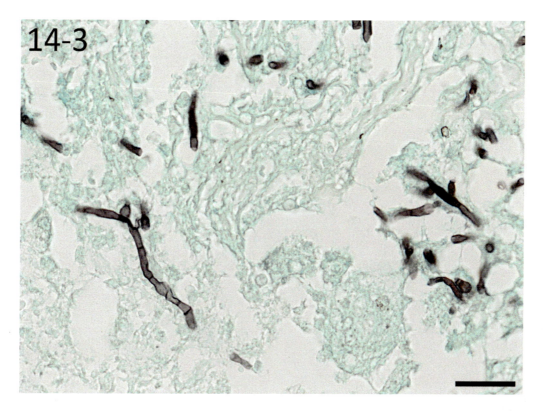

Figure 14.3 Chronic, cerebral apostematous phaeohyphomycosis. The outline of the septate hyphae is clearly visible in Grocott's methenamine silver-stained sections. However, this stain masks the brown colour of the fungal elements. GMS. Bar = 30 μm.

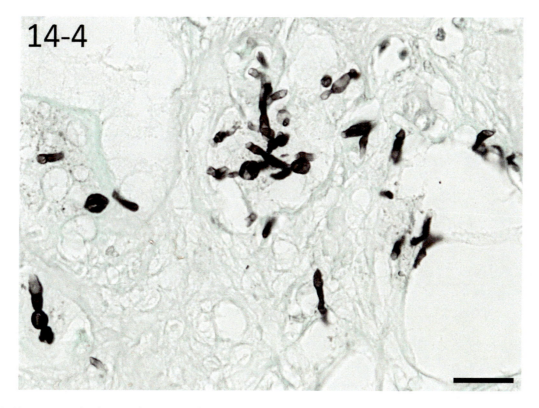

Figure 14.4 Chronic, cerebral, granulomatous phaeohyphomycosis. The outline of the pseudohyphae, some of which have bulbous contours, is clearly visible in Grocott's methenamine silver-stained sections. However, the stain masks the brown colour of the fungal elements. GMS. Bar = 30 μm.

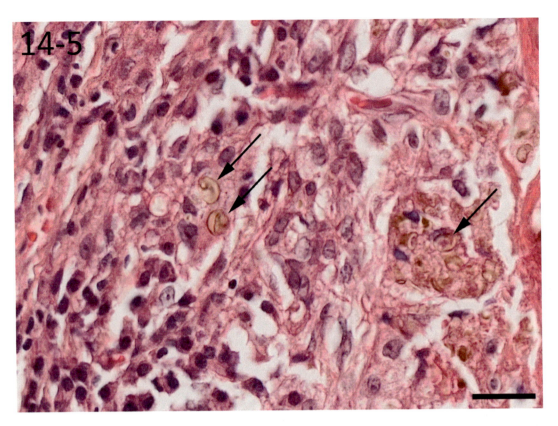

Figure 14.5 Chronic granulomatous lymphadenitis due to phaeohyphomycosis. The fungal elements are mainly present as yeast-like elements (arrows) in haematoxylin and eosin-stained sections. HE. Bar = 20 μm.

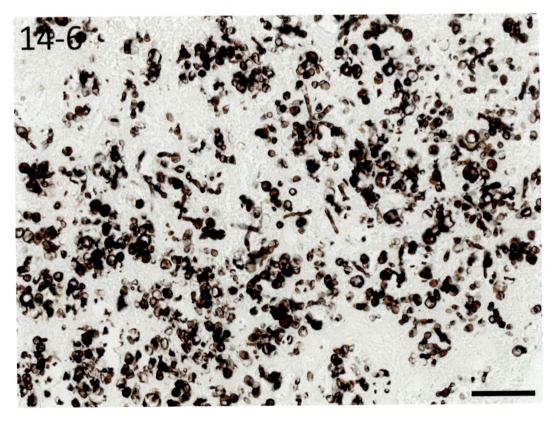

Figure 14.6 Chronic granulomatous lymphadenitis due to phaeohyphomycosis. Many different forms of fungal element are visible in Grocott's methenamine silver-stained sections. These include yeast cells, pseudohyphae, and hyphae. GMS. Bar = 60 μm.

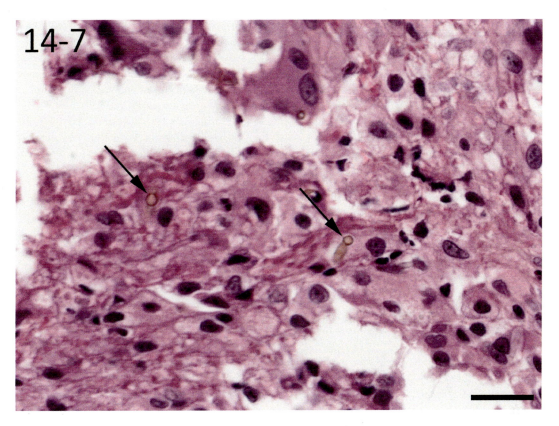

Figure 14.7 Chronic subcutaneous pyogranulomatous phaeohyphomycosis. In lesions with few fungal elements, the brown-stained fungal elements (arrows) may be difficult to detect. HE. Bar = 30 μm.

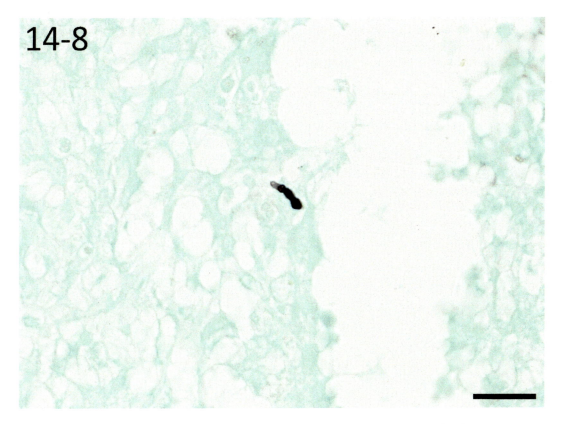

Figure 14.8 Chronic subcutaneous pyogranulomatous phaeohyphomycosis. In lesions with few fungal elements, Grocott's methenamine silver stain helps to visualize the fungal elements, although it masks the brown colour. GMS. Bar = 30 μm.

in phaeohyphomycosis lesions. Because of the presence of dematiaceous fungal elements, phaeohyphomycosis lesions should not be mistaken for those caused by hyaline fungi.

REFERENCES

1. Revankar SG. 2015. Phaeohyphomycosis: Infection due to dark (dematiaceous) molds. In: Diagnosis and Treatment of Fungal Infections. 2nd ed. Hospenthal DR, Rinaldi MGR, Eds. Springer, pp. 151–157.

2. Adeyemi O. 2007. Woman with multiple brain abscesses. Clin Infect Dis, 45, 1397–1399.

3. Arakaki O, Asato Y, Yagi N, Taira K, Yamamoto YI et al. 2010. Phaeohyphomycosis caused by *Exophiala jeanselmei* in a patient with polymyalgia rheumatica. J Dermatol, 37, 367–373.

4. Aranegui B, Feal C, García CP, Batalla A, Abalde T et al. 2013. Subcutaneous phaeohyphomycosis caused by *Exophiala jeanselmei* treated with wide surgical excision and posaconazole: Case report. Int J Dermatol, 52, 255–256.

5. Bonatti H, Lass-Flörl C, Zelger B, Lottersberger C, Singh N et al. 2007. *Alternaria alternata* soft tissue infection in a forearm transplant recipient. Surg Infect (Larchmt), 8, 539–544.

6. Bouljihad M, Lindeman CJ, Hayden DW. 2002. Pyogranulomatous meningoencephalitis associated with dematiaceous fungal (*Cladophialophora bantiana*) infection in a domestic cat. J Vet Diagn Invest, 14, 70–72.

7. Chen YC, Su YC, Tsai CC, Lai NS, Fan KS et al. 2014. Subcutaneous phaeohyphomycosis caused by *Exophiala jeanselmei*. J Microbiol Immunol Infect, 47, 546–549.

8. Elies L, Balandraud V, Boulouha L, Crespeau F, Guillot J. 2003. Fatal systemic phaeohyphomycosis in a cat due to *Cladophialophora bantiana*. J Vet Med A, 50, 50–53.

9. McGinnis MR. 1983. Chromoblastomycosis and phaeohyphomycosis: New concepts, diagnosis, and mycology. J Am Acad Dermatol, 8, 1–16.

10. Gomes J, Vilarinho C, Duarte MDL, Brito C. 2011. Cutaneous phaeohyphomycosis caused by *Alternaria alternata* unresponsive to itraconazole treatment. Case Rep Dermatol Med, 2011, 1–3.

11. Hussey SM, Gander R, Southern P, Hoang M. 2005. Subcutaneous phaeohyphomycosis caused by *Cladophialophora bantiana*. Arch Pathol Lab Med, 129, 794–797.

12. Schieffelin JS, Garcia-Diaz JB, Loss GE, Beckman EN, Keller RA et al. 2014. Phaeohyphomycosis fungal infections in solid organ transplant recipients: Clinical presentation, pathology, and treatment. Transpl Infect Dis, 16, 270–278.

13. Harrison DK, Moser S, Palmer CA. 2008. Central nervous system infections in transplant recipients by *Cladophialophora bantiana*. South Med J, 101, 292–296.

14. Ferreira IDS, Teixeira G, Abecasis M. 2013. *Alternaria alternata* invasive fungal infection in a patient with Fanconi's anemia after an unrelated bone marrow transplant. Clin Drug Investig, 33, 33–36.

15. Nomura M, Maeda M, Seishima M. 2010. Subcutaneous phaeohyphomycosis caused by *Exophiala jeanselmei* in collagen disease patient. J Dermatol, 37, 1046–1050.

16. Xu X, Low DW, Palevsky HI, Elenitsas R. 2001. Subcutaneous phaeohyphomycotic cysts caused by *Exophiala jeanselmei* in a lung transplant patient. Dermatol Surg, 27, 343–346.

17. Mckay JS, Cox CL, Foster AP. 2001. Cutaneous alternariosis in a cat. J Small Anim Pract, 42, 75–78.

18. Dicken M, Munday JS, Archer RM, Mayhew IG, Pandey SK. 2010. Cutaneous fungal granulomas due to *Alternaria* spp. infection in a horse in New Zealand. N Z Vet J, 58, 319–320.

19. Genovese LM, Whitbread TJ, Campbell C. 2001. Cutaneous nodular phaeohyphomycosis in five horses associated with *Alternaria alternata* infection. Vet Rec, 148, 55–56.

20. Frank C, Vemulapalli R, Lin T. 2011. Cerebral phaeohyphomycosis due to *Cladophialophora bantiana* in a Huacaya alpaca (*Vicugna pacos*). J Comp Pathol, 145, 410–413.

21. Cardoso SV, Campolina SS, Guimarães ALS, Faria PR, Costa EMDC et al. 2007. Oral phaeohyphomycosis. J Clin Pathol, 60, 204–205.

15

Chromoblastomycosis

INTRODUCTION

Chromoblastomycosis is a chronic infection of the skin and subcutaneous tissues, which occurs worldwide. However, infections are particularly common in countries with a tropical or subtropical climate (1, 2). Infections are often the result of traumatic injuries and implantation of a particular group of dematiaceous fungi (1). The organisms that are generally responsible for these infections include *Fonsecaea pedrosoi*, *Phialophora verrucosa*, *Cladophialophora carrionii* (*Cladosporium carrionii*), and, less frequently, *Rhinocladiella aquaspersa* (2, 3).

EPIDEMIOLOGY

The disease occurs predominantly in humid tropical and subtropical areas of America (e.g., Central and South America), Asia (e.g., Japan and China), India, and sub-Saharan Africa (4, 5). By contrast, few cases have occurred in Europe and Australia (1, 6, 7). In most countries, infections are particularly common among men working in rural regions (3). The various fungi that cause chromoblastomycosis generally occur within decomposing organic matter in the soil and water (1). Lesions develop slowly, sometimes over several years (3).

PATHOLOGY

Chromoblastomycosis lesions are mainly restricted to the skin and are generally similar to those caused by other subcutaneous mycoses. However, they are often accompanied by epidermal changes, including hyperkeratosis and pseudoepitheliomatous hyperplasia (3, 8, 9). In the dermal and subcutaneous tissues, non-specific pyogranulomatous inflammatory reactions occur, with infiltration of polymorphonuclear cells (e.g., neutrophils and eosinophils), lymphocytes, plasma cells, macrophages, and macrophage-derived cells, such as epithelioid cells and multinucleate giant cells (especially the Langhans type) (Figs. 15.1 and 15.2) (3, 9–12). Several animal models of chromoblastomycosis have been

developed in mice (13, 14) and rats (15). The lesions that develop in these models are similar to those that occur in spontaneous infections in humans (13–15). Very rarely, the disease may spread to other tissues, such as submucosal nasal tissues, muscles, bones, lungs, and the brain (2, 16, 17).

FUNGAL HISTOMORPHOLOGY

The histological diagnosis of chromoblastomycosis involves staining tissue sections with hematoxylin and eosin to identify sclerotic bodies, which are spherical/polyhedral, dark, thick-walled, muriform fungal cells that are 6–12 μm in diameter (2, 18). Ziehl-Neelsen and Wade-Fite stains have also been used to identify sclerotic bodies, with variable success (18–20). In the medical mycology literature, sclerotic bodies have been called Medlar bodies, fumagoid cells, chlamydospores, and copper pennies (2). Within lesions, the sclerotic bodies may be found inside macrophages (Figs. 15.1 and 15.2) or multinucleate giant cells, as well as outside cells (Fig. 15.3) (2). The different aetiologies of infection cannot be determined from the morphology of the sclerotic bodies, which are often produced by planate division (Fig. 15.4), although triradiate and quadraradiate division figures may be present (18). However, budding from sclerotic bodies has occasionally been reported (2). Periodic acid-Schiff, Grocott's methenamine silver, and Fontana-Mason stains are not used on sections because these would mask the colour of the fungi and the inflammatory reaction (1, 18).

DIFFERENTIAL DIAGNOSIS

The sclerotic bodies that characterize chromoblastomycosis are diagnostically important. However, these may be mistaken for the yeast-like cells present in phaeohyphomycosis because both groups of fungi are dematiaceous. However, in cases of phaeohyphomycosis, the yeast cells are often associated with fungal elements that grow as pseudohyphae and/or true hyphae (see the chapter on phaeohyphomycosis). Such elements are never present in chromoblastomycosis lesions.

DOI: 10.1201/9781003306177-15

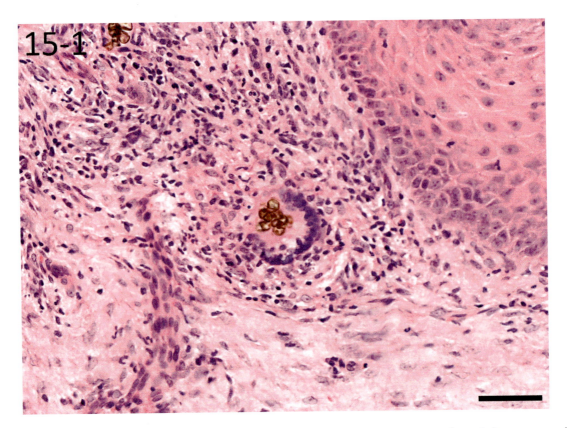

Figure 15.1 Chronic subcutaneous pyogranulomatous chromoblastomycosis. Dematiaceous fungal elements are clearly visible in tissue sections stained with hematoxylin and eosin. HE. Bar = 35 μm.

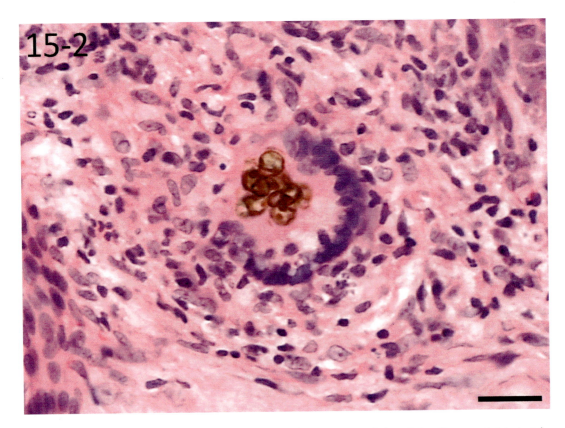

Figure 15.2 Chronic subcutaneous pyogranulomatous chromoblastomycosis. Sclerotic bodies are visible inside a Langhans-type multinucleate giant cell. Same case as in Fig. 15.1. HE. Bar = 15 μm.

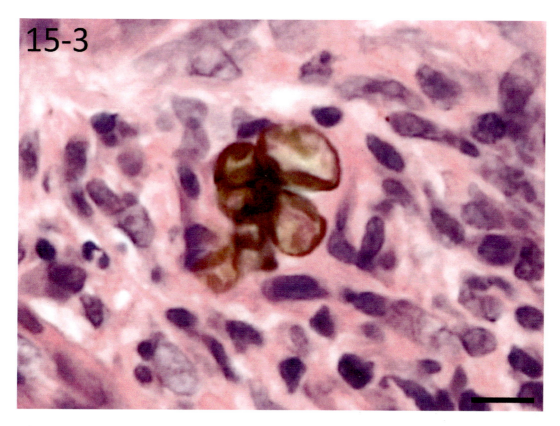

Figure 15.3 Chronic subcutaneous pyogranulomatous chromoblastomycosis. The brown-stained sclerotic bodies are located extracellularly. HE. Bar = 8 μm.

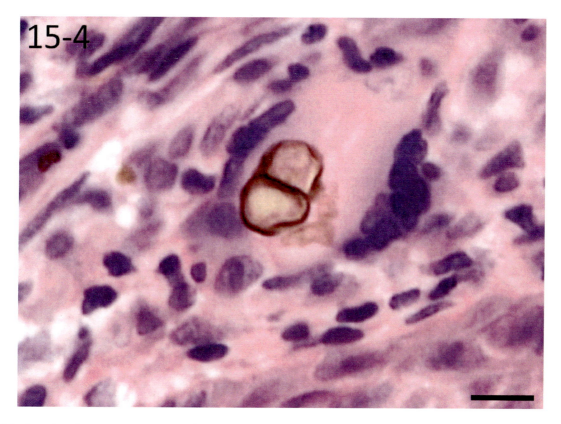

Figure 15.4 Chronic subcutaneous pyogranulomatous chromoblastomycosis. Fission of sclerotic bodies (stained brown) inside a Langhans-type multinucleate giant cell. HE. Bar = 8 μm.

REFERENCES

1. Krzyściak PM, Pindycka-Piaszczyńska M, Piaszczyńsnki M. 2014. Chromoblastomycosis. Postępy Dermatol Alergol, 31, 310–321.

2. McGinnis MR. 1983. Chromoblastomycosis and phaeohyphomycosis: New concepts, diagnosis, and mycology. J Am Acad Dermatol, 8, 1–16.

3. Correia RTM, Valente NYS, Criado PR, Martins JEDC. 2010. Chromoblastomycosis: Study of 27 cases and review of medical literature. An Bras Dermatol, 85, 448–454.

4. McDaniel P, Walsh DS. 2010. Chromoblastomycosis in western Thailand. Am J Trop Med Hyg, 83, 448.

5. Miyagi H, Yamamoto YI, Kanamori S, Taira K, Asato Y et al. 2008. Case of chromoblastomycosis appearing in an Okinawa patient with a medical history of Hansen's disease. J Dermatol, 35, 354–361.

6. Deb Roy A, Das D, Deka M. 2013. Chromoblastomycosis – A clinical mimic of squamous carcinoma. Australas Med J, 6, 458–460.

7. Weedon D, Van Deurse M, Allison S, Rosendahl C. 2013. Chromoblastomycosis in Australia: An historical perspective. Pathology, 45, 489–491.

8. Silva AAL, Criado PR, Nunes RS, da Silva WLF, Kanashiro-Galo L et al. 2014. In situ immune response in human chromoblastomycosis – A possible role for regulatory and Th17 T cells. PLoS Negl Trop Dis, 8, 3162–3162.

9. Uribe JF, Zuluaga AI, Leon W, Restrepo A. 1989. Histopathology of chromoblastomycosis. Mycopathologia, 105, 1–6.

10. Avelar-Pires C, Simoes-Quaresma JA, Moraes-de Macedo GM, Brasil-Xavier M, Cardoso-de Brito A. 2013. Revisiting the clinical and histopathological aspects of patients with chromoblastomycosis from the Brazilian Amazon region. Arch Med Res, 44, 302–306.

11. Krishna S, Shenoy MM, Pinto M, Saxena Y. 2016. Two cases of axillary chromoblastomycosis. Indian J Dermatol Venereol Leprol, 82, 455–456.

12. Minotto R, Edelweiss MIA, Scroferneker ML. 2017. Study on the organization of cellular elements in the granulomatous lesion caused by chromoblastomycosis. J Cutan Pathol, 44, 915–918.

13. Machado AP, Freymuller E, Fischman O. 2009. Experimental murine chromoblastomycosis obtained from *Fonsecaea pedrosoi* isolate cultured for a long period. J Venom Anim Toxins Incl Trop Dis, 15, 680–695.

14. Machado AP, Regis Silva MR, Fischman O. 2011. Local phagocytic responses after murine infection with different forms of *Fonsecaea pedrosoi* and sclerotic bodies originating from an inoculum of conidiogenous cells. Mycoses, 54, 202–211.

15. Xie Z, Zhang J, Xi L, Li X, Wang L et al. 2010. A chronic chromoblastomycosis model by *Fonsecaea monophora* in Wistar rat. Med Mycol, 48, 201–206.

16. Penjor D, Khizuan AK, Chong AW, Wong KT. 2014. A case of nasal chromoblastomycosis causing epistaxis. J Laryngol Otol, 128, 1117–1119.

17. Hofmann H, Choi SM, Wilsmann-Theis D, Horré R, De Hoog GS et al. 2005. Invasive chromoblastomycosis and sinusitis due to *Phialophora verrucosa* in a child from northern Africa. Mycoses, 48, 456–461.

18. Chavan SS, Kulkarni MH, Makannavar JH. 2010. "Unstained" and "de stained" sections in the diagnosis of chromoblastomycosis: A clinico-pathological study. Indian J Pathol Microbiol, 53, 666–671.

19. Gopal KVT, Ramani TV, Rama Laxmi P. 2012. Disseminated chromoblastomycosis: Diffuse truncal involvement with hematogenous spread. Int J Heal Allied Sci, 1, 194–196.

20. Lokuhetty MDS, Alahakoon VS, Kularatne BDMU, De Silva MVC. 2007. Zeil Neelson and Wade-Fite stains to demonstrate medlar bodies of chromoblastomycosis. J Cutan Pathol, 34, 71–72.

16

Mycetomas

INTRODUCTION

Mycetomas have different names such as Madura foot, maduromycosis, and fungus disease of India (1). The mycetomas are defined by their clinicopathological and histopathological characteristics, as well as by their etiology. They may be caused by fungi (eumycetomas) or by filamentous bacteria (actinomycetomas) (2). Mycetomas are slowly progressing, often painless, swellings that are associated with draining sinus tracts, which open onto the surface of the skin and drain purulent material as well as coloured granules (containing fungal or bacterial colonies) (3). Lesions are restricted to the skin, subcutaneous tissues, underlying bones, and other structures (4). Hematogenous spread does not occur; however, in actinomycetomas, spread to regional lymph nodes may take place and cause lymphedema (4).

EPIDEMIOLOGY

Infections are predominantly established following traumatic injuries, where fungi (eumycetomas) or bacteria (actinomycetomas) are implanted (1). Eumycetomas mainly occur in Africa and India, whereas actinomycetomas occur in Central and South America, as well as in Mexico (5). In Europe, cases mainly occur in Mediterranean countries. However, cases may also be imported by travellers visiting endemic areas (4). Eumycetomas may be caused by more than 30 different fungal species; however, *Madurella mycetomatis*, *M. grisea*, *Leptosphaeria senegalensis*, and *Pseudallescheria boydii* (*Scedosporium apiospermum*) cause the majority of cases. In addition, several of the hyaline hyphae-forming fungi, which cause other mycoses such as *Fusarium* and *Aspergillus*, may also cause eumycetomas (4, 6–8). Actinomycetomas may also have several etiologies; however, these are predominantly caused by *Actinomadura madurae*, *A. pelletieri*, *Streptomyces somaliensis*, *Nocardia brasiliensis*, and other *Nocardia* spp. (4, 6, 7). All fungi and bacteria that cause mycetomas are normally present in soil and on plants, including on thorns (4).

PATHOLOGY

As with other entrenched infections, fistular tracks that drain purulent material to the surface are characteristic of mycetomas. Sometimes the purulent material contains granules of varying size and colour (1, 5, 7). In lesions, the granules are located centrally within the abscesses, and in eumycetomas the hyphae are embedded in an amorphous intercellular mass termed "cement," due to its concrete-like appearance (1, 9). For mycetomas, the tissue reaction is independent of etiology. Therefore, eumycetoma and actinomycetoma lesions are similar (4, 9). The pathological changes that occur in lesions can be separated into three types (1, 9, 10):

- *Type I*: The granules are surrounded by and interspersed with neutrophils in the inner zone. Beyond the zone containing neutrophils, there is granular tissue containing macrophages, lymphocytes, and plasma cells. The outermost part of the lesion is encapsulated by fibrous tissue (Figs. 16.1–16.4).
- *Type II*: The inner zone contains macrophages and multinucleate giant cells, which may contain fungal fragments. The other histological features are similar to those described for Type I lesions (Figs. 16.5 and 16.6).
- *Type III*: These are characterized by palisade epithelioid cells and the formation of granulomas, with Langhans-type multinucleate giant cells. The granulomas may contain remnants of the granules at their centre. The surrounding histological features are similar to those described for Type I lesions (Figs. 16.7 and 16.8).

Because fungal or bacterial colonies may not be equally distributed throughout lesions and blocks of tissue, multiple sections should be examined from suspected lesions (7).

FUNGAL AND BACTERIAL HISTOMORPHOLOGY

Within lesions, the central granules consist of aggregates of fungi or bacteria, interspersed with an amorphous extracellular mass termed "cement" (Fig. 16.8) (4, 5). In mycetomas, the granules vary in size (10 μm to 1–5 mm) and colour (black, brown, white, yellow, or a combination of these) and are often found at the centre of abscesses, although they may occur in the fibrous tissue (2–5, 9, 11). In eumycetomas, hyphae are usually 2–6 μm in diameter with focal dilatations (Figs. 16.9 and 16.10), whereas the filamentous bacteria

DOI: 10.1201/9781003306177-16

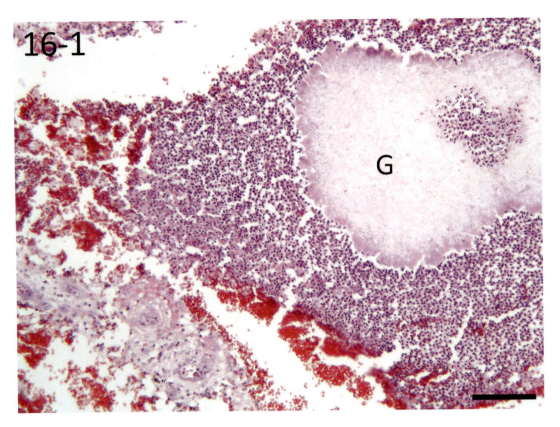

Figure 16.1 Eumycetoma due to *L. senegalensis*. A grain (G) is present centrally within an abscess (Type I). HE. Bar = 90 μm.

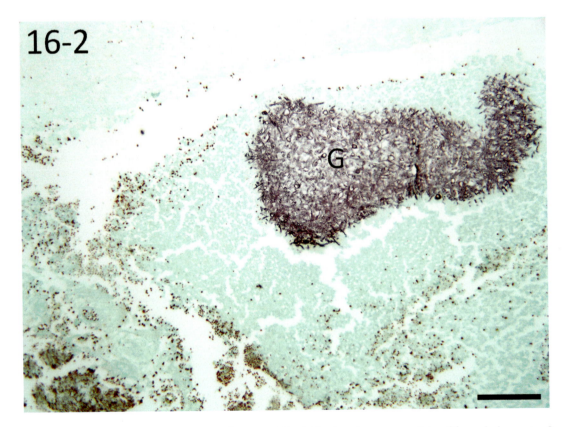

Figure 16.2 Eumycetoma due to *L. senegalensis*. The grain (G) within the abscess consists of fungal elements. Same case as in Fig. 16.1. GMS. Bar = 100 μm.

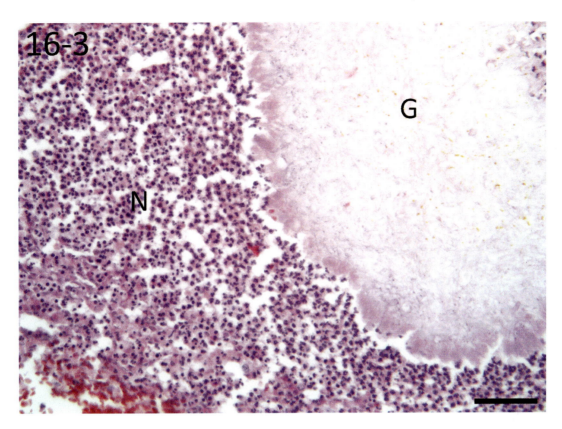

Figure 16.3 Eumycetoma due to *L. senegalensis.* The grain (G) is surrounded by neutrophils (N) (Type I). Same case as in Fig. 16.1. HE. Bar = 40 μm.

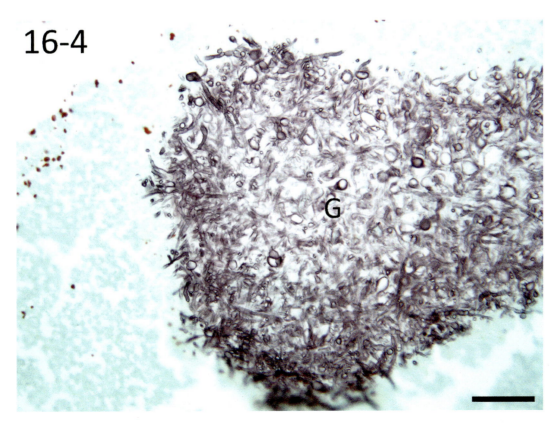

Figure 16.4 Eumycetoma due to *L. senegalensis.* The fungal elements within the grain (G) are morphologically diverse. Same case as in Fig. 16.1. GMS. Bar = 50 μm.

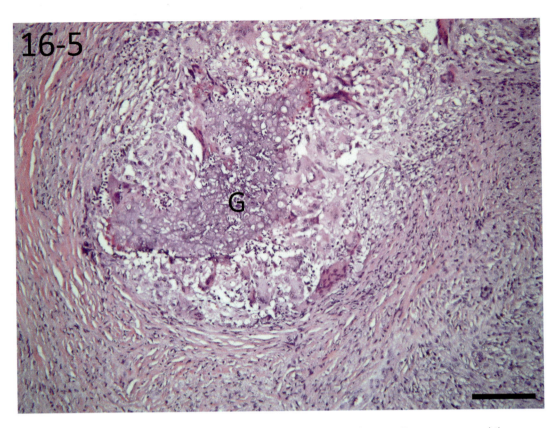

Figure 16.5 Eumycetoma due to *M. mycetomatis*. Around the centrally located grain (G), some neutrophils are present together with macrophages and multinucleate giant cells. The lesion is surrounded by fibrous tissue (Type II). HE. Bar = 80 μm.

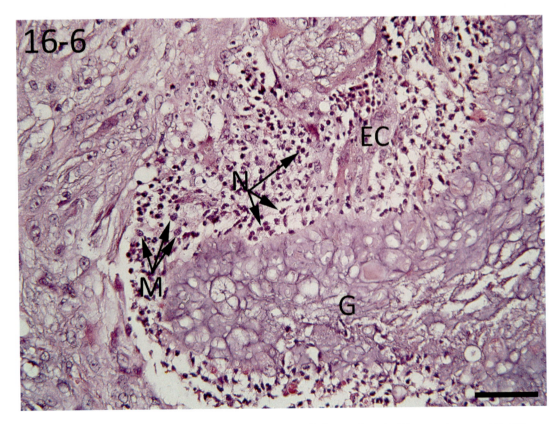

Figure 16.6 Eumycetoma due to *M. mycetomatis*. Around the centrally located grain (G), some neutrophils (N) are present together with macrophages (M) and epithelioid cells (EC). The lesion is surrounded by fibrous tissue (Type II). HE. Bar = 40 μm.

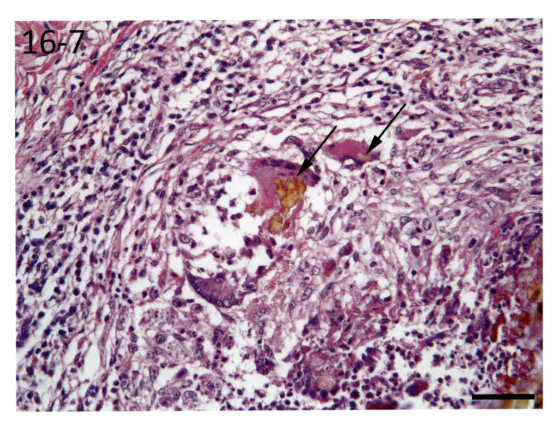

Figure 16.7 Eumycetoma due to *M. mycetomatis*. The granuloma contains several multinucleate giant cells, some of which have taken up hyphal elements and "cement" (arrows) (Type III). The lesion is surrounded by fibrous tissue. HE. Bar = 40 µm.

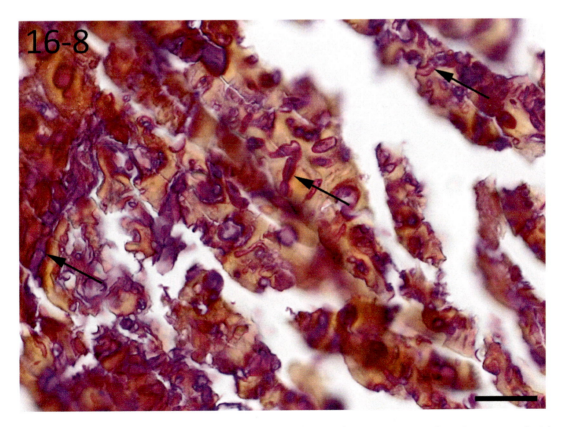

Figure 16.8 Eumycetoma of unknown etiology. Within the grain, hyphal fragments (arrows) are interspersed with golden coloured "cement" (Type III). HE. Bar = 30 µm.

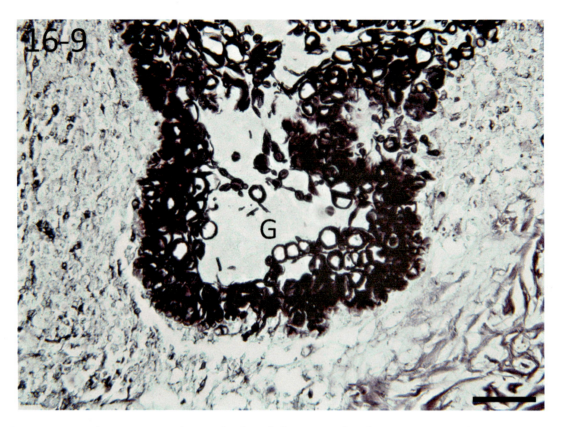

Figure 16.9 Eumycetoma due to *L. senegalensis*. The fungal elements within the grain (G) are only stained at the periphery. GMS. Bar = 30 μm.

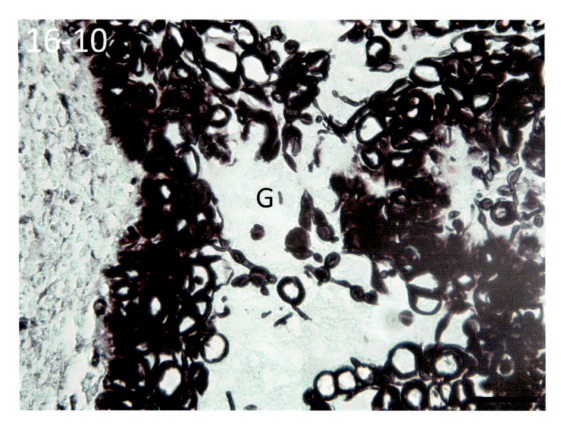

Figure 16.10 Eumycetoma due to *L. senegalensis*. The fungal elements at the periphery of the grain (G) are morphologically diverse and exhibit focal dilatations. GMS. Bar = 20 μm.

present in actinomycetomas are less than 1 µm in diameter (Figs. 16.11–16.13) (1, 5). Centrally located fungi and bacteria will often be surrounded by pink material, that is, the Splendore-Hoeppli phenomenon (Fig. 16.14) (4, 9).

For both eumycetomas and actinomycetomas, a tentative diagnosis to the genus level may be possible from the size, colour, and consistency of granules together with the histological appearance and histopathological reaction characteristics (2, 5, 9). In endemic areas, specialists can diagnose infections with a high degree of certainty (7). However, eumycetomas and actinomycetomas are easily distinguished histologically, due to differences in staining properties and the size of the pathogens (i.e., fungi versus bacteria) (10).

Grocott's methenamine silver (Fig. 16.15) and periodic acid-Schiff stains (Fig. 16.16) may be used to demonstrate the fungal etiology of eumycetomas. Fontana-Masson stain should be used to differentiate between melanin-pigmented (positive) and hyaline (negative) hyphae (4). In actinomycetoma cases, the Ziehl-Neelsen stain produces mostly a positive result for infections due to *Nocardia* spp., whereas *Actinomadura* spp. produce a negative result. However,

Actinomadura spp. produce a positive result with Gram stain (7, 10). Notably, *Nocardia* spp. and actinomycete species test positive with Grocott's methenamine silver stain.

Molecular diagnosis of the pathogen by direct sequencing of biopsy specimens may produce a rapid diagnosis and identify fungal or bacterial species. Such techniques are particularly valuable in culture-negative cases. The most commonly used methods are 16s RNA gene sequencing for the bacteria that cause actinomycetomas and pan-fungal polymerase chain reaction for cases of eumycetoma (12).

DIFFERENTIAL DIAGNOSIS

Draining abscesses caused by foreign bodies may constitute a differential diagnosis (7). However, histopathological examination of lesions should determine whether an infectious disease is present. If lesions do not have draining sinus tracts, then chromoblastomycosis, phaeohyphomycosis, and sporotrichosis may be mistaken for mycetomas (see the relevant chapters), as may other bacterial infections such as tuberculosis and botryomycosis (4).

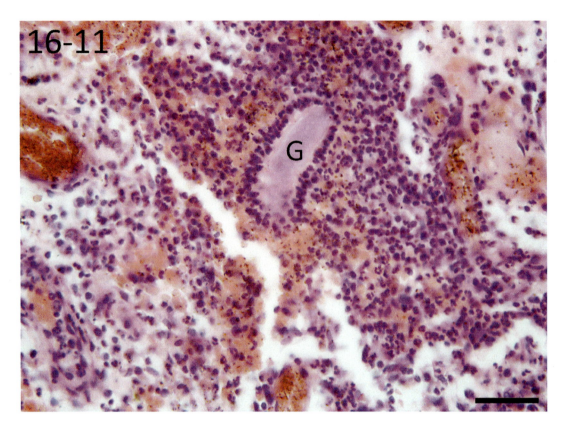

Figure 16.11 Actinomycetoma. A grain (G) formed by *N. brasiliensis* is situated centrally within an abscess. HE. Bar = 25 μm.

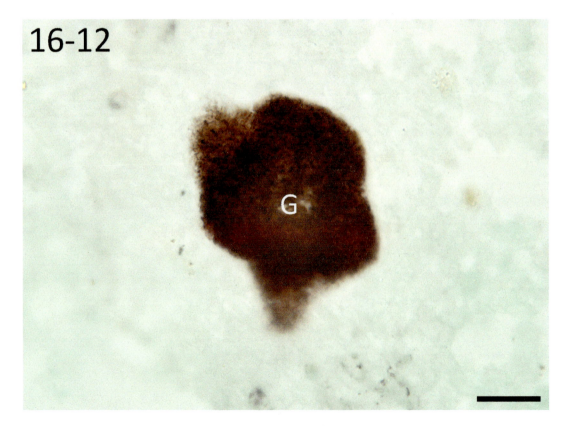

Figure 16.12 Actinomycetoma. Within a grain (G) formed by *N. brasiliensis*, the filamentous morphology of *Nocardia* is clearly visible after staining with Grocott's methenamine silver stain. GMS. Bar = 15 μm.

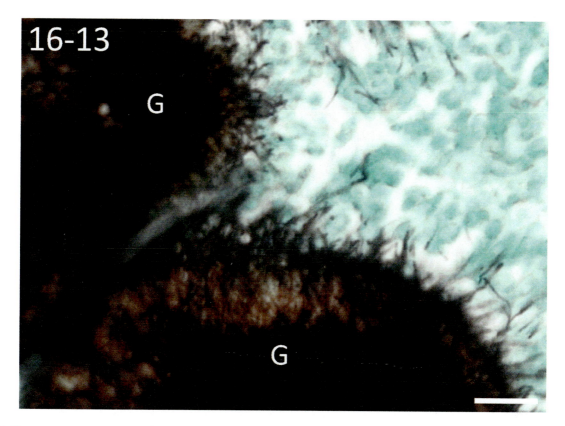

Figure 16.13 Actinomycetoma. The filamentous morphology of *Nocardia* is clearly visible at the periphery of a grain (G) of *N. brasiliensis* after staining with Grocott's methenamine silver stain. Same case as in Fig. 16.12. GMS. Bar = 8 μm.

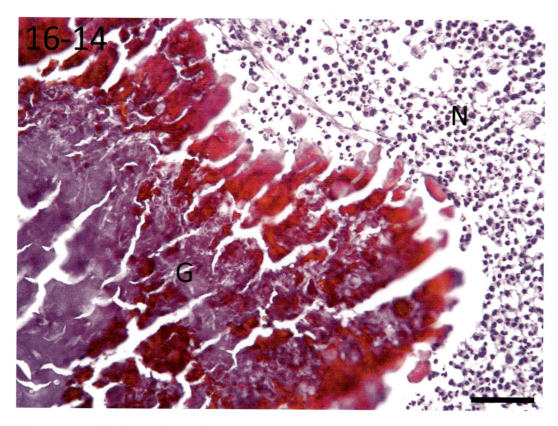

Figure 16.14 Eumycetoma. At the periphery of a grain (G) of unknown etiology, a large quantity of Splendore-Hoeppli material surrounds the neutrophils (N). HE. Bar = 40 μm.

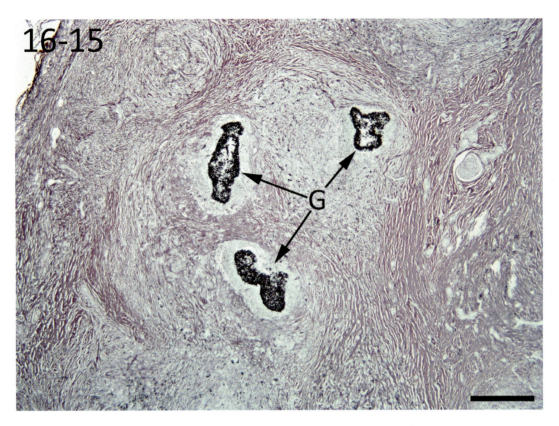

Figure 16.15 Eumycetoma. The grains (G) within the fibrous tissue are easily visible at low magnification in Grocott's methenamine silver-stained sections. GMS. Bar = 175 μm.

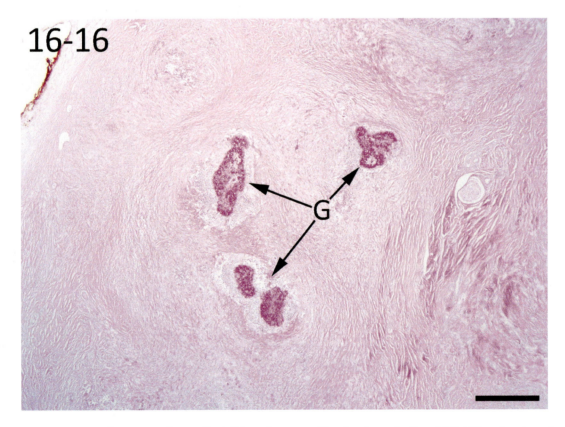

Figure 16.16 Eumycetoma. Grains are also easily visible at low magnification in periodic acid-Schiff-stained sections (same case as in Fig. 16.15). PAS. Bar = 175 μm.

REFERENCES

1. Queiroz-Telles F, Santos DW, Azevedo CMPS. 2015. Fungal infections of implantation (chromoblastomycosis, mycetoma, entomophthoramycosis, and lacaziosis). In: Diagnosis and Treatment of Fungal Infections. 2nd ed. Hospenthal DR, Rinaldi MG, Eds. Springer. pp 261–276.

2. Reis CMS, Reis-Filho EGM. 2018. Mycetomas: An epidemiological, etiological, clinical, laboratory and therapeutic review. An Bras Dermatol, 93, 8–18.

3. Venkatswami S, Sankarasubramanian A, Subramanyam S. 2012. The Madura foot: Looking deep. Int J Low Extrem Wounds, 11, 31–42.

4. Nenoff P, Sande WWJ, Fahal AH, Reinel D, Schöfer H. 2015. Eumycetoma and actinomycetoma – an update on causative agents, epidemiology, pathogenesis, diagnostics and therapy. J Eur Acad Dermatol Venereol, 29, 1873–1883.

5. Sampaio FMS, Wanke B, Freitas DFS, Coelho JMC, Galhardo MCG et al. 2017. Review of 21 cases of mycetoma from 1991 to 2014 in Rio de Janeiro, Brazil. PLoS Negl Trop Dis, 11, 1–18.

6. Karrakchou B, Boubnana I, Senouci K, Hassam B. 2020. Madurella mycetomatis infection of the foot: A case report of a neglected tropical disease in a non-endemic region. BMC Dermatol, 20, 1–7.

7. Sidding EE, Mhmoud NA, Bakhiet SM, Abdallah OB, Mekki SO et al. 2019. The accuracy of histopathological and cytopathological techniques in the identification of the mycetoma causative agents. PLoS Negl Trop Dis, 13, 1–19.

8. Alam K, Maheshwari V, Bhargava S, Jain A, Fatima U et al. 2009. Histological diagnosis of Madura foot (mycetoma): A must for definitive treatment. J Glob Infect Dis, 1, 64–67.

9. Relhan V, Mahajan K, Agarwal P, Garg VK. 2017. Mycetoma: An update. Indian J Dermatol, 62, 332–340.

10. Wang R, Yao X, Li R. 2019. Mycetoma in China: A case report and a review of the literature. Mycopathologia, 184, 327–334.

11. Siddig EE, Fahal AH. 2017. Histopathological approach in diagnosis of mycetoma causative agents: A mini review. J Cytol Histol, 8, 1–3.

12. Verma P, Jha A. 2019. Mycetoma: Reviewing a neglected disease. Clin Exp Dermatol, 44, 123–129.

Candidosis

INTRODUCTION

Candida spp. cause several different superficial infections, such as oropharyngeal, vaginal, nail, and cutaneous/mucocutaneous infections; they also cause invasive infections, which are described in this chapter (1, 2). Invasive candidosis is caused by several *Candida* spp., with *C. albicans* being the most important. Several other species also frequently cause candidosis, including *C. glabrata, C. krusei, C. parapsilosis,* and *C. tropicalis* (3). A variety of other species also cause candidosis occasionally, including *C. kefyr, C. lusitaniae, C. norvegensis, C. rugosa,* and *C. auris* (2, 3). These different species may be found on healthy skin, on mucocutaneous membranes, and in the environment (3).

EPIDEMIOLOGY

Risk factors for invasive candidosis include immunosuppression, the presence of vascular catheters (which may harbour biofilms), diabetes, renal failure, parenteral nutrition, and transplantation (1–3).

Invasive candidosis may occur in several organs or organ systems. Systemic, hematogenous spread of *Candida* spp. may cause lesions in almost any organ. However, the skin, eyes, meninges, central nervous system, muscles, kidneys, lungs, bone marrow, joints, spleen, and heart (endocarditis and myocarditis) are particularly vulnerable to infections (4–11). In addition to becoming established following hematogenous spread, invasive lesions of the kidneys and lungs may also become established following ascending spread and uptake via the airway, respectively. Occasionally candidosis may also cause placentitis, resulting in abortion. In these cases, the infection results from ascending or hematogenous spread (12–14). Problems with antifungal drug resistance have been reported for particular isolates of *C. glabrata, C. auris,* and *C. krusei* (1, 2).

PATHOLOGY

In acute lesions of invasive candidosis, the primary reaction is suppurative with infiltration of neutrophils (Figs. 17.1 and 17.2). Subsequently, lymphocytes and macrophages are also present in lesions (5, 6, 15, 16). Angioinvasion also occurs frequently, resulting in thrombosis and infarction and causing the hematogenous spread to other organs from the primary portal of entry (e.g., the gastrointestinal tract) (Figs. 17.3–17.5) (17). In chronic lesions, encapsulated abscesses may form, or the infection may result in areas of granulomatous inflammation containing macrophages, epithelioid cells, and multinucleate giant cells (Figs. 17.6–17.10) (6, 16).

FUNGAL HISTOMORPHOLOGY

Candida spp. are only weakly stained by haematoxylin and eosin, whereas they are clearly visible in periodic acid-Schiff and Grocott's methenamine silver-stained sections (18–20). In tissues, all *Candida* spp. grow by forming yeast cell buds (3–6 µm) (Figs. 17.11 and 17.12), and they often also form pseudohyphae (i.e., chains of yeast cells, where the cells remain attached end to end giving the impression of tubes with periodic constrictions), or true hyphae in the case of *C. albicans* (Fig. 17.13) (18, 21). The hyphae are 3–5 µm wide, septate, and have parallel walls (18, 21). In tissues, *C. glabrata* only grows as yeast cells that measure 2–5 µm in diameter (Fig. 17.14) (1, 18, 21).

DIFFERENTIAL DIAGNOSIS

The formation of blastospores along pseudohyphae (and hyphae) may be mistaken for branching (1). However, if present, the observation of both yeast-like elements (blastospores) in relation to pseudohyphae/hyphae will distinguish *Candida* from most other mycoses (Fig. 17.15).

In tissues, the morphology of *Candida* spp. is most often confused with the morphologies of *Trichosporon* spp. and *Aspergillus* spp. In some cases, *Candida* spp. may be misidentified as *Fusarium* spp., *Scedosporium* spp., or even the pathogens that cause mucormycosis (18). *Candida* spp. hyphae are generally narrower than those of *Aspergillus* spp. and those of other filamentous fungi (Fig. 17.16) (1, 18). Notably, however, treatment with antimycotics and necrosis can both induce swelling of hyphae (22). Furthermore, transverse sections containing *Aspergillus, Fusarium,* or *Scedosporium* hyphae may be misinterpreted as containing yeast cells. This is particularly problematic when only individual fungal elements are present within a section (18).

138

DOI: 10.1201/9781003306177-17

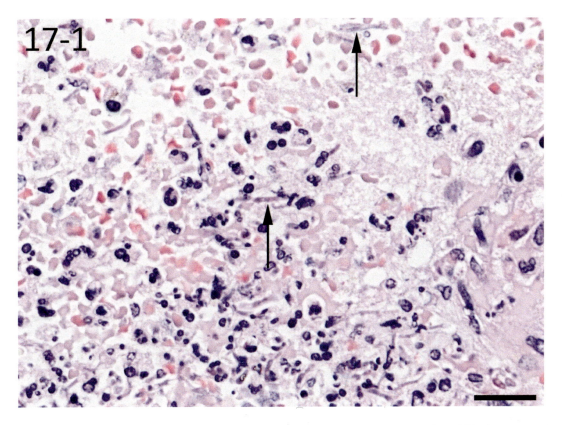

Figure 17.1 Acute, necrotizing, suppurative encephalitis. *Candida* elements (arrows) are often difficult to see in haematoxylin and eosin-stained sections. HE. Bar = 30 μm.

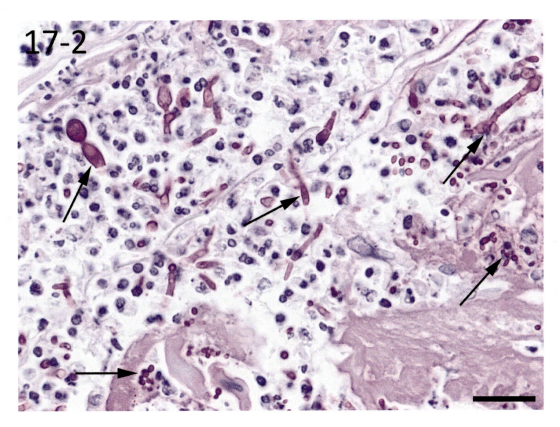

Figure 17.2 Acute, necrotizing, suppurative encephalitis. *Candida* elements (arrows) are easier to see in periodic acid-Schiff-stained sections. Same case as in Fig. 17.1. PAS. Bar = 30 μm.

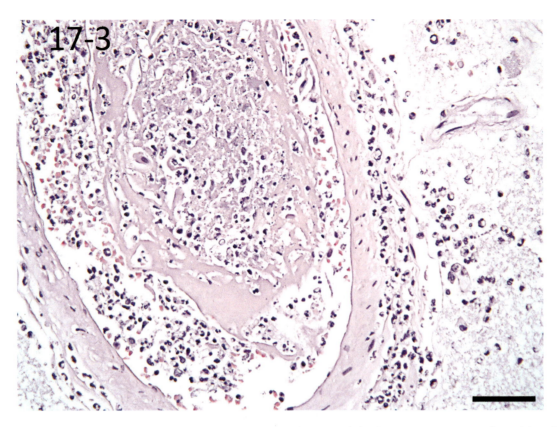

Figure 17.3 Acute, cerebral, suppurative, and thrombosing vasculitis. *Candida* elements are not usually visible in haematoxylin and eosin-stained sections. HE. Bar = 75 µm.

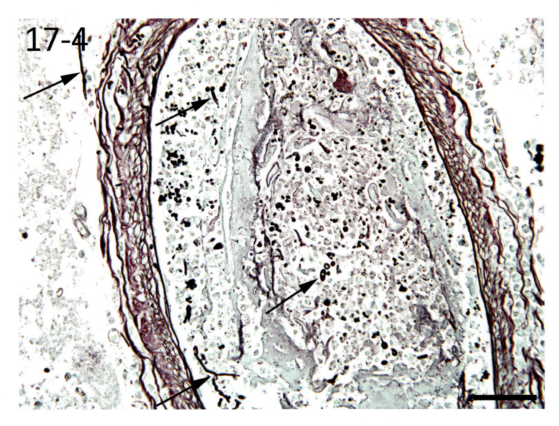

Figure 17.4 Acute, cerebral, suppurative, and thrombosing vasculitis. *Candida* elements are easily recognized both inside and outside the thrombosed vessel (arrows) in sections stained with Grocott's methenamine silver stain. Same case as in Fig. 17.3. GMS. Bar = 75 µm.

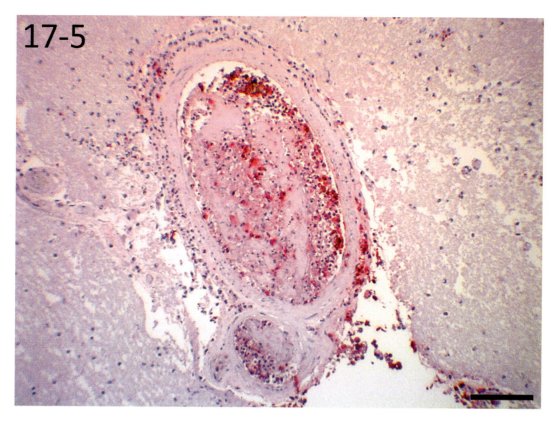

Figure 17.5 Acute, cerebral, suppurative, and thrombosing vasculitis. *Candida albicans* elements are stained red both inside and outside the thrombosed vessels, using a specific immunohistochemical staining procedure. IHC. Bar = 125 μm.

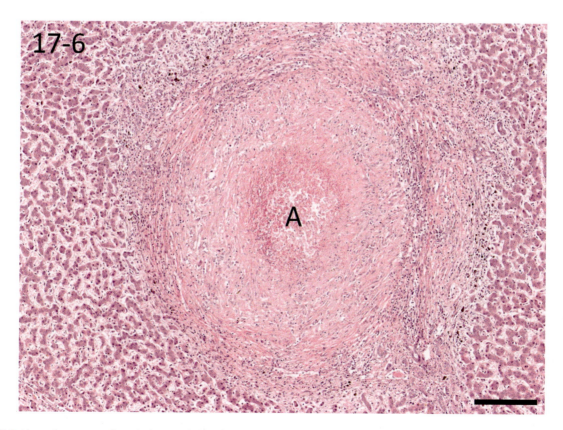

Figure 17.6 Hepatic, encapsulated abscess (A) with a necrotic centre caused by *C. albicans*. HE. Bar = 150 μm.

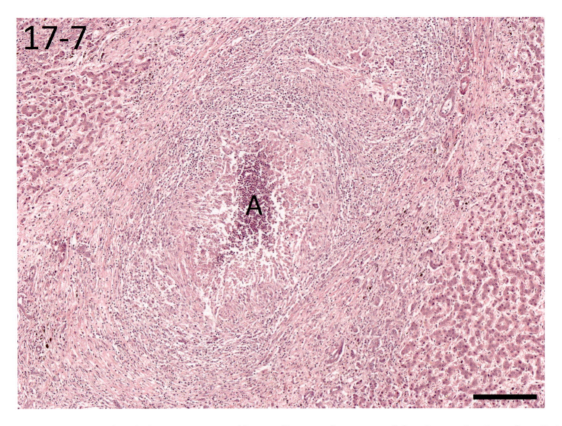

Figure 17.7 Hepatic, encapsulated abscess (A) caused by *C. albicans*. The centre of the abscess has been heavily infiltrated by neutrophils. HE. Bar = 150 μm.

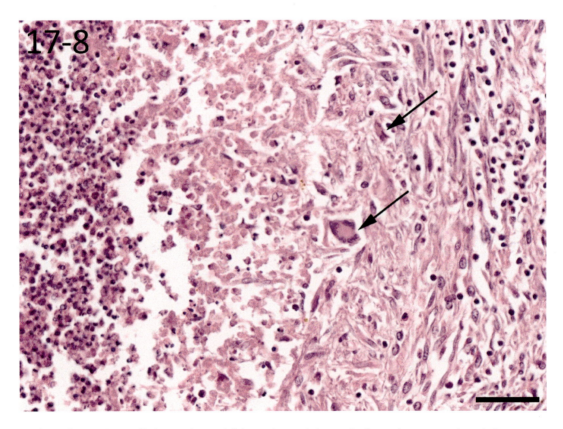

Figure 17.8 Multinucleate giant cells (arrows) are visible at the periphery of a hepatic, encapsulated abscess caused by *C. albicans*. Same case as in Fig. 17.7. HE. Bar = 60 μm.

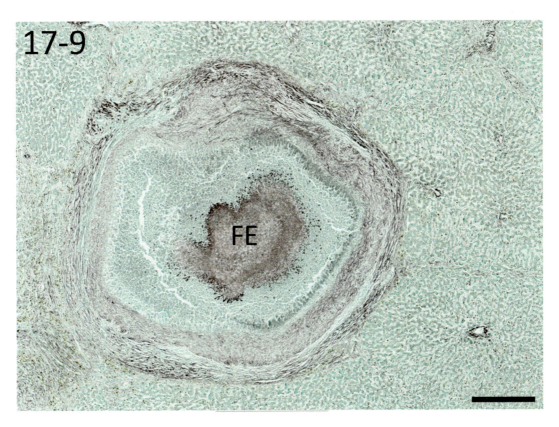

Figure 17.9 Hepatic, encapsulated abscess caused by *C. albicans*. The fungal elements (FE) are clearly visible at the centre, after Grocott's methenamine silver stain has been applied. Same case as in Fig. 17.7. GMS. Bar = 125 μm.

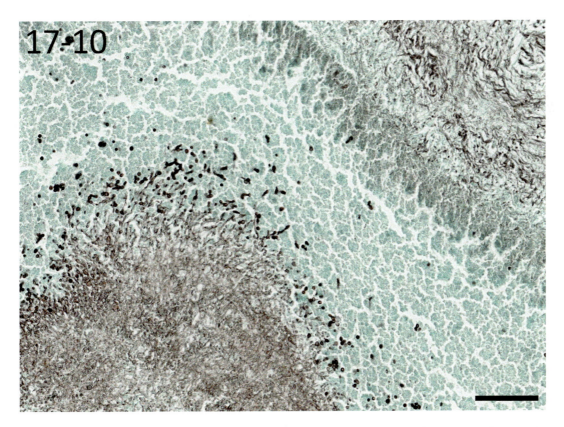

Figure 17.10 The fungal elements are strongly highlighted by Grocott's methenamine silver stain at the periphery of a hepatic, encapsulated abscess caused by *C. albicans*. Same case as in Fig. 17.7. GMS. Bar = 75 μm.

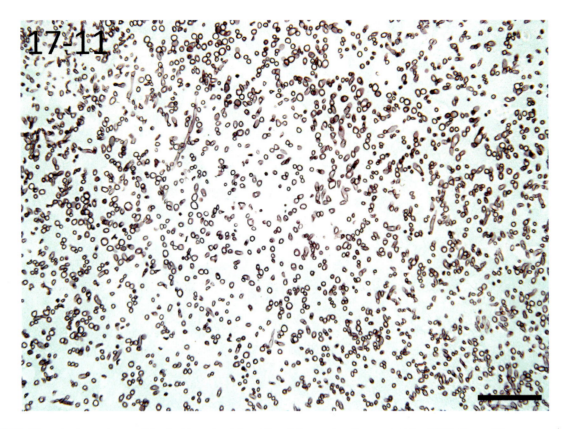

Figure 17.11 Chronic, hepatic candidosis. Many budding *Candida* yeast cells are visible. GMS. Bar = 50 μm.

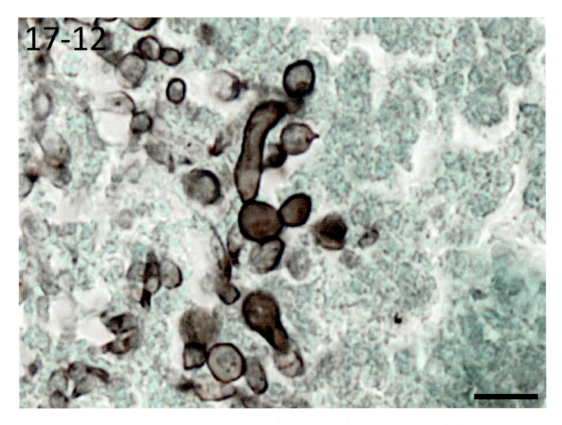

Figure 17.12 Chronic, hepatic candidosis. The budding *Candida* yeast cells have been magnified. Same case as in Fig. 17.11. GMS. Bar = 8 μm.

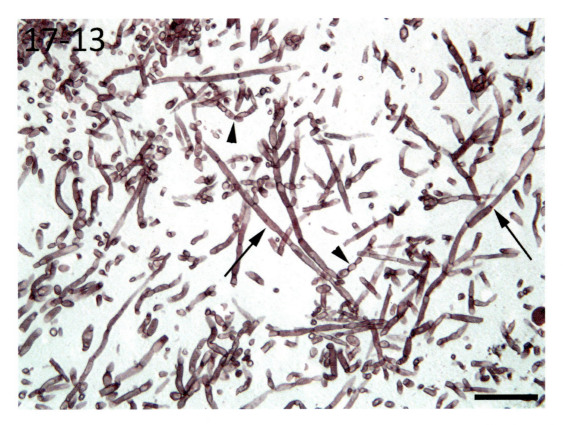

Figure 17.13 Chronic, pulmonary candidosis. Hyphae (arrows) and pseudohyphae (arrowheads) are often formed in lesions caused by *C. albicans*. GMS. Bar = 30 μm.

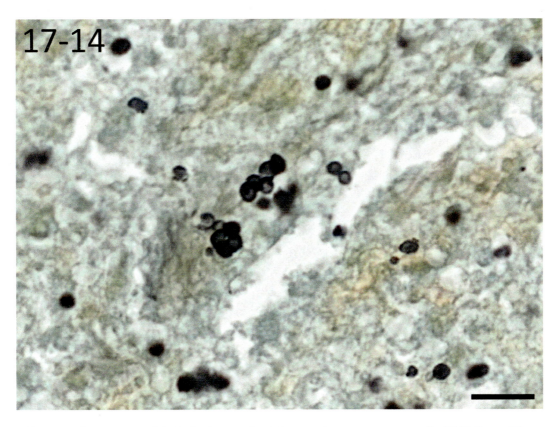

Figure 17.14 Chronic pulmonary candidosis. In tissues, *C. glabrata* only grows as yeast cells. GMS. Bar = 15 μm.

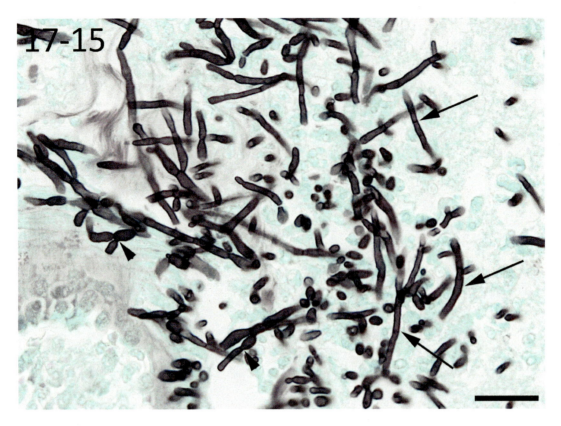

Figure 17.15 Chronic, cerebral candidosis. The presence of hyphae (arrows), pseudohyphae (arrowheads), and yeast cells is indicative of candidosis. GMS. Bar = 25 µm.

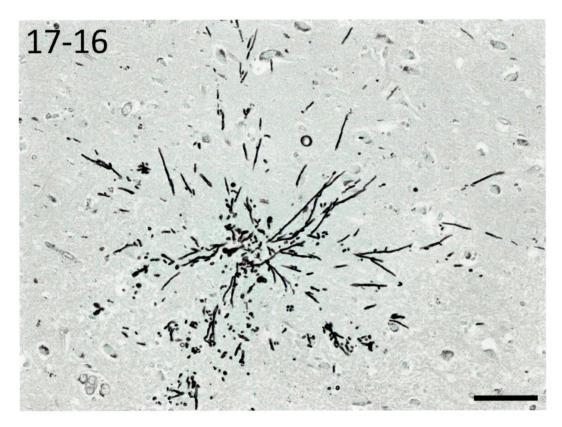

Figure 17.16 Chronic, cerebral candidosis. Identical thin *C. albicans* hyphae growing outward in a radial pattern from a cerebral vessel, following hematogenous spread. GMS. Bar = 100 µm.

Trichosporon spp. also form both yeast cells and pseudohyphae; however, the yeast cells produced by *Trichosporon* spp. are larger and more pleomorphic than those produced by *Candida*. Moreover, in contrast to *Candida*, *Trichosporon* spp. produce rectangular arthroconidia (see chapter on trichosporonosis).

Although the cells of *C. glabrata* are slightly larger than those of *H. capsulatum* var. *capsulatum*, they may be misidentified in regions where histoplasmosis is endemic. However, the characteristic granulomatous tissue reaction in histoplasmosis is important when evaluating the sections (1, 18–20). When endospores are located outside the spherule in cases of coccidioidomycosis, these may resemble *Candida* yeast cells. If only small yeast cells are present in cases of blastomycosis or paracoccidioidomycosis, these too may resemble *Candida* yeast cells. However, the characteristic tissue reactions and usually the simultaneous presence of the larger yeast cells will usually be sufficient for an accurate diagnosis (1, 18–20). In the lungs, *Candida* spp. may also need to be differentiated from elements of *Pneumocystis*. However, *Pneumocystis* and *Candida* spp. cells differ in shape and *Pneumocystis* causes a different inflammatory reaction (i.e., interstitial pneumonia), and no necrotizing lesions. In rare mycosis cases, such as those caused by *Trichosporonosis*, it may also be difficult to reach a tentative diagnosis based on histomorphology alone (see the chapter on trichosporonosis).

Therefore, in difficult cases, immunohistochemistry with commercially available monoclonal antibodies or polymerase chain reaction techniques should be applied to fresh or formalin-fixed, paraffin-embedded tissue samples (Fig. 17.5) (23, 24). Several specific DNA/RNA *in situ* hybridization probes are also available for differentiating *Candida* spp. from filamentous fungi that cause other infections, including aspergillosis and yeast infections (25).

REFERENCES

1. Guarner J, Brandt ME. 2011. Histopathologic diagnosis of fungal infections in the 21st century. Clin Microbiol Rev, 24, 247–280.
2. Richardson MD, Warnock, DW. 2003. Invasive candidosis. In: Fungal Infection. Diagnosis and Management. 3rd ed. Blackwell Publishing. pp 185–214.
3. Odds FC. 1988. *Candida* and Candidosis. 2nd ed. Bailliere Tindall.
4. Tauber SC, Eiffert H, Kellner S, Lugert R, Bunkowski S et al. 2014. Fungal encephalitis in human autopsy cases is associated with extensive neuronal damage but only minimal repair. Neuropathol Appl Neurobiol, 40, 610–627.
5. Carstensen H, Widding E, Storm K, Ostergaard E, Herlin T. 1990. Hepatosplenic candidiasis in children with cancer. Three cases in leukemic children and a literature review. Pediatr Hematol Oncol, 7, 3–12.
6. Kontoyiannis DP, Luna MA, Samuels BI, Bodey GP. 2000. Hepatosplenic candidiasis: A manifestation of chronic disseminated candidiasis. Infect Dis Clin North Am, 14, 721–739.
7. Mathai AM, Menezes RG, Naik R, Kanchan T, Kumar S et al. 2009. An autopsy case of renal candidiasis. J Forensic Leg Med, 16, 31–34.
8. Roden AC, Schuetz AN. 2017. Histopathology of fungal diseases of the lung. Semin Diagn Pathol, 34, 530–549.
9. Rao NA, Hidayat AA. 2001. Endogenous mycotic endophthalmitis: Variations in clinical and histopathologic changes in candidiasis compared with aspergillosis. Am J Ophthalmol, 132, 244–251.
10. Andriole VT, Kravetz HM, Roberts WC, Utz JP. 1962. *Candida* endocarditis: Clinical and pathologic studies. Am J Med, 32, 251–285.
11. Madakshira MG, Bal A, Shivaprakash RM, Vijayvegiya R. 2018. *Candida parapsilosis* endocarditis in an intravenous drug abuser: An autopsy report. Cardiovasc Pathol, 36, 30–34.
12. Garcia-Flores J, Cruceyra M, Canamares M, Garicano A, Nieto O et al. 2016. *Candida* chorioamnionitis: Report of two cases and review of literature. J Obstet Gynaecol, 36, 843–844.
13. Hood IC, Browning D, De Sa DJ, Whyte RK. 1985. Fetal inflammatory response in second trimester candidal chorioamnionitis. Early Hum Dev, 11, 1–10.
14. Rivasi F, Gasser B, Bagni A, Ficarra G, Negro RM et al. 1998. Placental candidiasis: Report of four cases, one with villitis. APMIS, 106, 1165–1169.
15. Haron E, Feld R, Tuffnell P, Patterson B, Hasselback R et al. 1987. Hepatic candidiasis: An increasing problem in immunocompromised patients. Am J Med, 83, 17–26.
16. Ihde DC, Roberts WC, Marr KC, Brereton HD, McGuire WP et al. 1978. Cardiac candidiasis in cancer patients. Cancer, 41, 2364–2371.
17. Cimbaluk D, Scudiere J, Butsch J, Jakate S. 2005. Invasive candidal enterocolitis followed shortly by fatal cerebral hemorrhage in immunocompromised patients. J Clin Gastroenterol, 39, 795–797.
18. Jensen HE, Chandler FW. 2005. Histopathological diagnosis of mycotic diseases. In: Topley and Wilson's Microbiology & Microbial Infections. Medical Mycology. 10th ed. Merz WG, Hay RJ, Eds. Hodder Arnold. pp 121–143.
19. O'Hara M. 1986. Histopathologic diagnosis of fungal diseases. Infect Control, 7, 78–84.
20. Kung VL, Chernock RD, Burnham CD. 2018. Diagnostic accuracy of fungal identification in histopathology and cytopathology specimens. Eur J Clin Microbiol Infect Dis, 37, 157–165.
21. Lombardi A, Croci GA, Brazzelli V, Vecchia M, Zuccaro V et al. 2017. Cutaneous septic emboli from *Candida glabrata* in a haematological patient. Am J Hematol, 92, 1111–1112.
22. Cronan J, Burrell M, Trepeta R. 1980. Aphthoid ulcerations in gastric candidiasis. Radiology, 134, 607–611.

23. Monteagudo C, Marcilla A, Mormeneo S, Llombart-Bosch A, Sentandreu R. 1995. Specific immuno-histochemical identification of *Candida albicans* in paraffin-embedded tissue with a new monoclonal antibody (1B12). Am J Clin Pathol, 103, 130–135.

24. Lau A, Chen S, Sorrell T, Carter D, Malik R et al. 2007. Development and clinical application of a panfungal PCR assay to detect and identify fungal DNA in tissue specimens. J Clin Microbiol, 45, 380–385.

25. Rickerts V, McCormick SI, Mousset S, Kommedal O, Fredricks DN. 2013. Deciphering the aetiology of a mixed fungal infection by broad-range PCR with sequencing and fluorescence in situ hybridisation. Mycoses, 56, 681–686.

18

Trichosporonosis

INTRODUCTION

Infection with species of the genus *Trichosporon* is mostly associated with skin lesions termed white piedra (1). However, systemic invasive infections occur in immunosuppressed patients, where *T. asahii* and *T. inkin* are the main causes of systemic trichosporonosis (2–4).

EPIDEMIOLOGY

As with *Candida* spp., *Trichosporon* species occur throughout the environment (in soil, in water, and on plants), as well as on the skin and mucocutaneous membranes including within the gastrointestinal tract (1). Infections may occur via gastrointestinal invasion or colonization of catheters and have a high mortality rate (50–80%); immunocompromised individuals, patients with hematologic neoplasms, and individuals receiving treatment with broad-spectrum antibiotics are susceptible to these infections (2–4). Following the invasion, the pathogens may spread hematogenously.

PATHOLOGY

The skin, eyes, central nervous system, spleen, lungs, and heart may be affected, following hematogenous spread. As with candidosis, hepatosplenic trichosporonosis may also result from dissemination (5, 6). The initial lesions are predominantly necrotic (5).

FUNGAL HISTOMORPHOLOGY

Trichosporon hyphae, which are septate, are only weakly stained by hematoxylin and eosin, whereas the arthroconidia (arthrospores) are basophilic (Fig. 18.1). Both elements are easily visible after periodic acid-Schiff or Grocott's methenamine silver stains are applied (5, 7). In trichosporonosis lesions, rectangular/oval arthroconidia (arthrospores) are present together with pseudohyphae and true hyphae with thin walls (Figs. 18.2–18.4). The spores are 3–8 μm wide and attached by a narrow single bud (Fig. 18.3), and the pseudohyphae/hyphae are 3–5 μm wide (Figs. 18.3 and 18.4).

DIFFERENTIAL DIAGNOSIS

The fungal elements of *Trichosporon* are easily confused with those of *Candida* spp. However, *Trichosporon* spp. tend to produce more true hyphae (Fig. 18.4) than *Candida* spp. Moreover, staining with Grocott's methenamine silver stain suggests that *Trichosporon* spp. exhibit less reactivity than *Candida* spp. (1). Due to the overlap in histomorphology, especially between *Candida* spp. and *Trichosporon* spp., a diagnosis of trichosporonosis must be determined carefully based on the results of histopathological staining and pathomorphology. Ideally, the diagnosis should be confirmed by polymerase chain reaction or by using immunohistochemical techniques that are designed to differentiate between *Trichosporon* and other fungi (1, 7–9). Such techniques will also exclude *Trichoderma* spp., which may also resemble species of *Trichosporon* in tissues.

DOI: 10.1201/9781003306177-18

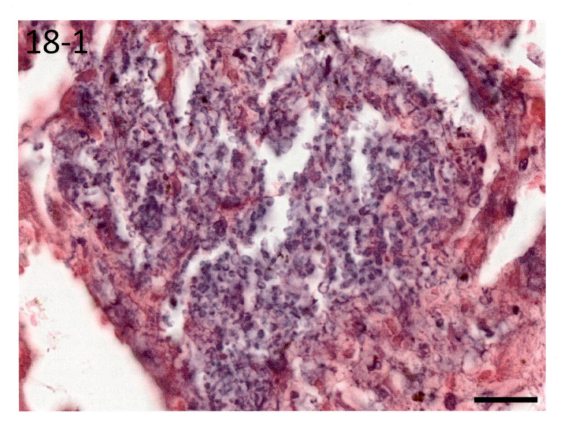

Figure 18.1 Pulmonary trichosporonosis due to *T. asahii*. In hematoxylin and eosin-stained sections, the arthroconidia are slightly basophilic, whereas hyphal elements are difficult to see. HE. Bar = 30 μm.

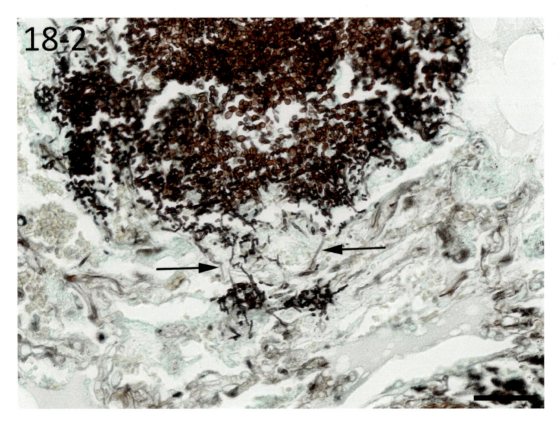

Figure 18.2 Pulmonary trichosporonosis due to *T. asahii*. Arthroconidia and pseudohyphae are clearly visible at the centre of the lesion. There are hyphae (arrows) at the periphery, growing into the surrounding tissue. GMS. Bar = 60 μm.

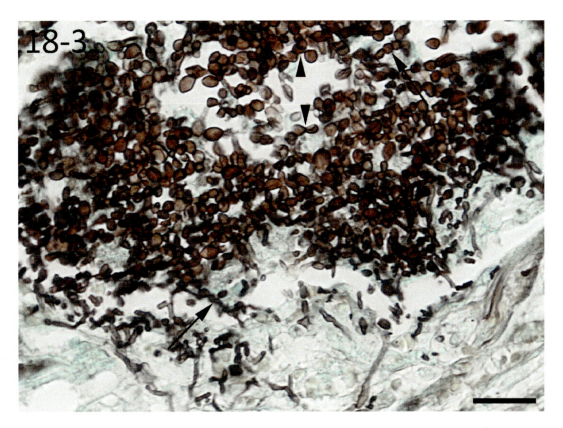

Figure 18.3 Pulmonary trichosporonosis due to *T. asahii*. Both pseudohyphae (arrows) and arthroconidia are visible at the centre of the lesion. Note the rectangular/oval shape of the arthroconidia, some of which have single buds (arrowheads). GMS. Bar = 30 μm.

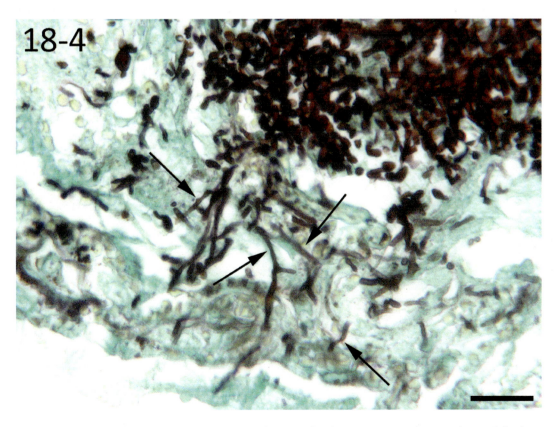

Figure 18.4 Pulmonary trichosporonosis due to *T. asahii*. There are hyphae (arrows) at the periphery of the lesion, growing out into the surrounding tissue. GMS. Bar = 30 μm.

REFERENCES

1. Obana Y, Sano M, Jike T, Homma T, Nemoto N. 2010. Differential diagnosis of trichosporonosis using conventional histopathological stains and electron microscopy. Histopathology, 56, 372–383.

2. Garcia JCV, Grajeda LAG, Burbano JCS, Aguilar LE. 2018. Infeccio por *Trichosporon asahii*. Caso Clinico, 2018, 63, 138–141.

3. Krzisch D, Camus V, David M, Gargala G, Lepretre S. 2019. Fatal invasive trichosporonosis caused by *Trichosporon inkin* after allogeneic stem cell transplant for very severe idiopathic aplastic anemia. J Bacteriol Parasitol, 10, 1–3.

4. Ruan S-Y, Chien J-Y, Hsueh, PR. 2009. Invasive trichosporonosis caused by *Trichosporon asahii* and other unusual *Trichosporon* species at a medical center in Taiwan. Clin Infect Disease, 49, 11–17.

5. Salazar J, Hardin KA, Wiederhold NP, Thompsom GR. 2020. Trichosporonosis presenting as an exophytic cutaneous mass lesion. Mycopathologia, 185, 705–708.

6. Richardson MD, Warnock, DW. 2003. Trichosporonosis. In: Fungal Infection. Diagnosis and Management. 3rd ed. Blackwell Publishing. pp 349–353.

7. Jensen HE, Chandler FW. 2007. Histopathological diagnoses of mycoses. In: Topley and Wilson's Microbiology & Microbial Infections. Medical Mycology. 10th ed. Merz WG, Hay RJ Eds. Hodder Arnold. pp 121–142.

8. Fukuzawa M, Inaba H, Hayama M, Sakaguchi N, Sano K et al. 1995. Improved detection of medically important fungi by immunoperoxidase staining with polyclonal antibodies. Virchows Arch, 427, 407–414.

9. Sadamoto S, Shinozaki M, Nagi M, Nihonyanagi Y, Ejima K et al. 2020. Histopathological study on the prevalence of trichosporonosis in formalin-fixed and paraffin-embedded tissue autopsy sections by in situ hybridization with peptide nucleic acid probe. Med Mycol, 58, 460–468.

19

Cryptococcosis

INTRODUCTION

Cryptococcosis is caused by a number of species within the genus *Cryptococcus*: *C. neoformans* var. *grubii* (serotype A), *C. gattii* (serotypes B and C), *C. neoformans* var. *neoformans* (serotype D), and *C. neoformans* (serotype AD). These are further subdivided into several molecular types (1). Recently, two new complexes, which include several hybrids, have been established: *C. neoformans* species complex and *C. gattii* species complex (2). Cryptococcosis due to either *Cryptococcus laurentii* or *Cryptococcus albidus* is rare (3). Cryptococcosis affects both humans and animals and has been diagnosed in various wild and domestic animals (4–16). Moreover, several distinct cryptococcosis models have been developed in different laboratory animals (17).

EPIDEMIOLOGY

The different species of *Cryptococcus* predominantly occur in different locations. *C. neoformans* var. *grubii* occurs worldwide, whereas *C. gattii* is typically found in tropical and subtropical regions. In Europe, *C. neoformans* var. *neoformans* is often isolated from lesions (4–6). The fungi are generally present in the environment, but are typically found in different places; serotypes A and D are often associated with pigeons, whereas serotypes B and C are associated with tropical and subtropical trees, including eucalyptus (18). Infections predominantly occur following inhalation of the fungus, but traumatic implantation and infection of the gastrointestinal tract may also occur. Following inhalation, the organisms often spread hematogenously, especially to the meninges and/or the central nervous system. Almost any organ may be infected by dissemination, but the skin, bones, liver, heart, and eyes are particularly susceptible (1, 19–25). Although cryptococcosis frequently affects immunocompromised individuals, the outbreak on Vancouver Island showed that *C. gattii* can infect immunocompetent individuals as well (19, 26).

PATHOLOGY

For cryptococcosis, the host reaction apparently depends on both the host's immune status and the virulence of the fungus (e.g., the presence of a capsule, melanin production,

growth characteristics at 37°C, and the response to oxidative stress) (1). In some cases, there may be granulomatous reactions, with macrophages, epithelioid cells, and multinucleate giant cells, as well as necrosis and fibrosis, whereas in other cases the inflammatory reaction may be sparse (Figs. 19.1–19.3) (22, 23, 27). In lesions, the pathogens are present outside cells and within macrophages and multinucleate giant cells (Figs. 19.2 and 19.3) (1). Neutrophils are not usually present in cryptococcosis lesions but may occur in cryptococcal cellulitis lesions (20).

FUNGAL HISTOMORPHOLOGY

The fungal elements are usually visible in haematoxylin and eosin-stained sections (Fig. 19.3), but they are more readily observed in sections stained with Grocott's methenamine silver, periodic acid-Schiff, or combined haematoxylin and eosin and Grocott's methenamine silver stains (Figs. 19.2 and 19.4) (1, 28, 29). The melanin in the yeast cell walls can be visualized by the Fontana-Masson staining technique (1, 28, 29). In haematoxylin and eosin and Grocott's methenamine silver-stained sections, fungal cells are typically surrounded by an unstained mucinous capsule (an empty halo) (Figs. 19.3 and 19.4). In rare cases, pseudohyphae may be formed (Fig. 19.5) (28, 29). If the cryptococci present in lesions have a capsule, this can be visualized using polysaccharide stains such as Alcian blue and Mayer's mucicarmine stain (Figs. 19.6–19.8). However, these stains will produce negative results in infections with capsule-deficient ("dry variants") cryptococci. *Cryptococcus* spp. have circular/oval yeast-like cells that vary in size (diameters: 2–20 μm, with most being 4–10 μm) that exhibit narrow-based budding (usually only single budding) (Figs. 19.4 and 19.6) (1, 28, 29).

DIFFERENTIAL DIAGNOSIS

Notably, *Blastomyces dermatitidis* and *Rhinosporidium seeberi* cells also have capsules that are stained by mucicarmine, although to a lesser degree. However, the morphology of these pathogens is quite different (see chapters on blastomycosis and rhinosporidiosis). Where capsules are absent, it is particularly important to distinguish the pathogens from those that cause histoplasmosis and candidosis (especially *C. glabrata*). In such cases, Fontana-Masson stain may be

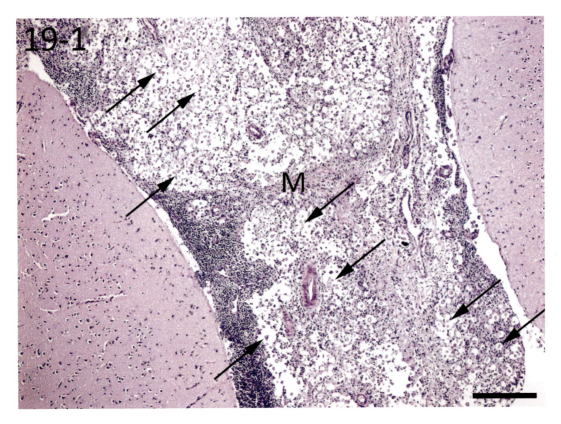

Figure 19.1 Chronic, meningeal cryptococcosis. A diffuse, non-suppurative inflamed region is present within the meninges (M). Numerous fungal cells (arrows) are visible in the inflamed region. HE. Bar = 200 μm.

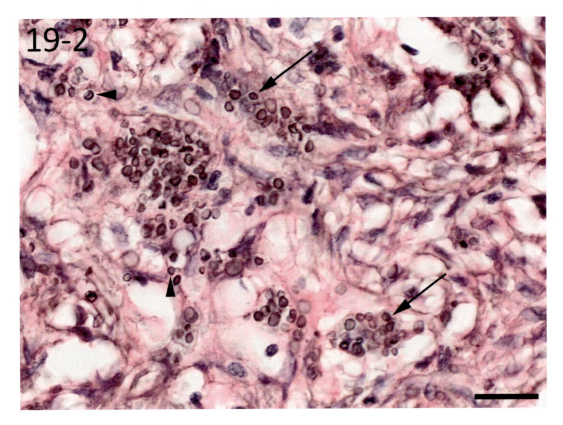

Figure 19.2 Chronic, pulmonary granulomatous cryptococcosis. The inflammatory reaction is dominated by fibrosis and macrophages. The *Cryptococcus* cells are visible both within macrophages (arrows) and outside cells (arrowheads). GMS and HE. Bar = 35 μm.

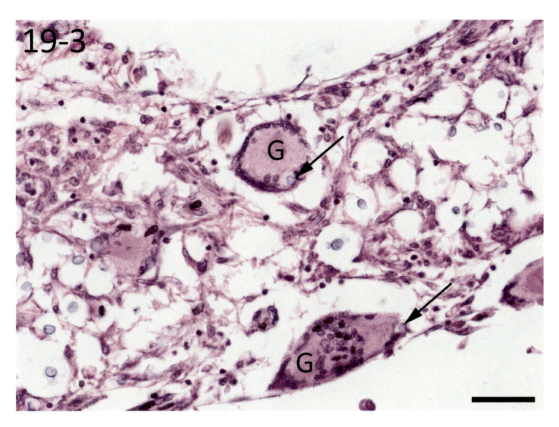

Figure 19.3 Chronic, meningeal granulomatous cryptococcosis. More multinucleate giant cells (G) are present. Two of the multinucleate giant cells contain blue-stained *Cryptococcus* cells (arrows). Both intracellular and extracellular fungal cells are surrounded by a halo (empty space). HE. Bar = 40 μm.

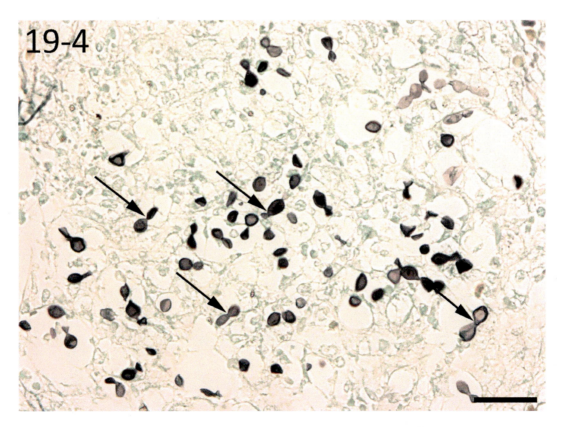

Figure 19.4 Acute, hepatic cryptococcosis. The characteristic narrow-based budding of *Cryptococcus* is visible in several cells (arrows). GMS. Bar = 35 μm.

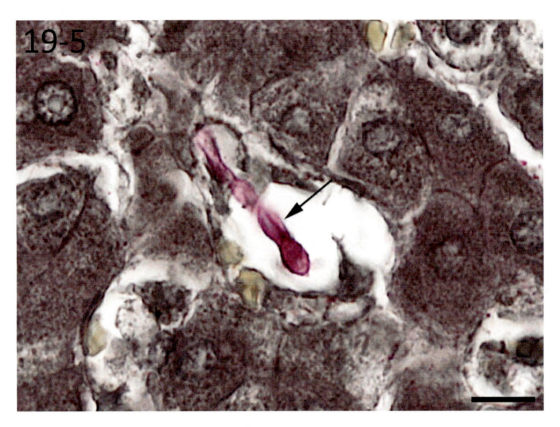

Figure 19.5 Acute, hepatic cryptococcosis. A cryptococcal pseudohypha is visible (arrow). Mucicarmine. Bar = 12 μm.

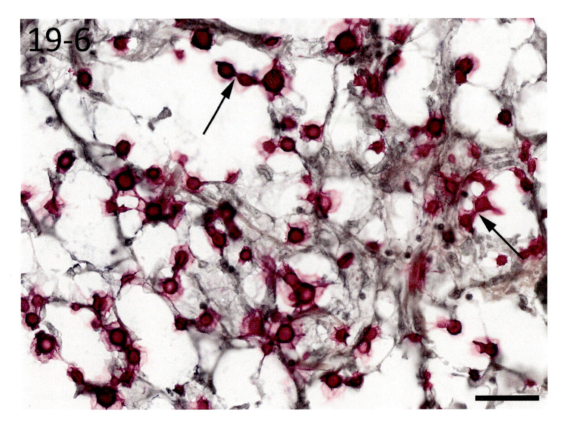

Figure 19.6 Chronic, meningeal cryptococcosis. The mucinous capsular material of *Cryptococcus* clearly highlights the fungal cells, some of which are budding (arrows). Mucicarmine. Bar = 25 μm.

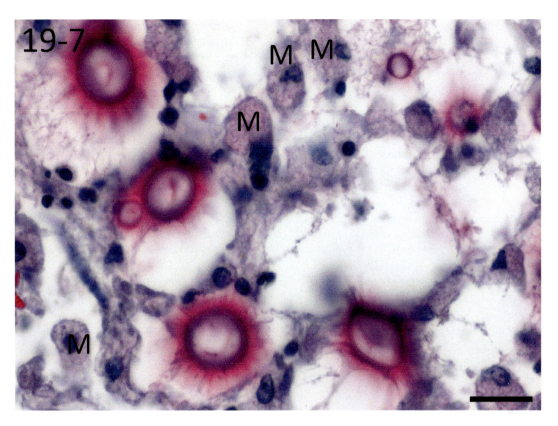

Figure 19.7 Chronic, meningeal cryptococcosis. The mucinous capsular material of *Cryptococcus* exhibits a radiating pattern. Positively stained mucinous material has been taken up by the surrounding macrophages (M). Mucicarmine. Bar = 6 µm.

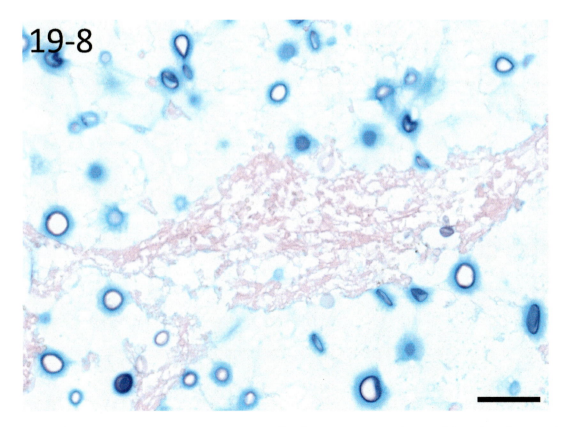

Figure 19.8 Acute, hepatic cryptococcosis. *Cryptococcus* cells of various sizes are shown in blue when the capsular material is stained. Alcian blue. Bar = 15 µm.

used to make a diagnosis based on the melanin content of the *Cryptococcus* spp. cell walls. Several immunohistochemical, *in situ* hybridization, and polymerase chain reaction techniques are available for making a diagnosis of cryptococcosis (10, 12, 15, 25, 29).

REFERENCES

1. Maziarz EK, Perfect JR. 2015. Cryptococcosis. In: Diagnosis and Treatment of Fungal Infections. 2nd ed. Hospenthal DR, Rinaldi MG, Eds. Springer. pp 175–193.

2. Casadevall A, Freij JB, Hann-Soden C et al. 2017. Continental drift and speciation of the *Cryptococcus neoformans* and *Cryptococcus gattii* species complexes. mSphere,2, e00103–e00117.

3. Harris J, Lockhart S, Chillet T. 2012. *Cryptococcus gattii*: Where do we go from here? Med Mycol, 50, 113–129.

4. Hull CM, Heitman J. 2002. Genetics of *Cryptococcus neoformans*. Annu Rev Genet, 36, 557–615.

5. Perfect JR. 2005. *Cryptococcus neoformans*. In: Mandell, Douglas and Bennett's Principles and Practice of Infectious Diseases. 6th ed. Mandell GL, Bennett JE, Dolin R, Eds. Elsevier. pp 2997–3012.

6. Chen S, Sorrell T, Nimmo G, Speed B, Currie B et al. 2000. Epidemiology and host- and variety-dependent characteristics of infection due to *Cryptococcus neoformans* in Australia and New Zealand. Australian Cryptococcal Study Group. Clin Infect Dis, 31, 499–508.

7. Eshar D, Mayer J. 2010. Disseminated, histologically confirmed *Cryptococcus* spp. infection in a domestic ferret. J Am Vet Med Assoc, 236, 770–774.

8. Del Fava C, Levy FL, Scannapieco EM, Lara CCSH, Villalobos EMC et al. 2011. Cryptococcal pneumonia and meningitis in a horse. J Equine Vet Sci, 31, 693–695.

9. Headley SA, Di Santis GW, de Alcântara BK, Costa TC, da Silva EO et al. 2015. *Cryptococcus gattii*-induced infections in dogs from Southern Brazil. Mycopathologia, 180, 265–275.

10. Headley SA, Mota FCD, Lindsay S, de Oliveira LM, Medeiros AA et al. 2016. *Cryptococcus neoformans* var. *grubii*-Induced arthritis with encephalitic dissemination in a dog and review of published literature. Mycopathologia, 181, 595–601.

11. Livet V, Javard R, Alexander K, Girard C, Dunn M. 2015. Cryptococcal nasopharyngeal polypoid mass in a cat. J Feline Med Surg Open Rep, 1, 1–6.

12. Magalhães GM, Saut JPE, Beninati T, Medeiros AA, Queiroz GR, Tsuruta SA et al. 2012. Cerebral cryptococcomas in a cow. J Comp Pathol, 147, 106–110.

13. Mischnik A, Stockklausner J, Hohneder N, Jensen HE, Zimmermann S et al. 2014. First case of disseminated cryptococcosis in a *Gorilla gorilla*. Mycoses, 57, 664–671.

14. Molter CM, Zuba JR, Papendick R. 2014. *Cryptococcus gattii* osteomyelitis and compounded itraconazole treatment failure in a Pesquet's parrot (*Psittrichas fulgidus*). J Zoo Wildl Med, 45, 127–133.

15. Riet-Correa F, Krockenberger M, Dantas AFM, Oliveira DM. 2011. Bovine cryptococcal meningoencephalitis. J Vet Diagn Invest, 23, 1056–1060.

16. Ropstad EO, Leiva M, Peña T, Morera N, Martorell J. 2011. *Cryptococcus gattii* chorioretinitis in a ferret. Vet Ophthalmol, 14, 262–266.

17. Jensen HE. 2021. Animal models of invasive mycoses. APMIS, 1–9. doi: 10.1111/apm.13110.

18. Galanis E, MacDougall L. 2010. Epidemiology of *Cryptococcus gattii*, British Colombia, Canada, 1999-2007. Emerg Infect Dis, 16, 251–257.

19. Mitchell TG, Perfect JR. 1995. Cryptococcosis in the era of AIDS-100 years after the discovery of *Cryptococcus neoformans*. Clin Microbiol Rev, 8, 15–48.

20. Akbary S, Ramirez J, Fivenson D. 2017. Cryptococcal cellulitis: A rare entity histologically mimicking a neutrophilic dermatosis. J Cutan Pathol, 45, 90–93.

21. Sandhu J, Sandhu JS, Puri HK, Munjal M. 2017. Laryngeal cryptococcus: A rare cause of hoarseness in renal allograft recipient. J Nephropharmacol, 6, 27–29.

22. Kanjanapradit K, Kosjerina Z, Tanomkiat W, Keeratichananont W, Panthuwong S. 2017. Pulmonary cryptococcosis presenting with lung mass: Report of 7 cases and review of literature. Clin Med Insights Pathol, 10, 1–5.

23. Flowers A, Gu X, Herrera GA, Gibson S, King J. 2018. A case of HIV associated cryptococcal nephritis: Ultrastructural findings and literature review. Ultrastruc Pathol, 42, 193–197.

24. Hayashida MZ, Seque CA, Pasin VP, Enokihara MMSS, Porro AM. 2017. Disseminated cryptococcosis with skin lesions: Report of a case series. An Bras Dermatol, 92, 69–72.

25. Hurtado JC, Castillo P, Fernandes F, Navarro M, Lovane L et al. 2019. Mortality due to *Cryptococcus neoformans* and *Cryptococcus gattii* in low-income settings: An autopsy study. Nature Sci Rep, 9, 1–10.

26. Kidd SE, Hagen F, Tscharke RL, Huynh M, Bartlett KH et al. 2004. A rare genotype of *Cryptococcus gattii* caused the cryptococcosis outbreak on Vancouver Island (British Columbia, Canada). Proc Natl Acad Sci USA, 101, 17258–17263.

27. Banshodani M, Marubayashi S, Shintaku S, Moriishi M, Tsuchiya S et al. 2019. Isolated pulmonary cryptococcosis confused with lung tumor 5 years after kidney transplantation: A case report. Transplant Proc, 51, 561–564.

28. Jensen HE, Chandler FW. 2007. Histopathological diagnoses of mycoses. In: Topley and Wilson's Microbiology & Microbial Infections. Medical Mycology. 10th ed. Merz WG, Hay RJ, Eds. Hodder Arnold. pp 121–143.

29. Jensen HE. 2021. Histopathology in the diagnosis of invasive fungal diseases. Curr Fungal Infect Rep, 15, 23–31.

20

Blastomycosis

INTRODUCTION

Blastomycosis is caused by *Blastomyces dermatitidis*, which is the imperfect (asexual) yeast stage of *Ajellomyces dermatitidis* (i.e., the teleomorph form) (1, 2). *B. dermatitidis* can be subdivided into several genotypes (1). In both humans and animals, it is the lungs that are primarily affected by lesions after inhalation of conidia (3). Often, the presence of pneumonia will result in the secondary hematogenous spread of the pathogens to different organs, particularly the skin, bones, genitals, urinary organs, and the central nervous system (1, 3–8).

EPIDEMIOLOGY

Infections with *B. dermatitidis* are generally restricted to particular geographic locations. These include the eastern United States, where *B. dermatitidis* is endemic in states such as Mississippi, Kentucky, Tennessee, and Arkansas. Infections are also common in parts of Africa and India, but rarely occur in Europe (1, 2, 9–11). The microhabitat of the fungus is unclear, but *B. dermatitidis* apparently prefers moist, warm soil that contains organic material (1, 2). The infection is not opportunistic; however, immunodeficiency will result in more serious complications (12–14). Blastomycosis has reportedly occurred in several species of wild and domestic animals, most frequently in dogs (15–20). Although the majority of infections are acquired via the airway, infections may also occur via traumatic implantation into the skin (21, 22). Several laboratory animal models of blastomycosis have been developed and applied in therapeutic studies (23).

PATHOLOGY

The pathology of lesions in humans and animals is similar. Acute lesions are predominantly suppurative. Chronic lesions are characterized by mixed inflammatory reactions such as pyogranulomas that involve macrophages, epithelioid cells, multinucleate giant cells (granulomatous inflammation), and neutrophils (Figs. 20.1–20.3) (9, 24). Caseous necrosis may also be observed in lesions. Chronic cutaneous lesions often exhibit marked pseudoepitheliomatous hyperplasia of the epidermis, which may resemble squamous or basal cell carcinomas (2).

FUNGAL HISTOMORPHOLOGY

B. dermatitidis yeast cells are multinucleate and resemble vacuoles in haematoxylin and eosin-stained sections (Fig. 20.3). Grocott's methenamine silver and periodic acid-Schiff stains may be used to reveal the thick capsule and cytoplasm (Figs. 20.4–20.6) (9, 25). Cells of *B. dermatitidis* may also to a variable extent be stained by the mucin stains. Spherical *B. dermatitidis* yeast cells are 7–15 μm in diameter; however, microforms (diameter 2–4 μm) and filamentous forms may also be present (Fig. 20.5) (9, 24, 26, 27). A key diagnostic characteristic is single broad-based budding, during which the daughter cell becomes almost as large as the parent cell while still attached via a broad base (Figs. 20.3–20.6) (13, 24, 26, 28). *B. dermatitidis* yeast cells are found outside cells, as well as within macrophages and multinucleate giant cells (1).

DIFFERENTIAL DIAGNOSIS

Several different mycotic elements may be confused with those of blastomycosis. *Histoplasma capsulatum* var. *duboisii* is similar in size and shape to *B. dermatitidis*. However, *H. capsulatum* var. *duboisii* is restricted to Africa and it exhibits a characteristic "hour-glass" shape when budding (see the chapter on histoplasmosis duboisii). In addition, coccidioidomycosis may also be confused with blastomycosis, especially when only a few immature fungal elements are present in, for example, biopsies. However, if spherules are present together with the absence of budding in coccidioidomycosis, it should not be confused with blastomycosis, despite these diseases occurring in overlapping endemic areas within the United States. In capsule-deficient cryptococcosis lesions, the yeast cells may resemble *B. dermatitidis*. However, the cryptococci exhibit narrow-based budding in contrast to the broad-based budding of *B. dermatitidis* cells (see the chapter on cryptococcosis). Moreover, Fontana-Masson staining of melanin within cells can be used to correctly diagnose cases of cryptococcosis. When many budding *Paracoccidioides* spp. cells occur in the shape of a "steering wheel," these should not be confused with blastomycosis yeast cells; however, when only non-budding *Paracoccidioides* spp. cells are present, the two mycoses are difficult to distinguish, and *in situ* molecular techniques

DOI: 10.1201/9781003306177-20

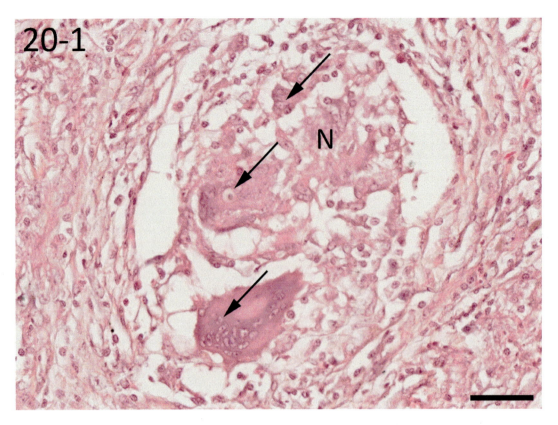

Figure 20.1 Chronic, necrotizing, granulomatous blastomycotic dermatitis due to *B. dermatitidis*. Within the lesion, multinucleate giant cells with fungal elements (arrows) are visible next to the necrotic area (N). HE. Bar = 75 μm.

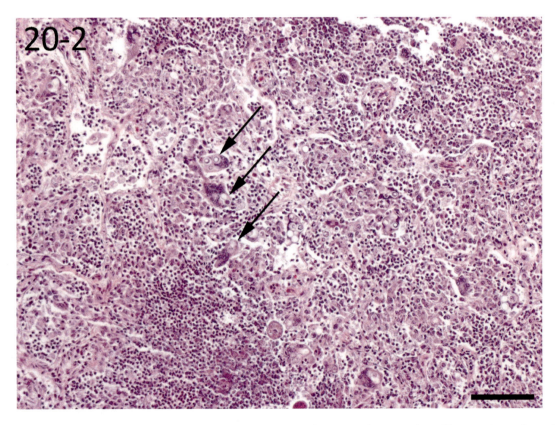

Figure 20.2 Chronic, pyogranulomatous blastomycotic pneumonia due to *B. dermatitidis*. Infiltration by multinucleate giant cells, mononuclear cells, and neutrophils is visible. Fungal cells are visible within some of the multinucleate giant cells (arrows). HE. Bar = 150 μm.

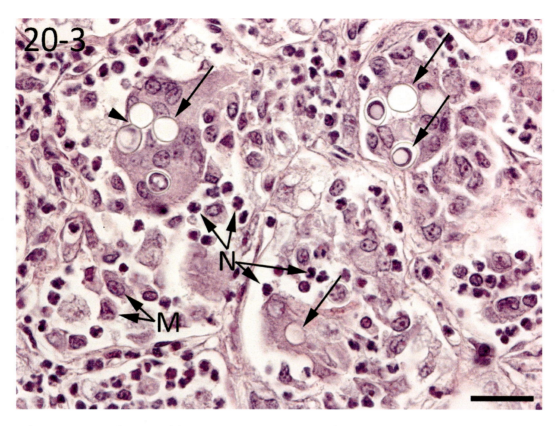

Figure 20.3 Chronic, pyogranulomatous blastomycotic pneumonia. *B. dermatitidis* cells that resemble vacuoles (arrows) have been engulfed by multinucleate giant cells. Broad-based budding is occurring (arrowhead) in one of them. Macrophages (M) and neutrophils (N) are interspersed with the multinucleate giant cells. HE. Bar = 15 μm.

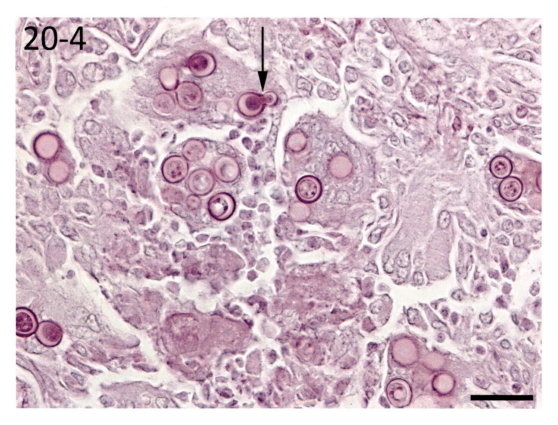

Figure 20.4 Chronic, pyogranulomatous blastomycotic pneumonia caused by *B. dermatitidis*. Single broad-based budding is visible (arrow) within a multinucleate giant cell. PAS. Bar = 35 μm.

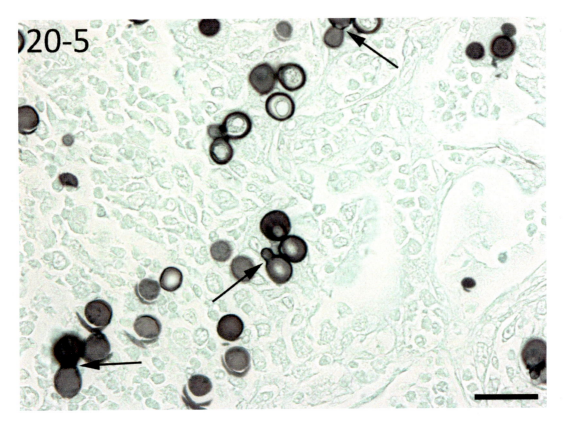

Figure 20.5 Chronic, pyogranulomatous blastomycotic pneumonia. *B. dermatitidis* cells of different sizes are visible within the lesion. Buds (arrows) are present on some of these cells. GMS. Bar = 15 µm.

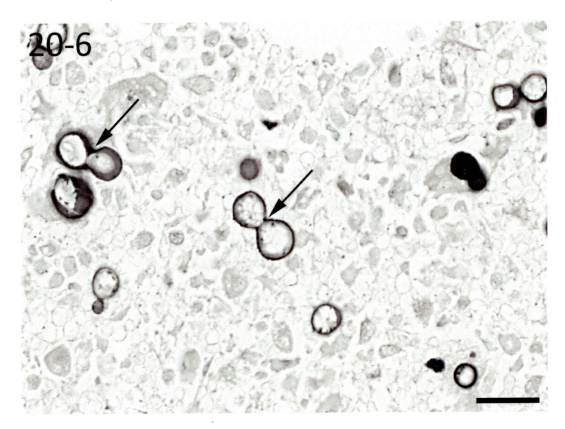

Figure 20.6 Chronic, pyogranulomatous blastomycotic pneumonia. A key diagnostic characteristic is broad-based budding of *B. dermatitidis* cells, during which the daughter cell often becomes as large as the parent cell while still attached (arrows). GMS. Bar = 15 µm.

should be applied (see the chapter on paracoccidioidomy-cosis). In addition, lacaziosis lesions may resemble blasto-mycosis skin lesions. However, *Lacazia loboi* cells form long chains, which should confirm a lacaziosis diagnosis (see the chapter on lacaziosis). Finally, single cells of the algae *Prototheca* and *Chlorella* may also resemble single cells of *B. dermatitidis*; however, the algae do not bud but reproduce by irregular fission.

Recently, several immunohistochemical and *in situ* hybridization techniques have been developed and applied, together with polymerase chain reaction techniques, to obtain accurate *in situ* diagnoses of blastomycosis (11, 27, 29).

REFERENCES

1. Saccente M, Woods GL. 2010. Clinical and laboratory update on blastomycosis. Clin Microbiol Rev, 23, 367–381.
2. Sullivan DC, Nolan RL. 2015. Blastomycosis. In: Diagnosis and Treatment of Fungal Infections. 2nd ed. Hospenthal DR, Rinaldi MG, Eds. Springer. pp 195–204.
3. Lemos LB, Guo M, Baliga M. 2000. Blastomycosis: Organ involvement and etiologic diagnosis. A review of 123 patients from Mississippi. Ann Diagn Pathol, 4, 391–406.
4. Craig J, Al Habeeb A, Leis JA. 2015. Budding issues: Blastomycosis. Am J Med, 128, 1182–1185.
5. Dobre MC, Smoker WRK, Kirby P. 2011. A case of solitary *Blastomyces dermatitidis* meningitis. Clin Neurol Neurosurg, 113, 665–667.
6. Hadjipavlou AG, Mader JT, Nauta HJ, Necessary JT, Chaljub G et al. 1998. Blastomycosis of the lumbar spine: Case report and review of the literature, with emphasis on diagnostic laboratory tools and management. Eur Spine J, 7, 416–421.
7. Hankins CL. 2009. Blastomycotic hand infections. Scand J Plast Reconstr Surg Hand Surg, 43, 166–170.
8. Jain R, Sing K, Lamzabi I, Harbhajanka A, Gattuso P et al. 2014. Blastomycosis of bone. Am J Clin Pathol, 142, 609–616.
9. Miceli MH, Castillo CG, Kauffman CA. 2016. Diagnosis of midwestern endemic mycoses. Curr Fungal Infect Rep, 10, 87–95.
10. Rao GR, Narayan BL, Durga Prasad BK, Amareswar A, Sridevi M et al. 2013. Disseminated blastomycosis in a child with a brief review of the Indian literature. Indian J Dermatol Venereol Leprol, 79, 92–96.
11. Guarner J, Brandt, ME. 2011. Histopathologic diagnosis of fungal infections in the 21st century. Clin Microbiol Rev, 24, 247–280.
12. Jehangir W, Tadepalli GS, Sen S, Regevik N, Sen P. 2015. Coccidioidomycosis and blastomycosis: Endemic mycotic co-infections in the HIV patient. J Clin Med Res, 7, 196–198.
13. Patel AJ, Gattuso P, Reddy VB. 2010. Diagnosis of blastomycosis in surgical pathology and cytopathology: Correlation with microbiologic culture. Am J Surg Pathol, 34, 256–261.
14. Sarkar PK, Malhotra P, Sriram PS. 2014. Rapid progression of pulmonary blastomycosis in an untreated patient of chronic lymphocytic leukemia. Case Rep Med, 2014, 1–5.
15. Ahasan SA, Chowdhury EH, Khan MAH, Parvin R, Azam SU et al. 2013. Histopathological investigation of blastomycosis in animals at Dhaka Zoo. Bangl J Vet Med, 11, 81–85.
16. Baron ML, Hecht S, Westermeyer HD, Mankin JM, Novak JM et al. 2011. Intracranial extension of retrobulbar blastomycosis (*Blastomyces dermatitidis*) in a dog. Vet Ophthalmol, 14, 137–141.
17. Chang SC, Hsuan SL, Lin CC, Lee WC, Chien MS et al. 2013. Probable *Blastomyces dermatitidis* infection in a young rat. Vet Pathol, 50, 343–346.
18. Dykstra JA, Rogers LL, Mansfield SA, Wünschmann A. 2012. Fatal disseminated blastomycosis in a free-ranging American black bear (*Ursus americanus*). J Vet Diagn Invest, 24, 1125–1128.
19. Funiciello B, Scandella M, Roccabianca P, Caniatti M, Martino PA et al. 2014. Cutaneous blastomycosis in a horse. Equine Vet Edu, 26, 458–463.
20. Imai DM, McGreevey N, Anderson JL, Meece JK. 2014. Disseminated *Blastomyces dermatitidis*, genetic group 2, infection in an alpaca (*Vicugna pacos*). J Vet Diagn Invest, 26, 442–447.
21. Harris JR, Blaney DD, Lindsley MD, Zaki SR, Paddock CD et al. 2011. Blastomycosis in man after kinkajou bite. Emerg Infect Dis, 17, 268–270.
22. Salem MB, Hamouda M, Mohamed M, Aloui S, Letaiel A et al. 2017. *Blastomyces dermatitidis* in renal transplant recipient: A case report. Transplant Proc, 49, 1583–1586.
23. Jensen HE. 2021. Animal models of invasive mycoses. APMIS, 1–9. doi: 10.1111/apm.13110.
24. López-Martínez R, Méndéz-Tovar LJ. 2012. Blastomycosis. Clin Dermatol, 30, 565–572.
25. Saeed AI, Williams AL, Bradley RF, Barker JA. 2009. Bronchoscopic view of pulmonary blastomycosis. J Bronchology Interv Pulmonol, 16, 266–269.
26. Jensen HE, Chandler FW. 2007. Histopathological diagnoses of mycoses. In: Topley and Wilson's Microbiology & Microbial Infections. Medical Mycology. 10th ed. Merz WG, Hay RJ, Eds. Hodder Arnold. pp 121–143.
27. Jensen HE. 2021. Histopathology in the diagnosis of invasive fungal diseases. Curr Fungal Infect Rep, 15, 23–31.
28. Mukhopadhyay S. 2011. Role of histology in the diagnosis of infectious causes of granulomatous lung disease. Curr Opin Pulm Med, 17, 189–196.
29. Abbott JJ, Hamacher KL, Ahmed I. 2006. In situ hybridization in cutaneous deep fungal infections: A valuable diagnostic adjunct to fungal morphology and tissue cultures. J Cutan Pathol, 33, 426–432.

21

Histoplasmosis capsulati

INTRODUCTION

Histoplasmosis capsulati is caused by the dimorphic fungus *Histoplasma capsulatum* var. *capsulatum* and occurs worldwide. However, there are several endemic regions, where many people are infected regularly. The disease is particularly common in Central and South America, but also in some of the eastern states of the United States (1). The disease is also endemic in particular regions of Asia and Africa, whereas it is rarely reported in Europe unless the infected persons or animals have visited endemic regions (2).

EPIDEMIOLOGY

In endemic regions, histoplasmosis is often diagnosed in both wild and domestic animals (1, 3–6). The fungus is present in soil, and infections occur as a result of inhaling conidia. The majority of infections are asymptomatic and resolve spontaneously without dissemination (1, 7). However, the pathogens may spread from primary lung lesions to regional lymph nodes and hematogenously to almost any organ. The phagocytic-mononuclear system is often affected, which includes pulmonary alveolar macrophages, fixed macrophages in the bone marrow, and spleen together with Kupffer cells in the liver (1, 3, 8). The adrenals, skin, eyes, and central nervous system are also often infected (3, 9–12). Several distinct animal models have been developed to study the disease (13).

PATHOLOGY

Histoplasmosis lesions are predominantly granulomatous, with heavy infiltration of macrophages and the production of epithelioid cells and multinucleate giant cells (Figs. 21.1–21.3) (1, 14–16). However, in patients with acquired immune deficiency syndrome (AIDS), granulomas may be absent (Figs. 21.4 and 21.5). Chronic histoplasmosis lesions typically exhibit necrosis with surrounding fibrosis, occasionally accompanied by calcification (1, 17). In pulmonary lesions, histoplasmosis has also been associated with the development of spindle cell pseudotumors (18).

FUNGAL HISTOMORPHOLOGY

H. capsulatum var. *capsulatum* cells are spherical/oval and measure 2–4 μm in diameter (2, 19, 20). They occur in lesions of various organs and are often present in clusters within macrophages (Figs. 21.1–21.3) or sometimes within multinucleate giant cells (21). They have a thin capsule, exhibit single budding, and the buds have narrow necks (Fig. 21.6) (2, 20). In very rare cases, pseudohyphae may be produced due to double budding (Fig. 21.6) (20). Although they are stained by haematoxylin and eosin, the yeast cells are best visualized by Grocott's methenamine silver and periodic acid-Schiff stains (Figs. 21.3, 21.5, and 21.6) (15, 19, 20).

DIFFERENTIAL DIAGNOSIS

H. capsulatum var. *capsulatum* yeast cells may be confused with several other types of yeast cells, both large and small, in tissue sections. Among the large yeast cells, the minor variants of *B. dermatitidis* and endospores of *Coccidioides* spp. may resemble *H. capsulatum* var. *capsulatum*. However, *B. dermatitidis* cells bud with broad bases, and they have a thicker capsule. With respect to coccidioidomycosis, the presence of spherules or fragments of such will help in the differentiation. Cryptococcosis due to capsule-deficient *Cryptococcus* variants and cells of *Candida glabrata* may be impossible to differentiate from *H. capsulatum* var. *capsulatum*. In addition, cells of *Pneumocystis jirovecii*, which are also intracellularly located, may constitute a challenge in the diagnosis on a morphological basis. However, the inflammatory reaction that occurs in pneumocystosis differs from the one that occurs in histoplasmosis. Parasitic infections such as toxoplasmosis, trypanosomiasis, and leishmaniasis may also resemble histoplasmosis. However, the corresponding pathogens are not stained by silver stains such as Grocott's methenamine silver stain (21), and they have bar-shaped kinetoplasts that are visible in haematoxylin and eosin-stained sections.

In situ hybridization techniques can identify *H. capsulatum* var. *capsulatum* within the tissue (22, 23), as can immunohistochemical techniques (5, 14, 24, 25). Polymerase chain reaction techniques have also been developed to identify *H. capsulatum* var. *capsulatum* in tissue specimens (8, 23).

DOI: 10.1201/9781003306177-21

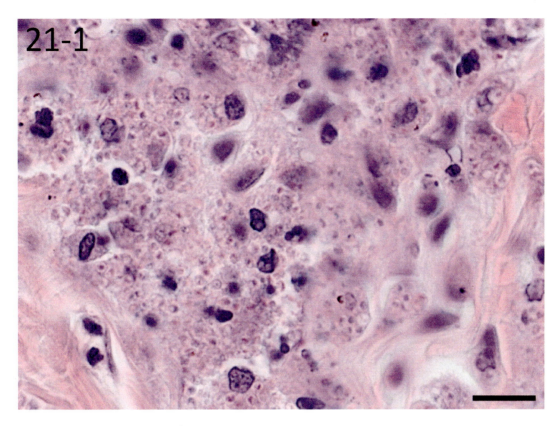

Figure 21.1 Chronic, granulomatous dermatitis due to *H. capsulatum* var. *capsulatum*. Numerous yeast-like cells are visible within the infiltrating macrophages. HE. Bar = 30 μm.

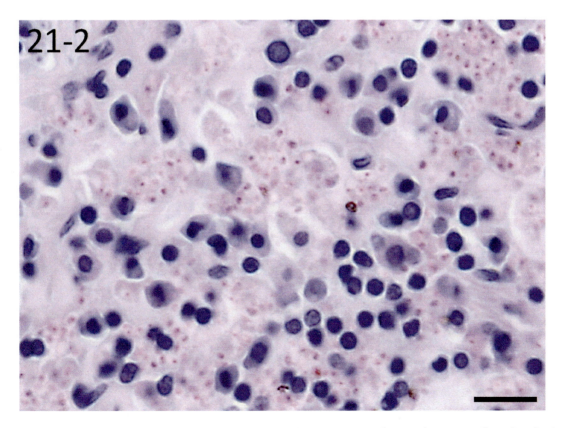

Figure 21.2 Chronic, granulomatous dermatitis due to *H. capsulatum* var. *capsulatum*. The yeast cells within the larger cells are visible as red dots when stained using the periodic acid-Schiff method. PAS. Bar = 30 μm.

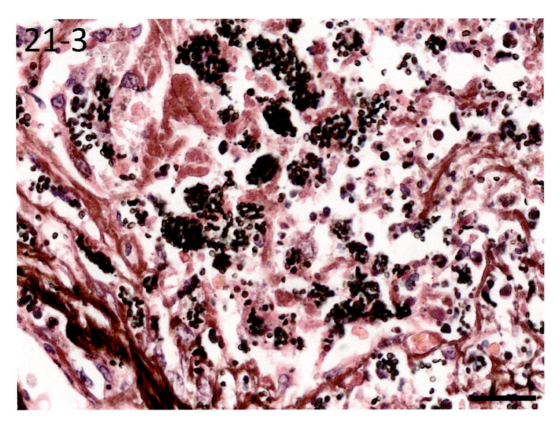

Figure 21.3 Chronic, granulomatous pneumonia due to *H. capsulatum* var. *capsulatum*. The clustering of the yeast cells within alveolar macrophages is apparent. GMS. Bar = 30 µm.

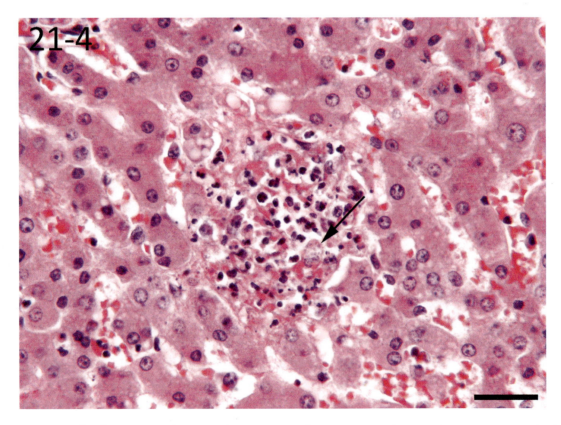

Figure 21.4 Subacute, focal, necrotizing hepatitis due to *H. capsulatum* var. *capsulatum*. In immunocompromised patients, the typical granulomatous inflammatory reaction may be absent. Fungal elements are visible within a macrophage (arrow). HE. Bar = 40 µm.

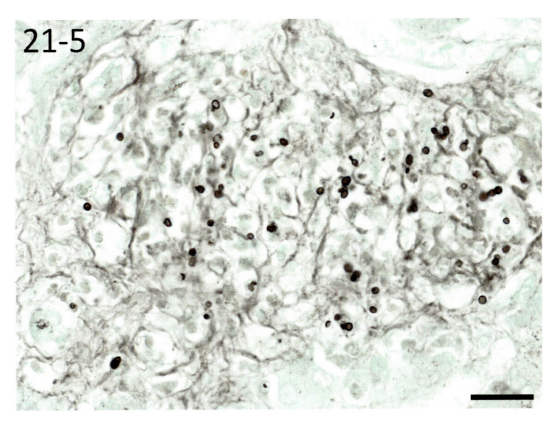

Figure 21.5 Subacute, focal, necrotizing hepatitis due to *H. capsulatum* var. *capsulatum*. Several different forms of *H. capsulatum* var. *capsulatum* yeast cell are visible when stained by Grocott's methenamine silver stain. GMS. Bar = 40 μm.

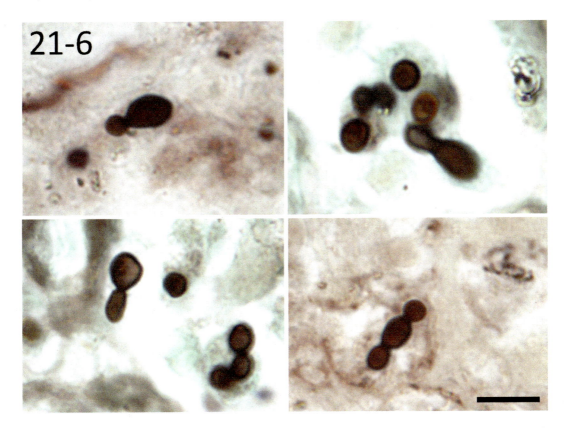

Figure 21.6 *H. capsulatum* var. *capsulatum* yeast cells in different tissue sections. The cells are typically reproduced by narrow-based single budding. However, in rare cases pseudohyphae may be present (lower right figure) due to double budding. GMS. Bar = 8 μm.

REFERENCES

1. Hage CA, Wheat LJ, Loyd J, Allen SD, Blue D et al. 2008. Pulmonary histoplasmosis. Semin Respir Crit Care Med, 29, 151–165.

2. Guarner J, Brandt, ME. 2011. Histopathologic diagnosis of fungal infections in the 21st century. Clin Microbiol Rev, 24, 247–280.

3. Highland MA, Chaturvedi S, Perez M, Steinberg H, Wallace R. 2011. Histologic and molecular identification of disseminated *Histoplasma capsulatum* in a captive brown bear (*Ursus arctos*). J Vet Diagn Invest, 23, 764–769.

4. Mavropoulou A, Grandi G, Calvi L, Passeri B, Volta A et al. 2010. Disseminated histoplasmosis in a cat in Europe. J Small Anim Pract, 51, 176–180.

5. Nishifuji K, Ueda Y, Sano A, Kadoya M, Kamei K et al. 2005. Interdigital involvement in a case of primary cutaneous canine histoplasmosis in Japan. J Vet Med Ser A Physiol Pathol Clin Med, 52, 478–480.

6. Pérez-Torres A, Rosas-Rosas A, Parás-García A, Juan-Sallés C, Taylor ML. 2009. Second case of histoplasmosis in a captive mara (*Dolichotis patagonum*): Pathological findings. Mycopathologia, 168, 95–100.

7. Mukhopadhyay S. 2011. Role of histology in the diagnosis of infectious causes of granulomatous lung disease. Curr Opin Pulm Med, 17, 189–196.

8. Chang P, Meaux T. 2015. Progressive disseminated histoplasmosis and HIV/AIDS: A dermatological perspective. Curr Fungal Infect Rep, 9, 213–219.

9. Bharti P, Bala K, Gupta N. 2015. Cutaneous manifestation of underlying disseminated histoplasmosis in an immunocompetent host of nonendemic area with reversible CD4 cell depletion and its recovery on antifungal therapy. Mycopathologia, 180, 223–227.

10. Escobar B, Maldonado VN, Ansari S, Sarria JC. 2014. Antigen negative gastrointestinal histoplasmosis in an AIDS patient. Am J Case Rep, 15, 90–93.

11. Iqbal F, Schifter M, Coleman HG. 2014. Oral presentation of histoplasmosis in an immunocompetent patient: A diagnostic challenge. Aust Dent J, 59, 386–388.

12. Rodriguez-Waitkus PM, Bayat V, George E, Sule N. 2013. Gastrointestinal histoplasmosis in a hepatitis C-infected individual. Mycopathologia, 176, 161–164.

13. Jensen HE. 2021. Animal models of invasive mycoses. APMIS, 1–9. doi: 10.1111/apm.13110.

14. Jung EJ, Park DW, Choi JW, Choi WS. 2015. Chronic cavitary pulmonary histoplasmosis in a non-HIV and immunocompromised patient without overseas travel history. Yonsei Med J, 56, 871–874.

15. Mukhopadhyay S, Doxtader EE. 2013. Visibility of *Histoplasma* within histiocytes on hematoxylin and eosin distinguishes disseminated histoplasmosis from other forms of pulmonary histoplasmosis. Hum Pathol, 44, 2346–2352.

16. Paulo LFB de, Rosa RR, Durighetto AF. 2013. Primary localized histoplasmosis: Oral manifestations in immunocompetent patients. Int J Infect Dis, 17, 139–140.

17. Mukhopadhyay S, Katzenstein ALA. 2010. Biopsy findings in acute pulmonary histoplasmosis: Unusual histologic features in 4 cases mimicking lymphomatoid granulomatosis. Am J Surg Pathol, 34, 541–546.

18. Gravdahl DJ, Gardetto JS, Hurley JR, Tazelaar HD, Koontz PW et al. 2011. Pulmonary histoplasmosis producing a spindle cell "pseudotumor." Am J Clin Pathol, 136, 410–415.

19. Ralph A, Raines M, Rode JW, Currie BJ. 2006. Histoplasmosis in two aboriginal patients from Australia's tropical Northern Territory. Trans R Soc Trop Med Hyg, 100, 888–890.

20. Jensen HE, Chandler FW. 2007. Histopathological diagnoses of mycoses. In: Topley and Wilson's Microbiology & Microbial Infections. Medical Mycology. 10th ed. Merz WG, Hay RJ, Eds. Hodder Arnold. pp 121–143.

21. Salfelder K. 1990. Atlas of Fungal Pathology. Kluwer Academic Publisher.

22. Abbott JJ, Hamacher KL, Ahmed I. 2006. In situ hybridization in cutaneous deep fungal infections: A valuable diagnostic adjunct to fungal morphology and tissue cultures. J Cutan Pathol, 33, 426–432.

23. Dial SM. 2007. Fungal diagnostics: Current techniques and future trends. Vet Clin North Am Small Anim Pract, 37, 373–392.

24. Reginato A, Giannuzzi P, Ricciardi M, De Simone A, Sanguinetti M et al. 2014. Extradural spinal cord lesion in a dog: First case study of canine neurological histoplasmosis in Italy. Vet Microbiol, 170, 451–455.

25. Romero-Martínez R, Curiel-Quesada E, Becerril-Luján B, Flores-Carreón A, Pérez-Torres A et al. 2007. Detection of constitutive molecules on *Histoplasma capsulatum* yeasts through single chain variable antibody fragments displayed in M13 phages. FEMS Immunol Med Microbiol, 50, 77–85.

22

Histoplasmosis duboisii

INTRODUCTION

African histoplasmosis is caused by *Histoplasma capsulatum* var. *duboisii*, a dimorphic fungus, and it is restricted to the African continent including Madagascar, where both humans and animals (especially baboons) may become infected (1, 2). A third species of *Histoplasma* (var. *farciminosum*) is particularly associated with infections in animals (equines, badgers (*Meles meles*), and dogs) (3, 4). In equines, the disease is named epizootic lymphangitis, and it predominantly causes lesions in the lymph vessels of the skin and regional lymph nodes (3). In badgers and dogs, ulcerating skin lesions often occur, but other organs may also be affected (4). The histopathology of the lesions caused by *H. capsulatum* var. *farciminosum* is similar to that of lesions caused by *H. capsulatum* var. *capsulatum*, as is the morphology of the yeast cells within lesions (3, 4).

EPIDEMIOLOGY

As with *H. capsulatum* var. *capsulatum*, infections with African histoplasmosis are generally acquired via the airway, but transcutaneous infections have also been reported (2, 5). Disseminated infections occur in immunodeficient individuals, especially patients with acquired immune deficiency syndrome (AIDS). However, African histoplasmosis also occurs in immunocompetent persons and often affects the bones, lymph nodes, and the skin (2, 5–9). Symptoms of African histoplasmosis may occur several decades after an individual has left the regions of Africa where the disease is endemic (2).

PATHOLOGY

A granulomatous reaction with abundant macrophages and multinucleate giant cells will be present in affected organs.

Fungal elements are present both within the macrophages and very large multinucleate giant cells, but they may also be present outside cells (Figs. 22.1–22.4) (5–7, 9). Lesions are characterized by varying degrees of fibrosis, whereas bone lesions tend to be osteolytic (2, 6).

FUNGAL HISTOMORPHOLOGY

The yeast cells that cause African histoplasmosis are much larger (6–12 μm in diameter) than those produced by *H. capsulatum* var. *capsulatum* and *H. capsulatum* var. *farciminosum*. The cells are round/oval and thick walled and reproduce by narrow- or broad-based single budding, with the daughter cells being similar in size to the parent cells and involving structures resembling an "hour-glass"; alternatively, chains of four or five cells may form (Figs. 22.3–22.6) (2, 5, 7, 10). The mononucleate yeast cells of *H. capsulatum* var. *duboisii* resemble vacuoles in hematoxylin and eosin-stained sections (Figs. 22.1 and 22.2), whereas they are strongly stained by both Grocott's methenamine silver stain and periodic acid-Schiff stain (Figs. 22.3–22.6) (2, 9).

DIFFERENTIAL DIAGNOSIS

Cells of *Blastomyces dermatitidis* may be confused with those of *H. capsulatum* var. *duboisii*; however, *B. dermatitidis* always buds via broad bases and is multinuclear. In skin lesions, *H. capsulatum* var. *duboisii* may resemble *Lacazia loboi* infections; however, *L. loboi* is characterized by long chains of cells and does not exhibit very large multinucleate giant cells containing multiple fungal elements which should help to state the correct diagnosis. A nested PCR has been developed for obtaining an accurate diagnosis of *H. capsulatum* var. *farciminosum* (3), and so has DNA sequencing of formalin-fixed, paraffin-embedded tissue been for identification of *H. capsulatum* var. *duboisii* (1).

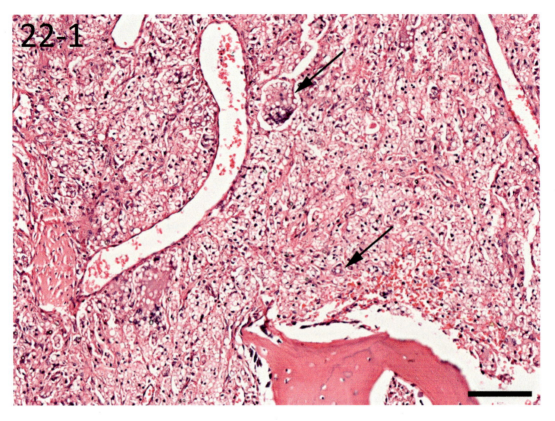

Figure 22.1 Chronic, granulomatous osteomyelitic histoplasmosis due to *H. capsulatum* var. *duboisii*. The medullary cavity has been heavily infiltrated by macrophages and multinucleate giant cells (arrows). HE. Bar = 160 μm.

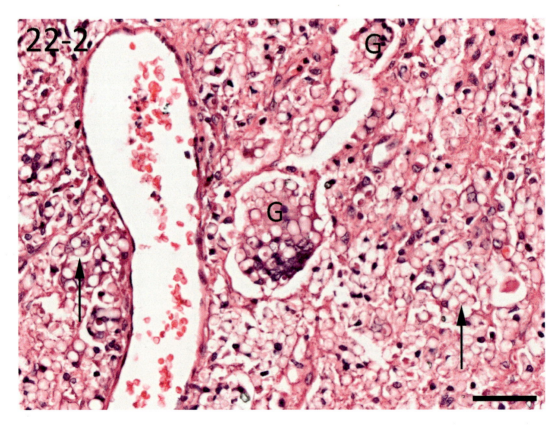

Figure 22.2 Chronic, granulomatous osteomyelitic histoplasmosis due to *H. capsulatum* var. *duboisii*. At higher magnification, the fungal cells resemble vacuoles within both macrophages (arrows) and multinucleate giant cells (G). HE. Bar = 60 μm.

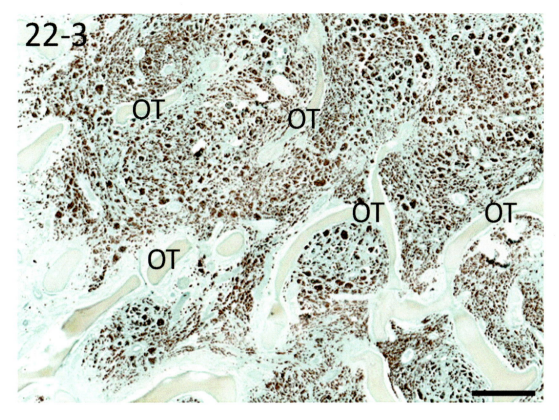

Figure 22.3 Chronic, granulomatous osteomyelitic histoplasmosis due to *H. capsulatum* var. *duboisii*. Black-stained yeast cells are visible between the osseous trabeculae (OT), even at low magnification. GMS. Bar = 160 µm.

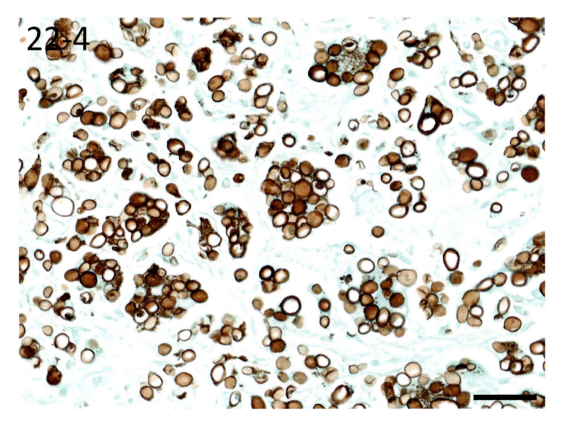

Figure 22.4 Chronic, granulomatous osteomyelitic histoplasmosis due to *H. capsulatum* var. *duboisii*. The outline of the yeast cells is clearly visible in Grocott's methenamine silver-stained sections. Note that most of the fungal cells are contained within macrophages and multinucleate giant cells. GMS. Bar = 40 µm.

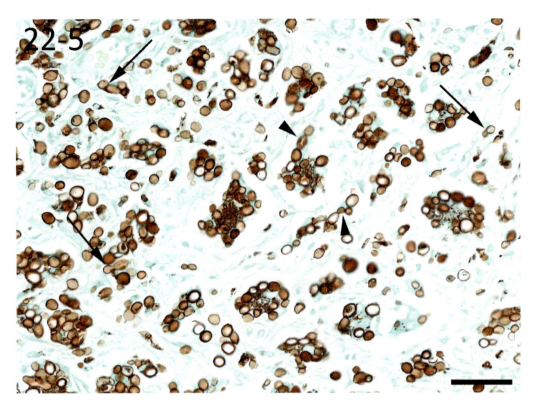

Figure 22.5 Chronic, granulomatous osteomyelitic histoplasmosis due to *H. capsulatum* var. *duboisii*. The size and arrangement of fungal cells vary extensively both inside and outside the phagocytes (i.e., the macrophages and multi-nucleate giant cells). Cells exhibiting narrow- and broad-based single budding (arrows) are visible, together with cells that have formed chains that are four to five cells long (arrowheads). GMS. Bar = 60 μm.

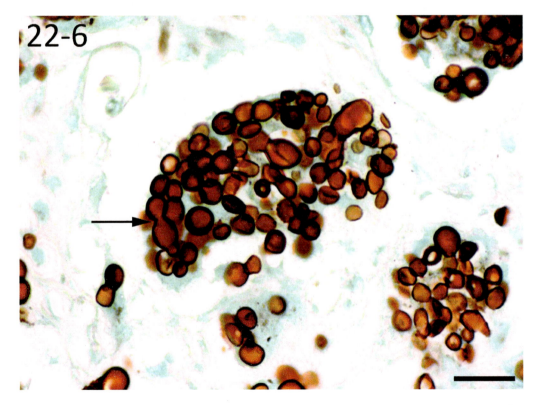

Figure 22.6 Chronic, granulomatous osteomyelitic histoplasmosis due to *H. capsulatum* var. *duboisii*. The fungal cells vary in size, and the typical "hour-glass" form of a budding cell is shown (arrow). GMS. Bar = 25 μm.

REFERENCES

1. Hensel M, Hoffmann, AR, Gonzales M, Owston MA, Dick EJ. 2019. Phylogenetic analysis of *Histoplasma capsulatum* var. *duboisii* in baboons from archived formalin-fixed, paraffin embedded tissues. Med Mycol, 57, 256–259.

2. Develoux M, Amona M, Hennequin C. 2021. Histoplamosis caused by *Histoplasma capsulatum* var. *duboisii*: A comprehensive review of cases from 1993–2019. Clin Infect Dis, 73, 543–549.

3. Hadush B, Michaelay M, Menghistu HT, Abebe N, Genzebu AT et al. 2020. Epidemiology of epizootic lymphangitis of carthorses in northern Ethiopia using conventional diagnostic methods and nested polymerase chain reaction. BMC Vet Res, 16, 375–381.

4. Eisenberg T, Seeger H, Kasuga T, Eskens U, Sauerwald C et al. 2013. Detection and characterization of *Histoplasma capsulatum* in a German badger (*Meles meles*) by ITS sequencing and multilocus sequencing analysis. Med Mycol, 51, 337–344.

5. Gugnani HC, Muotoe-Okafor F. 1997. African histoplasmosis: A review. Rev Iberoam Micol, 14, 155–159.

6. Loulergue P, Bastides F, Baudouin V, Chandenier J, Mariani-Kurkdjian P et al. 2007. Literature review and case histories of *Histoplasma capsulatum* var. *duboisii* infections in HIV-infected patients. Emerg Infect Dis, 13, 1647–1652.

7. Darré T, Saka B, Mouhari-Touré A, Dorkenoo AM, Amégbor K et al. 2017. Histoplasmosis by *Histoplasma capsulatum* var. *duboisii* observed at the laboratory of pathological anatomy of Lomé in Togo. Hindawi J Pathog. doi: 10.1155/2017/2323412.

8. Konan L, Drogba L, Brahima D, Mesfin FB. 2020. A case of *Histoplasma duboisii* brain abscess and review of the literature. Cureus. doi: 10.7759/cureus.6984.

9. Katchy AU, Eyesan SU, Awotunde TO, Adesina SA, Ayandele BO et al. 2019. *Histoplasma duboisii* of the femoral bone. J Res Med Sci, 24, 19–27.

10. Jensen HE, Chandler FW. 2007. Histopathological diagnoses of mycoses. In: Topley and Wilson's Microbiology & Microbial Infections. Medical Mycology. 10th ed. Merz WG, Hay RJ, Eds. Hodder Arnold. pp 121–143.

23

Paracoccidioidomycosis

INTRODUCTION

Paracoccidioidomycosis is caused by the dimorphic fungi *Paracoccidioides brasiliensis* (which contains three phylogenetically cryptic species) and *P. lutzii* (1–4). The *P. brasiliensis* fungi are endemic to particular regions of Central and South America (e.g., Brazil, Argentina, Venezuela, Peru, and Paraguay), whereas *P. lutzii* is mainly found in particular regions of Brazil (1–4). The habitat of *Paracoccidioides* spp. is obscure but these fungi probably inhabit soil. When paracoccidioidomycosis occurs outside endemic regions, there will usually be a history of previous visits to these areas (5). An unculturable type of *P. brasiliensis* (*P. brasiliensis* var. *ceti*) is the cause of cutaneous granulomas in dolphins (paracoccidioidomycosis ceti) (6). Lesions in dolphins are pathologically similar to human lesions caused by *L. loboi*, which is also unculturable (6). Therefore, *P. brasiliensis* var. *ceti* is included in the chapter on lacaziosis.

EPIDEMIOLOGY

The primary route of infection is the lungs following inhalation of spores (7, 8). The gastrointestinal tract is also frequently affected; however, the pathogenesis of gastrointestinal tract infections is controversial (9, 10). After the primary infection, lymphogenic spread often occurs to regional lymph nodes. Both immunocompetent and immunocompromised individuals frequently exhibit hematogenous spread to various organs (7, 11–13), especially the skin, mucocutaneous membranes, and the adrenal glands (8, 11, 14, 15). Reactivation of the infection years or decades after the initial infection has also been reported (9). Paracoccidioidomycosis lesions are rarely reported in animals (16–18); however, several animal models have been developed to study infections (19–22).

PATHOLOGY

Lesions are usually accompanied by necrosis. The inflammatory reaction may take several forms, from suppurative with abscesses to mixed granulomatous (pyogranulomatous) or pure granulomatous inflammation with the presence of a huge amount of macrophages, epithelioid cells, multinucleate giant cells, and plasma cells (Figs. 23.1 and 23.2) (6, 13, 23). In chronic lesions, an outer layer of fibrous tissue typically forms around necrotic foci that have epithelioid cells and multinucleate giant cells at the periphery (24).

FUNGAL HISTOMORPHOLOGY

P. brasiliensis and *P. lutzii* yeast cells are 5–60 µm in diameter and exhibit narrow-necked budding of daughter cells, which are typically smaller than the parent cells (24, 25). The presence of many buds around the parent cells ("pilot wheel") is pathognomonic for paracoccidioidomycosis; however, these may be absent or difficult to identify in some lesions (Figs. 23.3–23.6) (5, 24, 25). Usually, the yeast cells are visible in haematoxylin and eosin-stained sections, but the buds are often difficult to see (13). Therefore, as for all other fungal infections, Grocott's methenamine silver stain is indispensable (Figs. 23.3–23.6) (5, 8, 25, 26). The cells are present extracellularly (Figs. 23.3–23.6) and intracellularly (Fig. 23.2) within both macrophages and multinucleate giant cells (10, 14, 23). Deformed and degenerate yeast cells often occur at the periphery of necrotic areas (Fig. 23.3) (18).

DIFFERENTIAL DIAGNOSIS

If lesions do not exhibit the characteristic multiple peripheral budding patterns ("pilot wheel") of *P. brasiliensis* and *P. lutzii*, differentiating between these organisms and *Blastomyces dermatitidis* may be difficult or impossible (25). *Paracoccidioides* organisms may also be confused with immature endospores of *Coccidioides* spp. if the coccidioidomycosis lesions lack spherules and remnants of the spherules' capsular membranes (25). In difficult cases, the only way for obtaining a correct diagnosis is the application of *in situ* diagnostic techniques (16, 17, 23, 24, 27–29) and/or molecular tissue-based techniques like PCR (4, 16, 27).

DOI: 10.1201/9781003306177-23

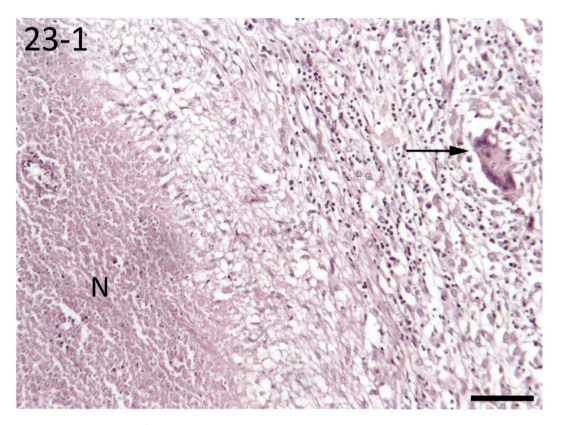

Figure 23.1 Chronic, pulmonary paracoccidioidomycosis. An area of necrosis (N) is bordered by a rim of mononuclear cells and a multinucleate giant cell (arrow) containing fungal elements. HE. Bar = 60 μm.

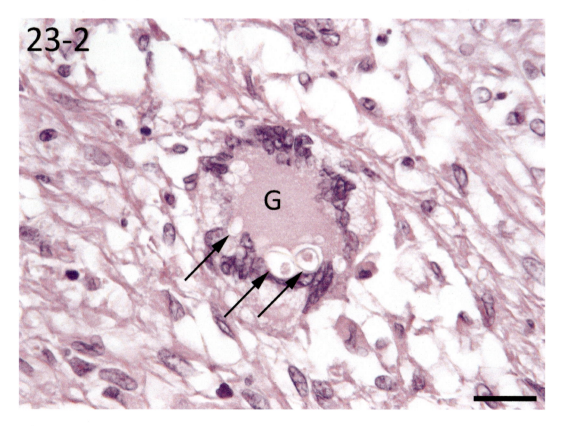

Figure 23.2 Chronic, pulmonary paracoccidioidomycosis. Elements of *P. brasiliensis* are visible (arrows) within a Langhans-type multinucleate giant cell (G). HE. Bar = 20 μm.

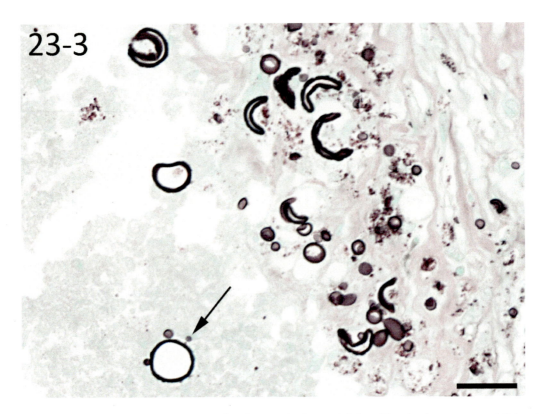

Figure 23.3 Chronic, adrenal, necrotizing paracoccidioidomycosis. Several *P. brasiliensis* elements are visible within and outside an area of necrosis. These vary in size and some have collapsed. Note the thin-base multiple budding of the spherule (arrow). GMS. Bar = 40 μm.

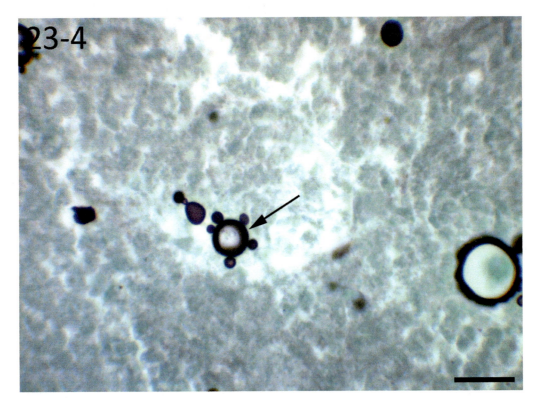

Figure 23.4 Chronic, adrenal, necrotizing paracoccidioidomycosis. Single budding is visible on one cell and multiple narrow-necked budding ("pilot wheel") is visible on another cell. The latter pattern of budding (arrow) is pathognomonic for paracoccidioidomycosis. GMS. Bar = 30 μm.

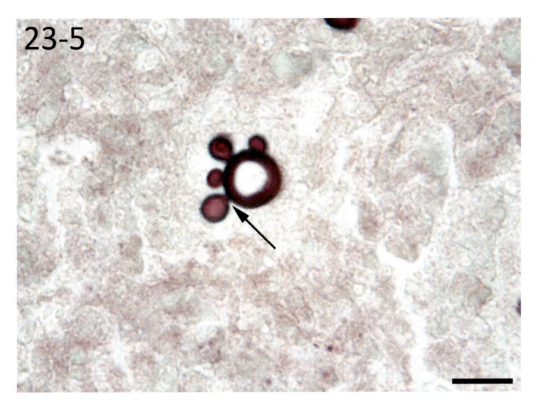

Figure 23.5 Chronic, adrenal, necrotizing paracoccidioidomycosis. The presence of multiple narrow-necked budding ("pilot wheel") cells is pathognomonic for paracoccidioidomycosis. In one of the buds, the thin base is visible (arrow). However, such manifestations may be rare or absent in paracoccidioidomycosis lesions. GMS. Bar = 20 μm.

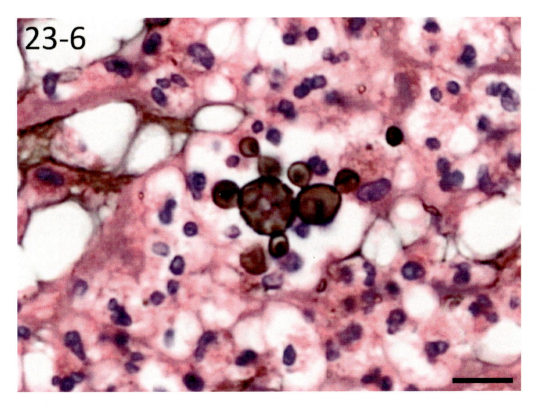

Figure 23.6 Chronic, pulmonary paracoccidioidomycosis. *P. brasiliensis* elements of varying size are present within the sediment of bronchial lavage material, together with the characteristic multiple budding "Mickey-mouse-like" form. GMS and HE. Bar = 20 μm.

REFERENCES

1. Matute DR, McEwen JG, Puccia R, Montes BA, San-Blas G et al. 2006. Cryptic speciation and recombination in the fungus *Paracoccidioides brasiliensis* as revealed by gene genealogies. Mol Biol Evol, 23, 65–73.

2. Desjardins CA, Champion MD, Holder JW, Muszewska A, Goldberg J et al. 2011. Comparative genomic analysis of human fungal pathogens causing paracoccidioidomycosis. PLoS Genet, 7. doi: org/10.1371/journal.pgen.1002345.

3. Teixeira MM, Theodoro RC, Oliveira FF, Machado GC, Hahn RC et al. 2014. *Paracoccidioides lutzii* sp. nov.: Biological and clinical implications. Med Mycol, 52, 19–28.

4. Pinheiro BG, Hahn RC, de Camargo ZP, Rodrigues AM. 2020. Molecular tools for detection and identification of *Paracoccidioides* species: Current status and future perspectives. J Fungi, 6. doi:10.3390/jof6040293

5. Walker SL, Pembroke AC, Lucas SB, Vega-Lopez F. 2008. Paracoccidioidomycosis presenting in the U.K. Br J Dermatol, 158, 624–626.

6. Vilela R, Mendoza L. 2018. Paracocidiomycosis ceti (Lacaziosis/Lobomycosis) in Dolphins. In: Emerging and Epizootic Fungal Infections in Animals. Seyedmousave S, de Hoog GS, Guillot J, Verweij PE, Eds. Springer. pp 177–196.

7. de Melo Braga G, Hessel G, Pereira RM, Escanhoela CAF. 2014. Hepatic involvement in paediatric patients with paracoccidioidomycosis: A histological study. Histopathology, 64, 256–262.

8. de Oliveira GR, Mariano FV, dos Santos Silva AR, Vargas PA, Lopes MA. 2012. Single oral paracoccidioidomycosis mimicking other lesions: Report of eight cases. Mycopathologia, 173, 47–52.

9. Benard G, Costa AN, Leopércio APS, Vicentini AP, Kono A et al. 2013. Chronic paracoccidioidomycosis of the intestine as single organ involvement points to an alternative pathogenesis of the mycosis. Mycopathologia, 176, 353–357.

10. Bravo EA, Zegarra AJ, Piscoya A, Pinto JL, De Los Rios RE et al. 2010. Chronic diarrhea and pancolitis caused by paracoccidioidomycosis: A case report. Case Rep Med, 2010, 1–4.

11. Muller SF, de Miranda MF. 2013. Sarcoid-like paracoccidioidomycosis presenting with perineural granuloma. An Bras Dermatol, 88, 994–995.

12. Pagliari C, Sotto MN. 2002. Correlation of factor XIIIa+ dermal dendrocytes with paracoccidioidomycosis skin lesions. Med Mycol, 40, 407–410.

13. Pereira GH, Santos AQ, Park M, Muller PR, Padua S et al. 2010. Bone marrow involvement in a patient with paracoccidioidomycosis: A rare presentation of juvenile form. Mycopathologia, 170, 259–261.

14. Pedreira RPG, Guimarães EP, de Carli ML, Magalhães EMS, Pereira AAC et al. 2014. Paracoccidioidomycosis mimicking squamous cell carcinoma on the dorsum of the tongue and review of published literature. Mycopathologia, 177, 325–329.

15. de Abreu SMÀ, Salum FG, Figueiredo MA, Lopes TG, da Silva VD et al. 2013. Interrelationship of clinical, histomorphometric and immunohistochemical features of oral lesions in chronic paracoccidioidomycosis. J Oral Pathol Med, 42, 235–242.

16. de Farias MR, Zeni Condas LA, Ribeiro MG, de Gimenes BSM, Muro MD et al. 2011. Paracoccidioidomycosis in a dog: Case report of generalized lymphadenomegaly. Mycopathologia, 172, 147–152.

17. Ricci G, Mota FT, Wakamatsu A, Serafim RC, Borra RC et al. 2004. Canine paracoccidioidomycosis. Med Mycol, 42, 379–383.

18. Trejo-Chávez A, Ramírez-Romero R, Ancer-Rodríguez J, Nevárez-Garza AM, Rodríguez-Tovar LE. 2011. Disseminated paracoccidioidomycosis in a southern two-toed sloth (*Choloepus didactylus*). J Comp Pathol, 144, 231–234.

19. Essayag SM, Landaeta ME, Hartung C, Magaldi S, Spencer L et al. 2002. Histopathologic and histochemical characterization of calcified structures in hamsters inoculated with *Paracoccidioides brasiliensis*. Mycoses, 45, 351–357.

20. Loth EA, Biazin SK, Paula CR, de Simão RCG, de Franco MF et al. 2012. Experimental model of arthritis induced by *Paracoccidioides brasiliensis* in rats. Mycopathologia, 174, 187–191.

21. Da Silva FC, Svidzinski TIE, Patussi EV, Cardoso CP, De Oliveira Dalalio MM et al. 2009. Morphologic organization of pulmonary granulomas in mice infected with *Paracoccidioides brasiliensis*. Am J Trop Med Hyg, 80, 798–804.

22. Jensen HE. 2021. Animal models of invasive mycoses. APMIS, 1–9. doi:10.1111/apm.13110.

23. de Carli ML, Cardoso BCB, Malaquias LCC, Nonogaki S, Pereira AAC et al. 2015. Serum antibody levels correlate with oral fungal cell numbers and influence the patients' response to chronic paracoccidioidomycosis. Mycoses, 58, 356–361.

24. Fernandez-Flores A, Saeb-Lima M, Arenas-Guzman R. 2014. Morphological findings of deep cutaneous fungal infections. Am J Dermatopathol, 36, 531–556.

25. Jensen HE, Chandler FW. 2007. Histopathological diagnoses of mycoses. In: Topley and Wilson's Microbiology & Microbial Infections. Medical Mycology. 10th ed. Merz WG, Hay RJ, Eds. Hodder Arnold. pp 121–143.

26. Jensen HE. 2021. Histopathology in the diagnosis of invasive fungal diseases. Curr Fungal Infect Rep, 15, 23–31.

27. De Brito T, Sandhu GS, Kline BC, Aleff RA, Sandoval MP et al. 1999. In situ hybridization in paracoccidioidomycosis. Med Mycol, 37, 207–211.

28. De Freitas RS, Dantas KC, Garcia RSP, Magri MMC, De Andrade HF. 2010. *Paracoccidioides brasiliensis* causing a rib lesion in an adult AIDS patient. Hum Pathol, 41, 1350–1354.

29. Arantes TD, Theodoro RC, Teixeira MM, Bagagli E. 2017. Use of fluorescent oligonucleotide probes for differentiation between *Paracoccidioides brasiliensis* and *Paracoccidioides lutzii* in yeast and mycelial phase. Mem Inst Oswaldo Cruz, 112, 140–145.

24

Sporotrichosis

INTRODUCTION

Sporotrichosis is a fungal infection that occurs worldwide. It is caused by phylogenetically distinct organisms within the *Sporothrix schenckii* species complex, which differ in their geographic distributions and virulence (1). Several different species are recognized as causal organisms, including *S. brasiliensis*, *S. globose*, *S. luriei*, *S. schenckii sensu stricto*, *S. albicans*, and *S. mexicana* (2, 3). In the vast majority of cases, sporotrichosis infections occur following small cuts in the skin, with the pathogen being implanted in the subcutaneous tissue (1, 4). However, infections may also occur following inhalation of the fungi (5, 6).

EPIDEMIOLOGY

The organisms that cause sporotrichosis are found in the environment in decaying wood, hay, vegetation, and moss (4). Severe zoonotic outbreaks have been reported in Rio de Janeiro and other areas of Brazil, where the transmission of *S. brasiliensis* from cats to humans has been particularly problematic (7–10). Most subcutaneous lesions involve spread along lymph vessels (Figs. 24.1–24.4), with the formation of satellite nodules in a chain-like pattern along the vessels (11). In rare cases, bones and joints may be affected too, sometimes as a result of hematogenous spread (12, 13). Disseminated infections are rare but have caused meningitis, hepatitis, and splenitis (1). In such cases, patients are typically immunodeficient. Wild and domestic animal species may also be spontaneously infected with *Sporothrix* spp., including cats, horses, dogs, and donkeys (8, 14–17). Sporotrichosis can also be easily introduced into various laboratory animals (18).

PATHOLOGY

Histologically, sporotrichosis lesions may exhibit suppurative and/or granulomatous inflammation. Epithelioid cells and multinucleate giant cells will also be present because the immunological reaction is apparently mediated by the T_H1 and T_H2 response (19, 20). In addition, plasma cells are present in chronic lesions (15). Liquefactive or caseous necrosis often accompanies the inflammatory reactions (Fig. 24.2). In some chronic cases, the Splendore-Hoeppli phenomenon may also occur around the fungal elements (21). *Sporothrix* yeast cells are often localized within the infiltrating inflammatory cells, especially in macrophages (Figs. 24.1 and 24.4) (7, 22).

FUNGAL HISTOMORPHOLOGY

The *S. schenckii* complex organisms are oval, circular, or cigar-shaped yeast cells that are 2–5 μm in diameter or 4–10 μm in length (Fig. 24.3) (22–24). Usually, they produce single narrow buds, although some may produce multiple buds (22). The organisms are barely visible in haematoxylin and eosin-stained sections (Fig. 24.1); however, they are easily visualized by using Grocott's methenamine silver stain (Figs. 24.2 and 24.3) and periodic acid-Schiff stain (Fig. 24.4) (23).

DIFFERENTIAL DIAGNOSIS

Sporotrichosis must be differentiated from some bacterial infections, including those caused by atypical mycobacteria (e.g., *Mycobacterium marinum*) and *Nocardia* spp. and protozoan parasites such as *Leishmania* spp.

Polymerase chain reaction probes that bind specifically to 18S ribosomal RNA sequences (1) and antibodies that can identify *Sporothrix* species (24–26) are available to make diagnoses from tissue samples.

DOI: 10.1201/9781003306177-24

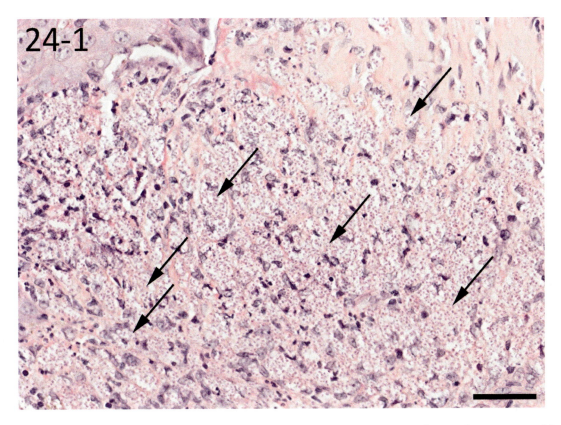

Figure 24.1 Chronic, subcutaneous sporotrichosis. Numerous circumscribed elements of *Sporothrix* sp. are visible within the macrophages (arrows). HE. Bar = 60 μm.

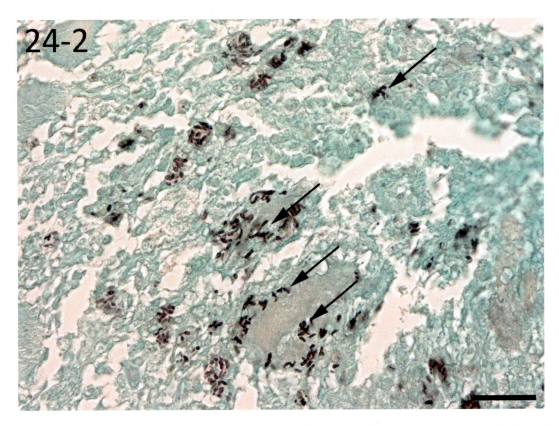

Figure 24.2 Chronic, subcutaneous sporotrichosis. The pleomorphic forms of *Sporothrix* sp. (arrows) within an abscess are visualized by applying Grocott's methenamine silver stain. GMS. Bar = 60 μm.

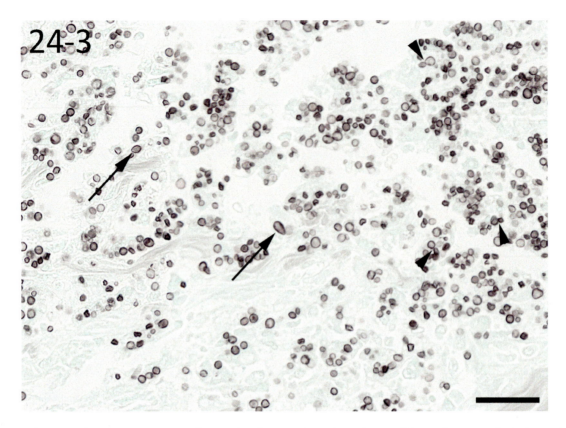

Figure 24.3 Chronic, subcutaneous sporotrichosis. The characteristic cigar shape of *Sporothrix* sp. cells is shown (arrows), together with budding yeast cells (arrowheads). GMS. Bar = 30 μm.

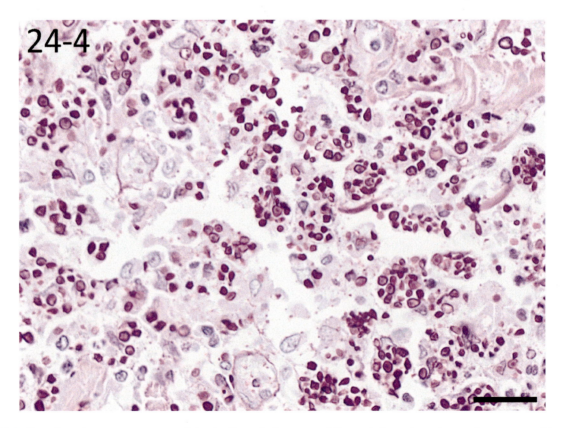

Figure 24.4 Chronic, subcutaneous sporotrichosis. Fungal elements of *Sporothrix* sp. have been phagocytosed by macrophages and multinucleate giant cells. PAS. Bar = 25 μm.

REFERENCES

1. Kaufmann CA. Sporotrichosis. 2015. In: Diagnosis and Treatment of Fungal Infections. 2nd ed. Hospenthal DR, Rinaldi MG, Eds. Springer. pp 237–244.

2. Rodrigues AM, Sybren de Hoog G, de Camargo ZP. 2015. Molecular diagnosis of pathogenic Sporotrix species. PLoS Negl Trop Dis, 1–22. doi: 10.1371/journal.pntd.0004190.

3. Rangel-Gamboa L, Martrinez-Hernandez F, Maravilla P, Arenas-Guzman R, Flisser A. 2016. Update of phylogenetic and genetic diversity of Soprotrix schenckii sensu lato. Med Mycol, 54, 248–255.

4. Guarner J, Brandt, ME. 2011. Histopathologic diagnosis of fungal infections in the 21st century. Clin Microbiol Rev, 24, 247–280.

5. Zhou CH, Asuncion A, Love GL. 2003. Laryngeal and respiratory tract sporotrichosis and steroid inhaler use. Arch Pathol Lab Med, 127, 893–894.

6. Lima RB, Jeunon-Sousa MAJ, Jeunon T, Oliveira JC, Oliveira MME, Zancope-Oliveira RM, Moraes ACS. 2017. Sporitrichosis masquerading as pyoderma gangrenosum. J Eur Acad Dermatol Venereol, 31, 539–541.

7. Quintella LP, Passos SRL, do Vale ACF, Galhardo MCG et al. 2011. Histopathology of cutaneous sporotrichosis in Rio de Janeiro: A series of 119 consecutive cases. J Cutan Pathol, 38, 25–32.

8. Pacheco Schubach TM, De Oliveira Schubach A, Cuzzi-Maya T, Okamoto T, Santos Reis R, Fialho Monteiro PC, Gutierrez-Galhardo MC, Wanke B. 2003. Pathology of sporotrichosis in 10 cats in Rio de Janeiro. Vet Rec, 152, 172–175.

9. Yegneswaran PP, Sripathi H, Bairy I, Lonikar V, Rao R, Prabhu S. 2009. Zoonotic sporotrichosis of lymphocutaneous type in a man acquired from a domesticated feline source: Report of a first case in southern Karnataka, India. Int J Dermatol, 48, 1198–1200.

10. Brandolt TM, Madrid IM, Poester VR, Sanchotene KO, Basso RP, Klafke GB, Roderigues ML, Xavier MO. 2019, Human sporotrichosis: A zoonotic outbreak in southern Brazil, 2012-2017. Med Mycol, 57, 527–533.

11. Vaishampayan S, Borde P. 2013. An unusual presentation of sporotrichosis. Indian J Dermatol, 58, 409.

12. Fujii H, Tanioka M, Yonezawa M, Arakawa A, Matsumura Y, Kore-Eda S, Miyachi Y, Tanaka S, Mochizuki T. 2008. A case of atypical sporotrichosis with multifocal cutaneous ulcers. Clin Exp Dermatol, 33, 135–138.

13. Gordhan A, Ramdial PK, Morar N, Moodley SD, Aboobaker J. 2001. Disseminated cutaneous sporotrichosis: A marker of osteoarticular sporotrichosis masquerading as gout. Int J Dermatol, 40, 717–719.

14. Crothers SL, White SD, Ihrke PJ, Affolter VK. 2009. Sporotrichosis: A retrospective evaluation of 23 cases seen in northern California (1987-2007). Vet Dermatol, 20, 249–259.

15. de Miranda LHM, Quintella LP, dos Santos IB, Menezes RC, Figueiredo FB, Gremião IDF, Okamoto T, de Oliveira RVC, Pereira SA, Tortelly R, Schubach TMP. 2009. Histopathology of canine sporotrichosis: A morphological study of 86 cases from Rio de Janeiro (2001-2007). Mycopathologia, 168, 79–87.

16. Miranda LHM, Conceição-Silva F, Quintella LP, Kuraiem BP, Pereira SA, Schubach TMP. 2013. Feline sporotrichosis: Histopathological profile of cutaneous lesions and their correlation with clinical presentation. Comp Immunol Microbiol Infect Dis, 36, 425–432.

17. Gremiao IDF, Menezes RC, Schubach TMP, Figueiredo ABF, Cavalcant MCH, Pereira SA. 2015. Feline sporotrichosis: Epidemiological and clinical aspects. Med Mycol, 53, 15–21.

18. Arrillaga-Moncrieff I, Capilla J, Mayayo E, Marimon R, Mariné M, Gené J, Cano J, Guarro J. 2009. Different virulence levels of the species of Sporothrix in a murine model. Clin Microbiol Infect, 15, 651–655.

19. Chang S, Hersh AM, Naughton G, Mullins K, Fung MA, Sharon VR. 2013. Disseminated cutaneous sporotrichosis. Dermatol Online J, 19, 1–3.

20. Vasquez-del-Mercado E, Arenas R, Padilla-Desgarenes C. 2012. Sporotrichosis. Clin Dermatol, 30, 437–443.

21. Rodríguez G, Sarmiento L. 1998. The asteroid bodies of sporotrichosis. Am J Dermatopathol, 20, 246–249.

22. Zhang YQ, Xu XG, Zhang M, Jiang P, Zhou XY, Li ZZ, Zhang MF. 2011. Sporotrichosis: Clinical and histopathological manifestations. Am J Dermatopathol, 33, 296–302.

23. Bonifaz A, Vázquez-González D. 2013. Diagnosis and treatment of lymphocutaneous sporotrichosis: What are the options? Curr Fungal Infect Rep, 7, 252–259.

24. Chelladurai V, Lakshmi Y, Srinivasan C, Karthik S. 2017. A case report of rare fungal lesions. Int J Cur Res Rev, 9, 13–15.

25. Marques ME, Coelho KI, Sotto MN, Bacchi CE. 1992. Comparison between histochemical and immunohistochemical methods for diagnosis of sporotrichosis. J Clin Pathol, 45, 1089–1093.

26. Miranda LHM, Quintella LP, Menezes RC, dos Santos IB, Oliveira RVC, Figueiredo FB, Lopes-Bezerra LM, Schubach TMP. 2011. Evaluation of immunohistochemistry for the diagnosis of sporotrichosis in dogs. Vet J, 190, 408–411.

25

Talaromycosis

INTRODUCTION

Talaromyces marneffei (formerly *Penicillium marneffei*) is a dimorphic fungus and the cause of talaromycosis. *T. marneffei* is endemic to Thailand, China, Hong Kong, Vietnam, and Indonesia (1–3). Although the fungus has been isolated from species of bamboo rat (*Rhizomys* and *Cannomyces*), contaminated soil is generally the cause of infections (2, 4). When talaromycosis is diagnosed outside endemic areas, patients have typically travelled to these areas (4, 5).

EPIDEMIOLOGY

Infections are rare in immunocompetent persons. They have been diagnosed most frequently in Asian patients with acquired immune deficiency syndrome (AIDS) (1, 6). However, other immunocompromising conditions such as hematologic malignancies, autoimmune diseases, malnutrition, or debilitating infections may increase an individual's susceptibility to talaromycosis (7, 8). *T. marneffei* infections often involve the skin, lungs, liver, or gastrointestinal tract, and may cause osteolytic lesions (1, 6–10). Dissemination can occur in only a few weeks and may rapidly result in death.

PATHOLOGY

Skin lesions are typically molluscum contagiosum-like umbilicated papules, necrotic nodules, or acneiform papules. Hyperkeratosis of the epidermis typically occurs, together with inflammatory infiltration of the dermis with histiocytes, lymphocytes, plasma cells, and nuclear debris, resulting in coagulative necrosis (Figs. 25.1 and 25.2) (4, 5). Disseminated infections usually affect the monocyte–macrophage system in multiple organs, including the lungs and the reticuloendothelial system. Systemic infections are characterized by lymphadenopathy, septicaemia, hepatosplenomegaly, and skin lesions. The pathogens infect the mononuclear phagocyte system and multiply within histiocytes, which become enlarged (1, 2). The inflammatory response may be granulomatous, suppurative, or mixed (3, 8, 10, 11). Pathological characteristics may vary in different organs, depending on host immunity status. A necrotizing tissue reaction is often observed in patients with AIDS, whereas granulomas rarely form in these patients (2).

Focal (lung) or disseminated (hepatic) infections occurred in mice that were exposed to *T. marneffei* by either respiratory or parenteral routes (12).

FUNGAL HISTOMORPHOLOGY

Histologically, *T. marneffei* infections may be difficult to identify, because the size and staining pattern of the yeast cells resemble those of cellular debris (Figs. 25.1 and 25.2). However, Grocott's methenamine silver and periodic acid-Schiff stains show the pathogens clearly (Figs. 25.3 and 25.4) (2–4, 7). The *T. marneffei* cells vary in size and have a characteristic spherical, oval, or elliptical yeast cell morphology. *T. marneffei* do not bud. Instead, they divide at their central septum by fission. The fungi are typically small (2.5 μm) and resemble *Histoplasma capsulatum*. Occasionally, elongated and/or curved forms with a central septum occur; these resemble short tubes with blunt ends (Figs. 25.5 and 25.6) (1, 7, 8, 11–13). These forms are sometimes called "pill capsule" or "sausage" shaped and measure up to 7 μm in length (14). The yeast cell-like organisms are scattered throughout the tissue or phagocytosed within distended histiocytes (1–4, 7). As the lesions expand, necrosis increases and the macrophages may lyse to release free organisms (3, 12, 13).

DIFFERENTIAL DIAGNOSIS

Most importantly, the characteristic septate forms (Figs. 25.5 and 25.6) and the absence of budding should distinguish the pathogens that cause talaromycosis from those that cause histoplasmosis, candidosis (especially *C. glabrata*), toxoplasmosis, trypanosomiasis, and other protozoan infections (11, 14, 15). However, *Toxoplasma gondii* and the *Trypanosoma* spp. are not stained by Grocott's methenamine silver technique, which may be used to identify *T. marneffei* (2). Polymerase chain reaction techniques have also been developed to identify these pathogens in tissue specimens (16).

DOI: 10.1201/9781003306177-25

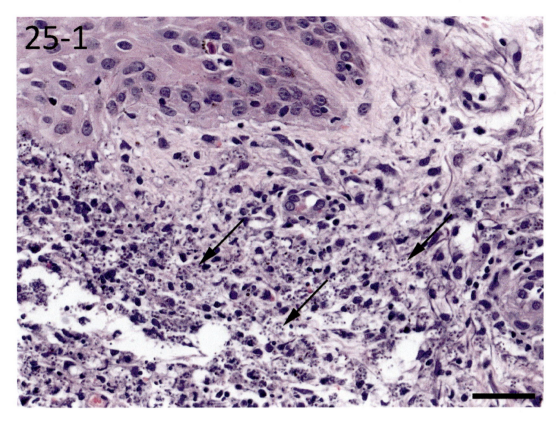

Figure 25.1 Chronic, subcutaneous talaromycosis. A mixed inflammatory reaction comprising predominantly macrophages that contain fungal elements is visible throughout the subcutaneous tissue (arrows). HE. Bar = 60 μm.

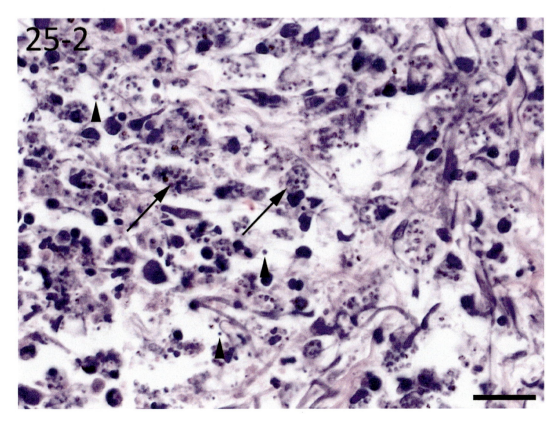

Figure 25.2 Chronic, subcutaneous talaromycosis. Magnified *T. marneffei* organisms are visible both within (arrows) and outside (arrowheads) the infiltrating macrophages. The same case as in Fig. 25.1. HE. Bar = 40 μm.

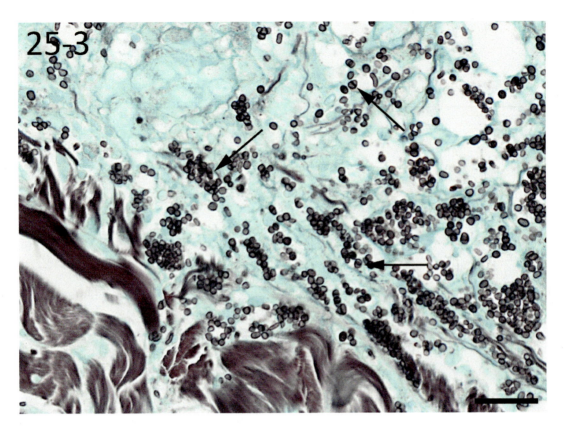

Figure 25.3 Chronic, subcutaneous talaromycosis. The yeast cells of *T. marneffei* are clearly visible after the application of Grocott's methenamine silver stain. Several cells exhibit a central septum (arrows). GMS. Bar = 40 µm.

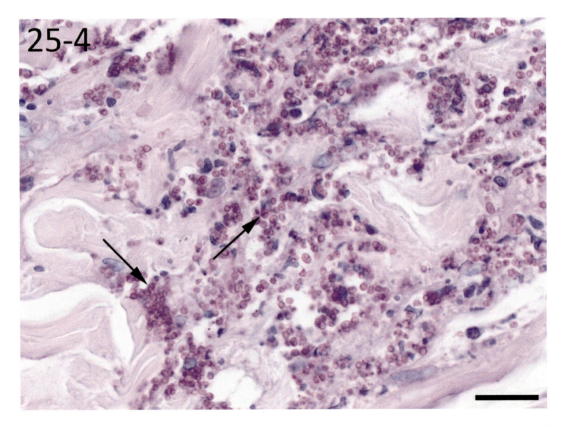

Figure 25.4 Chronic, subcutaneous talaromycosis. The yeast cells of *T. marneffei* are easily recognized in the subcutaneous tissue when the periodic acid-Schiff stain is applied. The central septum is also visible (arrows). PAS. Bar = 40 µm.

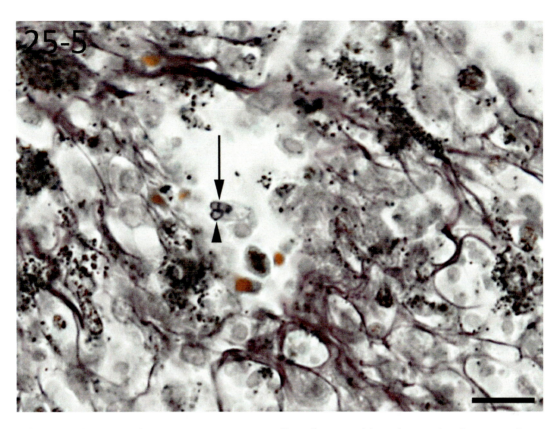

Figure 25.5 Chronic, pulmonary talaromycosis. Two *T. marneffei* cells are visible within an alveolar macrophage. One cell is spherical (arrowhead) and the other exhibits the characteristic "pill capsule form" with a central septum (arrow). GMS. Bar = 25 μm.

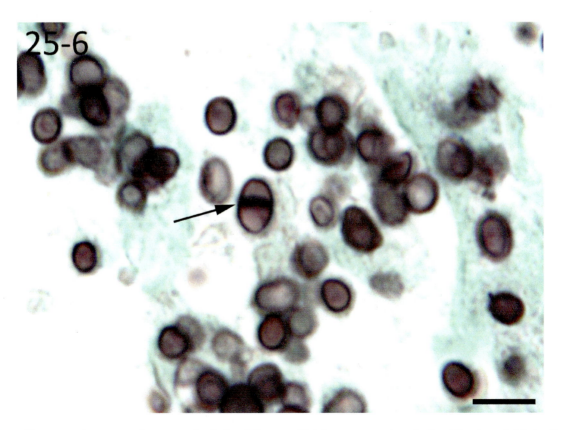

Figure 25.6 Chronic, pulmonary talaromycosis. Cells of *T. marneffei* do not reproduce by budding but divide by fission forming a single transverse septum (arrow). GMS. Bar = 10 μm.

REFERENCES

1. Borradori L, Schmit JC, Stetzkowski M, Dussoix P, Saurat JH et al. 1994. Penicilliosis marneffei infection in AIDS. J Am Acad Dermatol, 31, 843–846.

2. Wong SYN, Wong KF. 2011. *Penicillium marneffei* infection in AIDS. Pathol Res Int, 2011, 1–10.

3. Yousukh A, Jutavijittum P, Pisetpongsa P, Chitapanarux T, Thongsawat S et al. 2004. Clinicopathologic study of hepatic *Penicillium marneffei* in Northern Thailand. Arch Pathol Lab Med, 128, 191–194.

4. Sood N, Gugnani HC. 2010. Disseminated *Penicillium marneffei* infection in a Myanmar refugee from Mizoram state. Indian J Pathol Microbiol, 53, 361–363.

5. Nguyen K, Taylor S, Wanger A, Ali A, Rapini P. 2006. A case of *Penicillium marneffei* in a US hospital. J Am Acad Dermatol, 54, 730–732.

6. Chen R, Ye F, Luo Q, Zhou Y, Xie J et al. 2015. Disseminated penicilliosis marneffei in immunocompetent patients: A report of two cases. Indian J Med Microbiol, 33, 161–165.

7. Luo D-Q, Chen M-C, Liu J-H, Li Z, Li H-T. 2011. Disseminated *Penicillium marneffei* infection in an SLE patient: A case report and literature review. Mycopathologia, 171, 191–196.

8. Qiu Y, Zhang J, Liu G, Zhong X, Deng J et al. 2015. Retrospective analysis of 14 cases of disseminated *Penicillium marneffei* infection with osteolytic lesions. BMC Infect Dis, 15, 1–7.

9. Ko C, Hung C, Chen M, Hsueh P, Hsiao C et al. 1999. Endoscopic diagnosis of intestinal penicilliosis marneffei: Report of three cases and review of the literature. Gastrointest Endosc, 50, 111–114.

10. Lamps LW, Lai KKT, Milner DA. 2014. Fungal infections of the gastrointestinal tract in the immunocompromised host: An update. Adv Anat Pathol, 21, 217–227.

11. Wong KF. 2010. Marrow penicilliosis: A readily missed diagnosis. Am J Clin Pathol, 134, 214–218.

12. Liu Y, Huang X, Yi X, He Y, Mylonakis E et al. 2016. Detection of *Talaromyces marneffei* from fresh tissue of an inhalational murine pulmonary model using nested PCR. PLoS One, 11, 1–9.

13. Feng S, Wang X, Zhang X, Yang H, Wang Z. 2017. Pathological diagnosis of a rare intestinal *Penicillium marneffei* infection in an acquired immunodeficiency syndrome patient: A case report and literature review. Int J Clin Exp Pathol, 10, 3710–3715.

14. Yadav S, Gupta R, Anuradha S, Makkar AM. 2019. A rare case of disseminated penicilliosis - first of its kind from North India. Indian J Pathol Microbiol, 62, 156–158.

15. Hee CH, Pil CY, Cho KJ. 2017. *Penicillium marneffei* infection in a HIV-positive patient: A comparison of bronchial washing cytology and biopsy. J Cytol, 34, 45–48.

16. Tsunemi Y, Takahashi T, Tamaki T. 2003. *Penicillium marneffei* infection diagnosed by polymerase chain reaction from the skin specimen. J Am Acad Dermatol, 49, 344–346.

Pneumocystosis

INTRODUCTION

Pneumocystis jirovecii (formerly named *P. carinii*) is the cause of pneumocystosis in humans, whereas the animal-specific pathogens are still named *P. carinii* with a suffix to describe the animal species of origin (1–6). The pathogens generally cause pneumonia in immunodeficient (i.e., T-cell suppressed) humans and animals. Therefore, pneumocystosis is an important opportunistic infection that principally affects patients with acquired immune deficiency syndrome (AIDS), as well as domestic and wild animals that are co-infected with various viruses (4, 6–12).

EPIDEMIOLOGY

Infections only occur in immunocompromised individuals. In the absence of prophylaxis and/or therapy, this is one of the most frequent opportunistic infections that occurs in AIDS patients (1, 2). Infections may also occur in other immunodeficient patients, including patients who have had solid organ transplants and patients with neoplasia (2, 13, 14). Extrapulmonary *Pneumocystis* infections are only rarely reported (2, 15, 16). The *Pneumocystis* organisms are host species specific: the strains/species of *Pneumocystis* from any given animal host can only be transmitted to the same host species (2, 17). *Pneumocystis* organisms cannot be cultured, but may be propagated in cell cultures *in vitro*; they are highly prevalent in the general human population (18).

PATHOLOGY

Pneumocystis pneumonia is a typical interstitial pneumonia and is characterized by thickened interalveolar septa due to infiltration with mononuclear cells, such as macrophages, lymphocytes, and plasma cells. The alveolar spaces are filled with an eosinophilic foamy "bubble-like" material, which is a mixture of hyaline membranes, proteinaceous fluid, and fungal elements (1, 2, 15). The lesions that form in both humans and animals are similar (Figs. 26.1 and 26.2) (1, 2, 7, 9, 15, 17). In addition to the lung lesions typically associated with interstitial pneumonia, atypical lesions such as granulomas and interstitial fibrosis may occur (14, 19–21).

FUNGAL HISTOMORPHOLOGY

The *Pneumocystis* pathogens may be present in two forms. First, there are spherical thin-walled trophic forms (previously called trophozoites) with diameters of 2–10 µm. Second, there are thick-walled forms (cysts) with diameters of 4–6 µm (Figs. 26.3 and 26.4) (1–3, 15). These pathogens are surrounded by the foamy material within the alveolar spaces and are difficult to see in hematoxylin and eosin-stained sections. The pathogens are best visualized by applying Grocott's methenamine silver stain, but the toluidine blue method will also highlight them convincingly (Figs. 26.3–26.5) (1–3). When appropriately treated, the *Pneumocystis* organisms are birefringent (22). Black dots are visible within the cell walls and cytoplasm when sections are stained using the Grocott's methenamine silver technique (1, 2, 8). Broken and collapsed elements are frequently present alongside intact organisms. The collapsed organisms are crescent shaped.

DIFFERENTIAL DIAGNOSIS

Excluding the possible presence of *Histoplasma capsulatum* and *Candida glabrata* is important for differentiating pneumocystosis (1, 2, 20). However, in cases of histoplasmosis and candidosis, the pathogens do not exhibit black dots within the cell walls and cytoplasm. Moreover, *H. capsulatum* buds and *C. glabrata* produce blastospores (see the chapters on histoplasmosis and candidosis, respectively). For specific *in situ* diagnoses, immunohistochemical, *in situ* hybridization, and polymerase chain reaction techniques are available (Fig. 26.6) (5, 7, 15, 17, 18).

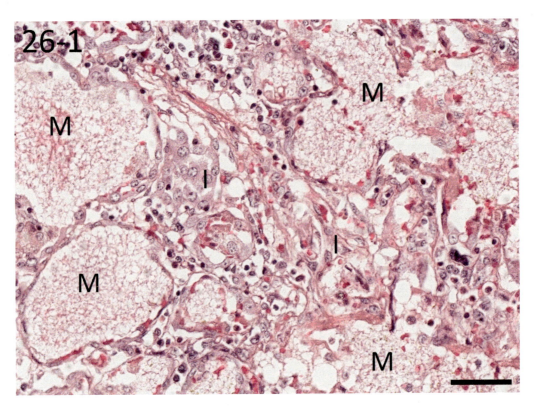

Figure 26.1 Chronic, pulmonary pneumocystosis. The large quantity of foamy material (M) within the alveoli, together with interstitial infiltration (I) of mononuclear cells, strongly suggests pneumocystosis. However, the *Pneumocystis* cells are not visible in hematoxylin and eosin-stained sections. HE. Bar = 55 μm.

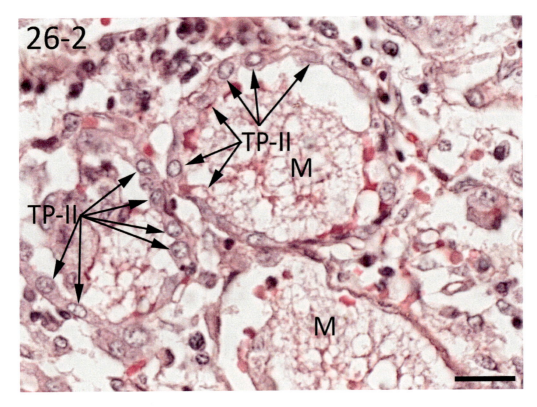

Figure 26.2 Chronic, pulmonary pneumocystosis. The large quantity of foamy material (M) within the alveoli, together with type II cell hyperplasia (TP-II), strongly suggests pneumocystosis. However, the *Pneumocystis* cells are not visible in hematoxylin and eosin-stained sections. HE. Bar = 35 μm.

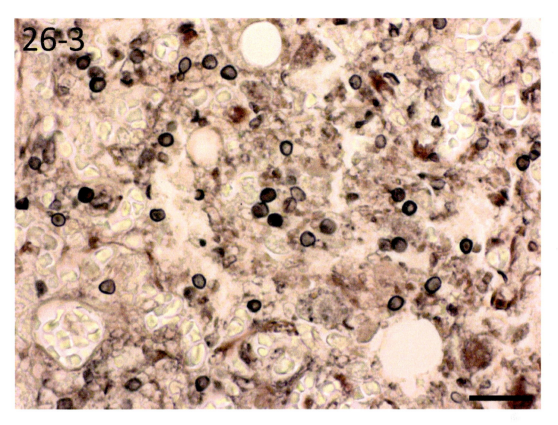

Figure 26.3 Chronic, pulmonary pneumocystosis. The outlines of *P. jirovecii* organisms among the foamy material within the alveoli are clearly visible in Grocott's methenamine silver-stained sections. GMS. Bar = 25 µm.

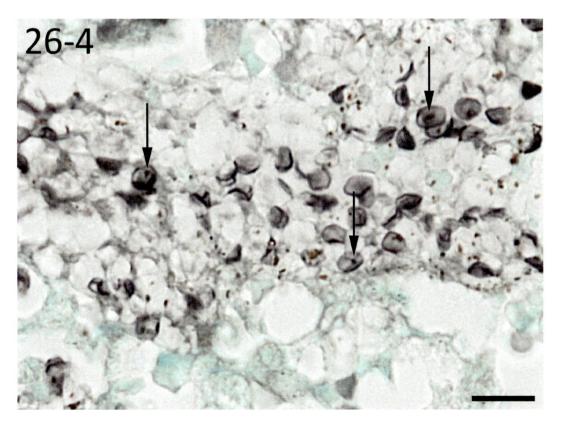

Figure 26.4 Chronic, pulmonary pneumocystosis. *P. jirovecii* organisms of various sizes and shapes (large, small, and collapsed cells) exhibit intracellular black dots (arrows). GMS. Bar = 12 µm.

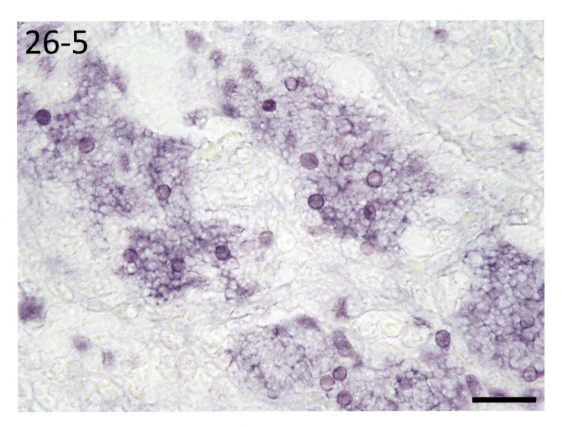

Figure 26.5 Chronic, pulmonary pneumocystosis. *P. jirovecii* organisms within the foam-filled alveolar spaces are highlighted by the toluidine blue (TB) staining technique. TB. Bar = 20 μm.

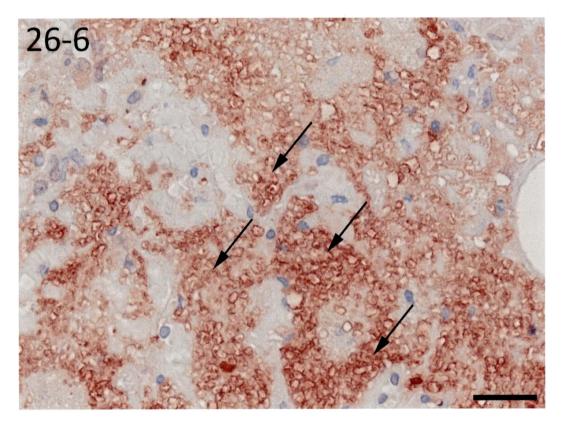

Figure 26.6 Chronic, pulmonary pneumocystosis. *P. jirovecii* organisms within the foam-filled alveolar spaces (arrows) may be identified using specific immunohistochemical staining techniques. IHC. Bar = 30 μm.

REFERENCES

1. Guarner J, Brandt, ME. 2011. Histopathologic diagnosis of fungal infections in the 21st century. Clin Microbiol Rev, 24, 247–280.

2. Gigliotti F, Wright TW. 2015. Pneumocystosis. In: Diagnosis and Treatment of Fungal Infections. 2nd ed. Hospenthal DR, Rinaldi MG, Eds. Springer. pp 169–174.

3. Jensen HE. 2021. Histopathology in the diagnosis of invasive fungal diseases. Curr Fungal Infect Rep, 15, 23–31.

4. Sakakibara M, Shimizu C, Kadota K, Hatama S. 2013. *Pneumocystis carinii* Infection in a domestic goat (*Capra hircus domesticus*) with multibacillary paratuberculosis. J Vet Med Sci, 75, 671–674.

5. Vestereng VH, Bishop LR, Hernandez B, Kutty G, Larsen HH et al. 2004. Quantitative real-time polymerase chain-reaction assay allows characterization of *Pneumocystis* infection in immunocompetent mice. J Infect Dis, 189, 1540–1544.

6. Ueno T, Niwa H, Kinoshita Y, Katayama Y, Hobo S. 2014. *Pneumocystis* pneumonia in a thoroughbred racehorse. J Equine Vet Sci, 34, 333–336.

7. Binanti D, Mostegl MM, Weissenbacher-Lang C, Nedorost N, Weissenböck H. 2015. Detection of *Pneumocystis* infections by in situ hybridization in lung samples of Austrian pigs with interstitial pneumonia. J Music Ther, 52, 196–201.

8. Borba MR, Sanches EMC, Corrêa AMR, Spanamberg A, De Souza Leal J et al. 2011. Immunohistochemical and ultra-structural detection of *Pneumocystis* in wild boars (*Sus scrofa*) co-infected with porcine circovirus type 2 (PCV2) in Southern Brazil. Med Mycol, 49, 172–175.

9. Henderson KS, Dole V, Parker NJ, Momtsios P, Banu L et al. 2012. *Pneumocystis carinii* causes a distinctive interstitial pneumonia in immunocompetent laboratory rats that had been attributed to "Rat Respiratory Virus." Vet Pathol, 49, 440–452.

10. Kim KS, Jung JY, Kim JH, Kang SC, Hwang EK et al. 2011. Epidemiological characteristics of pulmonary pneumocystosis and concurrent infections in pigs in Jeju Island, Korea. J Vet Sci, 12, 15–19.

11. Kim HS, Do SI, Kim YW. 2014. Histopathology of *Pneumocystis carinii* pneumonia in immunocompetent laboratory rats. Exp Ther Med, 8, 442–446.

12. Sanches EMC, Pescador C, Rozza D, Spanamberg A, Borba MR et al. 2007. Detection of *Pneumocystis* spp. in lung samples from pigs in Brazil. Med Mycol, 45, 395–399.

13. Hagiya H, Miyake T, Kokumai Y, Murase T, Kuroe Y et al. 2013. Co-infection with invasive pulmonary aspergillosis and *Pneumocystis jirovecii* pneumonia after corticosteroid therapy. J Infect Chemother, 19, 342–347.

14. Kanemoto H, Morikawa R, Chambers JK, Kasahara K. 2015. Common variable immune deficiency in a Pomeranian with *Pneumocystis carinii* pneumonia. J Vet Med Sci, 77, 715–719.

15. Mahlakwane MS, Ramdial PK, Sing Y, Calonje E, Biyana S. 2008. Otic pneumocystosis in acquired immune deficiency syndrome. Am J Surg Pathol, 32, 1038–1043.

16. Kim B, Kim J, Paik SS, Pai H. 2018. Atypical presentation of *Pneumocystis jirovecii* infection in HIV infected patients: Three different manifestations. J Korean Med Sci, 33, 115–121.

17. Jensen TK, Boye M, Bille-Hansen V. 2001. Application of fluorescent in situ hybridization for specific diagnosis of *Pneumocystis carinii* pneumonia in foals and pigs. Vet Pathol, 38, 269–274.

18. Ponce CA, Gallo M, Bustamante R, Vargas SL. 2010. *Pneumocystis* colonization is highly prevalent in the autopsied lungs of the general population. Clin Infect Dis, 50, 347–353.

19. Foley NM, Miller RF, Griffiths MH. 1993. Histologically atypical *Pneumocystis carinii* pneumonia. Thorax, 48, 996–1001.

20. Hartel PH, Shilo K, Klassen-Fischer M, Neafie RC, Ozbudak IH et al. 2010. Granulomatous reaction to *Pneumocystis jirovecii*: Clinicopathologic review of 20 cases. Am J Surg Pathol, 34, 730–734.

21. Patel KB, Gleason JB, Diacovo MJ, Martinez-Galvez N. 2016. *Pneumocystis* pneumonia presenting as an enlarging solitary pulmonary nodule. Case Rep Infect Dis. doi: org/10.1155/2016/1873237.

22. An T, Tabaczka P. 2004. The use of polarization microscopy in the diagnosis of pneumocystis pneumonia. Arch Pathol Lab Med, 128, 363–364.

27

Lacaziosis

INTRODUCTION

Lacaziosis, formerly known as Lobo's disease or lobomycosis, is caused by *Lacazia loboi*. Jorge Lobo described the disease in 1931. Natural infections have only been reported in humans and dolphins; the skin and subcutaneous lesions that occur are similar in both hosts (1). To date, the infective organism in humans and dolphins has not been successfully cultured, despite many attempts (2, 3). During the years, several names have been applied to the pathogen causing the disease. However, from DNA sequences the pathogen in dolphins has recently been placed within the DNA sequences of the culturable *Paracoccidioides brasiliensis* (2). Therefore, the fungus causing the lesions in dolphins was named *P. brasiliensis* var. *ceti*, and the disease accordingly paracoccidioidomycosis ceti (2).

EPIDEMIOLOGY

Lacaziosis typically occurs in men living in rural areas, often close to water, and is associated with skin trauma (1, 4, 5). Paracoccidioidomycosis ceti is common among dolphins inhabiting the Gulf of Mexico, the Suriname River, the Indian River Lagoon, the coast of Brazil, and the Spanish–French border coast. Human infections have been reported in Central and South America, Africa, and Southeastern Europe (1, 6–9). Infections of people outside of these regions have also been reported, but have always been associated with travel to these regions (10, 11).

PATHOLOGY

Lesions of lacaziosis and paracoccidioidomycosis ceti are generally restricted to the epidermis and subcutis of the skin, although human lymph nodes (12) and dolphin muscle tissue have reportedly been affected (13). Skin lesions typically manifest as subcutaneous inflammation, which may disseminate within the subcutis by spreading contiguously or through lymph vessels (Figs. 27.1 and 27.2) (4). The epidermis above the lesions is usually atrophic, and fibrous tissue occupies the dermis (12). Lesions are histopathologically characterized by infiltration with macrophages, Langhans- and foreign body-type multinucleate giant cells, lymphocytes, and fungal cells (Figs. 27.3 and 27.4) (14). In addition, epithelioid cells and some eosinophils may be present (15). Dermal lesions may be lepromatous (1). Changes in the local microvasculature may interfere with the cell-mediated immune response, restricting lesions to the site of injury (16).

Lacaziosis has been introduced into laboratory animals (2, 10) such as mice, and lesions are reportedly similar to those that occur in humans and dolphins; however, the murine lesions are infiltrated with neutrophils (17), which does not occur in human or dolphin lesions (6). Both CD8+ and Th-17 cells may play important roles in the immune response to *L. loboi* (14, 18).

FUNGAL HISTOMORPHOLOGY

Cells of both *L. loboi* and *P. brasiliensis* var. *ceti* are weakly stained by haematoxylin and eosin and are negative for Mayers's mucicarmine stain, but they are clearly visible if the periodic acid-Schiff stain or Grocott's methenamine silver stain is applied (2, 13). The *P. brasiliensis* var. *ceti* cells present in lesions that occur in dolphins are reportedly smaller than those found in human lacaziosis lesions (6). The yeast cells are 5–12 μm in diameter (2, 3, 11, 13). In lesions, these round, thick-walled yeast cells reproduce by simple budding (Fig. 27.5). *L. loboi* and *P. brasiliensis* var. *ceti* cells are often found within multinucleate giant cells (Fig. 27.3) (4). Occasionally, these cells form chains that resemble strings of pearls, connected by isthmuses (13) (Fig. 27.6). The presence of these fungal chains may help to diagnose both lacaziosis and paracoccidioidomycosis ceti (Figs. 27.5 and 27.6).

DIFFERENTIAL DIAGNOSIS

If only a few *P. brasiliensis*, *P. lutzii*, or *Histoplasma capsulatum* cells are present (e.g., from biopsies), then distinguishing these pathogens from *L. loboi* may be difficult. However, *H. capsulatum* cells are smaller than *L. loboi* cells, and *Paracoccidioides* cells are larger than *L. loboi* cells and have thicker walls (7). Moreover, if the characteristic multibudding *Paracoccidioides* "Steering wheel" is visible, then *P. brasiliensis* can easily be distinguished from *L. loboi*. Therefore, a histopathological diagnosis of lacaziosis can

DOI: 10.1201/9781003306177-27

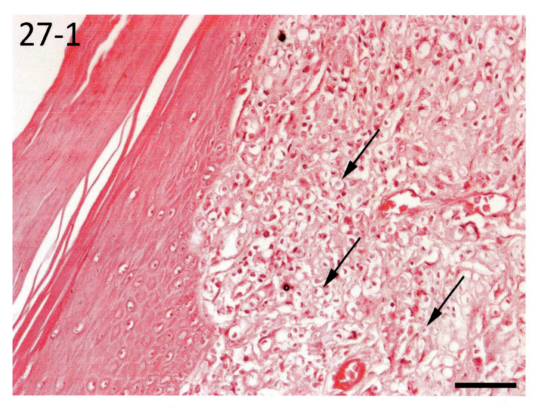

Figure 27.1 Skin biopsy from a chronic subcutaneous lacaziosis lesion. Within the fibrotic subcutaneous tissue, multiple elements of *L. loboi* are visible (arrows) both within macrophages and outside the cells. These elements are not clearly visible in haematoxylin and eosin-stained sections. HE. Bar = 50 μm.

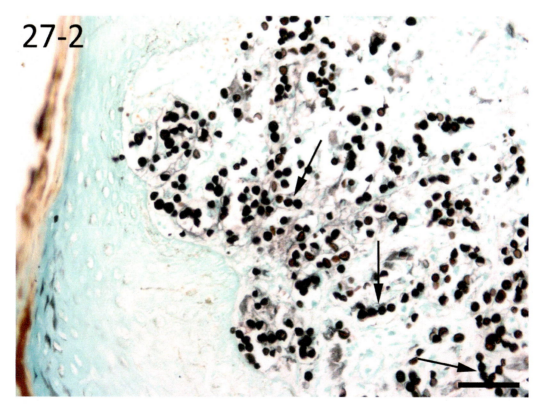

Figure 27.2 Skin biopsy from the same lacaziosis case as in Fig. 27.1. Within the fibrotic subcutaneous tissue, multiple *L. loboi* organisms are visible when Grocott's methenamine silver stain is applied. Some of the fungi have formed chains of cells (arrows). GMS. Bar = 50 μm.

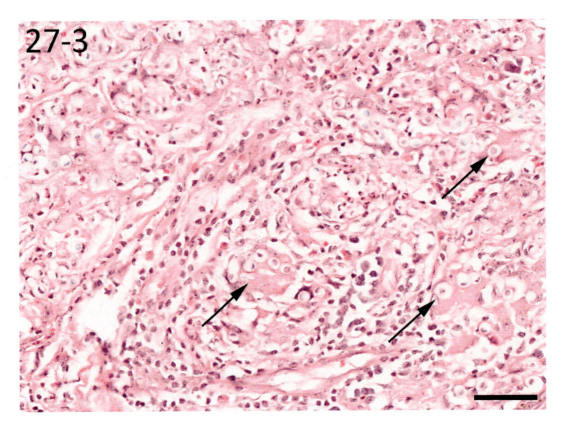

Figure 27.3 Chronic, subcutaneous lacaziosis. Within the fibrotic subcutaneous tissue, multiple macrophages and some multinucleate giant cells containing *L. loboi* cells are visible (arrows). HE. Bar = 50 μm.

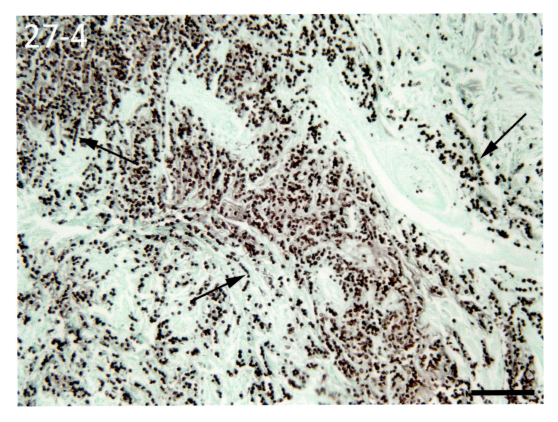

Figure 27.4 Chronic, subcutaneous lacaziosis. Many yeast-like cells are visible within the subcutaneous lesion. Some of these cells have formed a row (arrows). GMS. Bar = 250 μm.

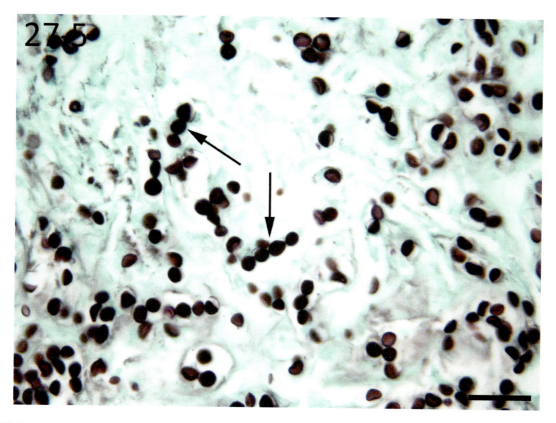

Figure 27.5 Chronic, subcutaneous lacaziosis. The *L. loboi* cells in this lesion have formed chains that resemble strings of pearls (arrows). This feature may help to diagnose lacaziosis. GMS. Bar = 40 μm.

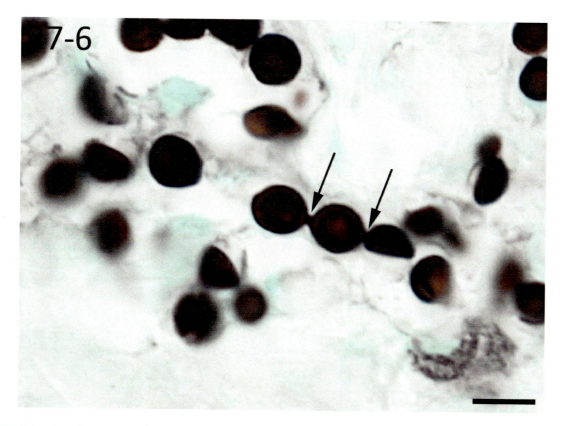

Figure 27.6 Chronic, subcutaneous lacaziosis. The *L. loboi* cells that are growing in chains are connected by isthmuses (arrows). GMS. Bar = 20 μm.

usually be made. However, in difficult cases, polymerase chain reaction techniques may be used to confirm lacaziosis diagnoses (11).

REFERENCES

1. Mondolfi AEP, Talhari C, Sander Hoffmann L, Connor DL, Talhari S et al. 2012. Lobomycosis: An emerging disease in humans and delphinidae. Mycoses, 55, 298–309.

2. Vilela R, Mendoza L. 2018. Paracocidioidomycosis ceti (Lacaziosis/Lobomycosis) in Dolphins. In: Emerging and Epizootic Fungal Infections in Animals. Seyedmousave S, de Hoog GS, Guillot J, Verweij PE, Eds. Springer. pp 177–196.

3. Schaefer AM, Reif JS, Guzmán EA, Bossart GD, Ottuso P et al. 2016. Toward the identification, characterization and experimental culture of *Lacazia loboi* from Atlantic bottlenose dolphin (*Tursiops truncatus*). Med Mycol, 54, 659–665.

4. Carneiro FP, Maia LB, Moraes MAP, de Magalhães AV, de Vianna LMS et al. 2009. Lobomycosis: Diagnosis and management of relapsed and multifocal lesions. Diagn Microbiol Infect Dis, 65, 62–64.

5. Cabrera-Salom C, González LF, Rolón M, Sánchez BF. 2017. Keloids on the ears. Internat J Dermatolog, 56, 819–821.

6. Haubold EM, Cooper CR, Wen JW, McGinnis MR, Cowan DF. 2000. Comparative morphology of *Lacazia loboi* (syn. *Loboa loboi*) in dolphins and humans. Med Mycol, 38, 9–14.

7. Al-Daraji WI, Husain E, Robson A. 2008. Lobomycosis in African patients. Br J Dermatol, 159, 234–236.

8. Papadavid E, Dalamaga M, Kapniari I, Pantelidaki E, Papageorgiou S et al. 2012. Lobomycosis: A case from southeastern Europe and review of the literature. J Dermatol Case Rep, 6, 65–69.

9. Reif JS, Mazzoil MS, McCulloch SD, Varela R, Goldstein JD et al. 2006. Lobomycosis in Atlantic bottlenose dolphins from the Indian River Lagoon, Florida. J Am Vet Med Assoc, 228, 104–108.

10. Elsayed S, Kuhn SM, Barber D, Church DL, Adams S et al. 2004. Human case of lobomycosis. Emerg Infect Dis, 10, 715–718.

11. Beltrame A, Danesi P, Farina C, Orza P, Perandin F et al. 2017. Case report: Molecular confirmation of lobomycosis in an Italian traveler acquired in the Amazon region of Venezuela. Am J Trop Med Hyg, 97, 1757–1760.

12. Talhari C, Oliveira CB, De Souza Santos MN, Ferreira LC, Talhari S. 2008. Disseminated lobomycosis. Int J Dermatol, 47, 582–583.

13. Sacristán C, Réssio RA, Castilho P, De Azevedo Fernandes NCC et al. 2016. Lacaziosis-like disease in *Tursiops truncates* from Brazil: A histopathological and immunohistochemical approach. Dis Aquat Organ, 117, 229–235.

14. Alexandre AF, Quaresma JAS, Barboza TC, De Brito AC, Xavier MB et al. 2017. The cytotoxic T cells may contribute to the in situ immune response in Jorge Lobo's Disease human lesions. Med Mycol, 55, 145–149.

15. Carneiro FRO, Fischer TRDC, Brandão CM, Pagliari C, Duarte MIS et al. 2015. Disseminated infection with *Lacazia loboi* and immunopathology of the lesional spectrum. Hum Pathol 46, 334–338.

16. Quaresma JAS, Brito MV, Sousa JR, Silva LM, Hirai KE et al. 2015. Analysis of microvasculature phenotype and endothelial activation markers in skin lesions of lacaziosis (lobomycosis). Microb Pathog, 78, 29–36.

17. Vilani-Moreno FR, Silva SMUR, Barbosa ASAA, Satori BGC, Barboza Pedrini SC et al. 2014. Study of murine experimental Jorge Lobo's disease by analysis of peritoneal lavage cells and footpad histopathology: Early versus chronic lesions. Med Mycol, 53, 378–386.

18. Kanashiro-Galo L, Pagliari C, Barboza TC, de Brito AC, Xavier MB et al. 2016. Th17 and regulatory T cells contribute to the in situ immune response in skin lesions of Jorge Lobo's disease. Med Mycol, 54, 23–28.

28

Coccidioidomycosis

INTRODUCTION

Coccidioides immitis and *C. posadasii* cause coccidioidomycosis. Both fungi are found in distinct desert regions, but these regions of fungal habitation may be extended considerably following rainfall. *C. posadasii* is found in Texas, Mexico, and Central and South America, whereas *C. immitis* predominantly occurs in California (1–3). *Coccidioides* spp. grow in soil and are largely restricted to areas of previous human or animal habitation (1, 2, 4, 5). The *Coccidioides* spp. are responsible for the same spectrum of diseases (6, 7).

EPIDEMIOLOGY

Coccidioidomycosis is rarely diagnosed outside the endemic regions. However, travellers who have visited these areas may have infections that lie dormant for several years, and low doses of prednisolone may trigger the reemergence of the disease in non-endemic areas (8, 9). Patients with diabetes or human immunodeficiency virus (HIV), or recipients of immunomodulatory or immunosuppressive drugs (including high doses of corticosteroids) are more susceptible to developing chronic pulmonary diseases or disseminated coccidioidomycosis lesions (3, 10–15). Several animal species have reportedly been infected with the fungi (7), and several animal models of coccidioidomycosis have been developed (16).

PATHOLOGY

Coccidioidomycosis is primarily a pulmonary disease, which may be transient or may develop into persistent pneumonia (2). Lesions are often necrotic, leading to cavity formation in the lungs. The target organs for disseminated lesions include the skin, bones, joints, and central nervous system/meninges (15, 17–19). Usually, the skin only becomes infected as a result of hematogenous spread (18), but it may also be the primary infection site following trauma (20). However, almost any organ or tissue may become infected (15, 17, 19). Although coccidioidomycosis is not contagious, it has reportedly been transmitted via organ transplantation (21). Granulomatous lesions are regularly formed in all affected tissues. These exhibit infiltration with macrophages, epithelioid cells, and lymphocytes, together with multinucleate giant cells that may contain fungal elements (Fig. 28.1) (17). In some cases, neutrophils are also present, resulting in the formation of pyogranulomas or abscesses (Fig. 28.2) (6, 20).

FUNGAL HISTOMORPHOLOGY

Several types of thick-walled yeast-like *Coccidioides* may be present in tissues. Spores that are released from ruptured spherules measure 2–5 µm in diameter and may also be found in tissues. The spores mature, and large yeast cells may measure up to 10–20 µm in diameter (Fig. 28.3) (22). The largest forms are those with endosporulating spherules, which measure 20–200 µm (Fig. 28.4). Lesions also contain ruptured empty "yeast-shells" (Figs. 28.5 and 28.6) (22). Occasionally, hyphae, arthroconidia, and budding yeast cells may be found in lung sections. These may grow better within cavity lesions due to the high levels of oxygen and humidity (10, 23). Haematoxylin and eosin usually stains *Coccidioides* fungal elements strongly, and fungal elements are also highlighted by Grocott's methenamine silver and periodic acid-Schiff stains (Figs. 28.1 and 28.4–28.6). Mixed inflammatory reactions occur in cases of coccidioidomycosis. Pyogranulomatous inflammation is present, and fungal elements may be found both inside and outside of multinucleate giant cells (17).

DIFFERENTIAL DIAGNOSIS

Many forms of yeast-like cells may be present following the release of endospores. Therefore, several alternative diagnoses must be excluded, especially if the large *Coccidioides* endospores that contain cells and their breakdown fragments are absent. Small endospores within the tissue may be confused with other small yeast cells, especially *Histoplasma capsulatum* var. *capsulatum* and *Candida glabrata* cells. In addition, smaller cells from species that are typically larger may be problematic, especially *Cryptococcus* spp., *Blastomyces dermatitidis*, *Paracoccidioides brasiliensis*, *P. lutzii*, and *H. capsulatum* var. *duboisii* cells. Finally, the pathogens that cause rhinosporidiosis may be confused with those that cause coccidioidomycosis.

DOI: 10.1201/9781003306177-28

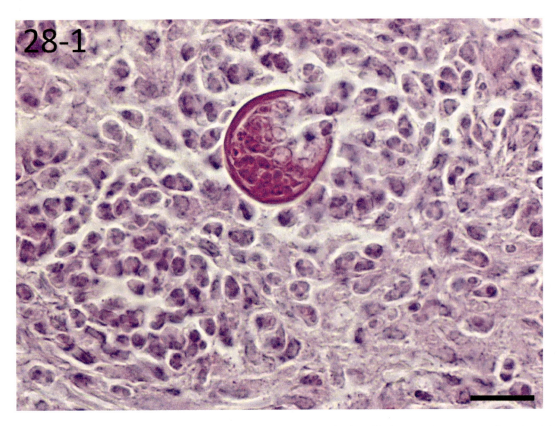

Figure 28.1 Chronic, granulomatous pulmonary coccidioidomycosis. A thick-walled open *C. immitis* spherule with endospores is visible, surrounded by macrophages and epithelioid cells. PAS. Bar = 40 μm.

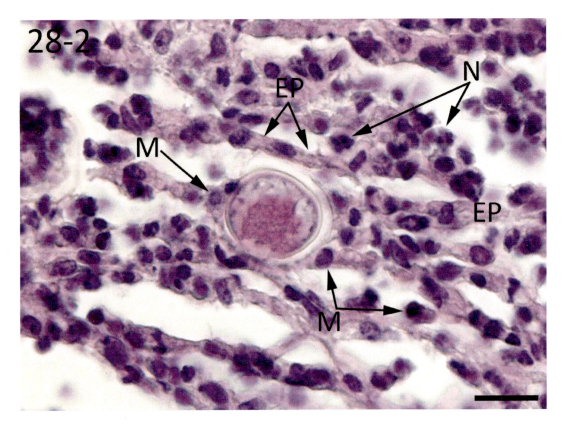

Figure 28.2 Chronic, pyogranulomatous pulmonary coccidioidomycosis. A thick-walled *C. immitis* spherule is visible, surrounded by neutrophils (N), macrophages (M), and epithelioid cells (EP). HE. Bar = 40 μm.

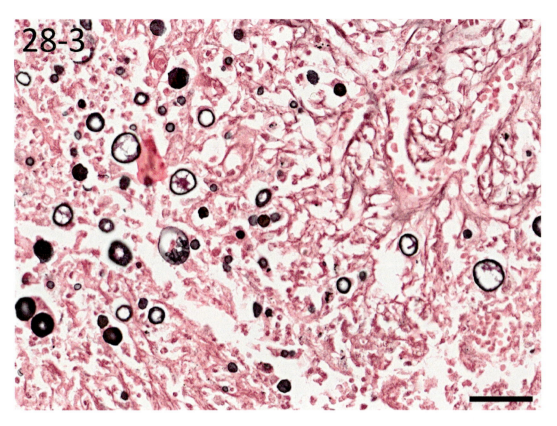

Figure 28.3 Chronic, granulomatous pulmonary coccidioidomycosis. *Coccidioides* elements of various sizes are visible. GMS and HE. Bar = 150 μm.

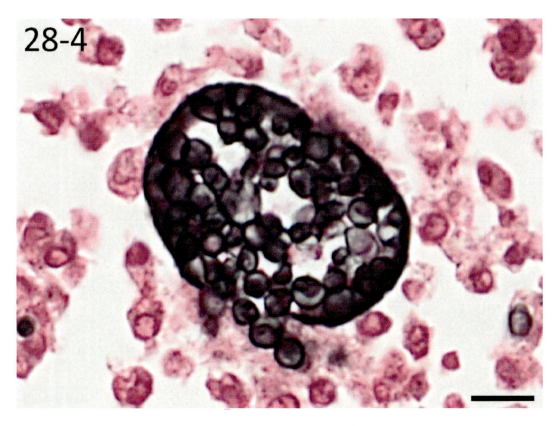

Figure 28.4 Chronic, granulomatous pulmonary coccidioidomycosis. A thick-walled *C. immitis* spherule releases its endospores into the surrounding tissue. GMS and HE. Bar = 15 μm.

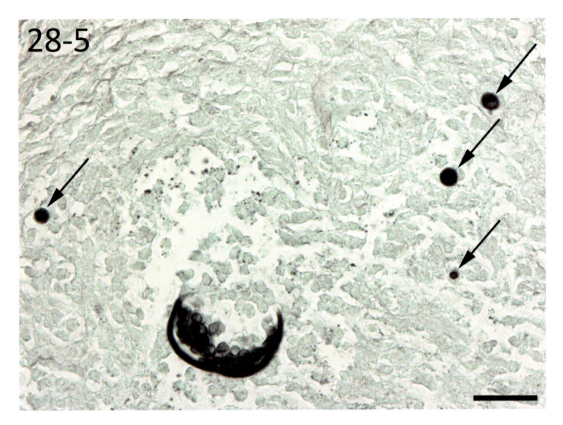

Figure 28.5 Chronic, granulomatous pulmonary coccidioidomycosis. A thick-walled *C. immitis* spherule immediately before endospore release. The endospores are visible within the tissue (arrows). GMS. Bar = 40 μm.

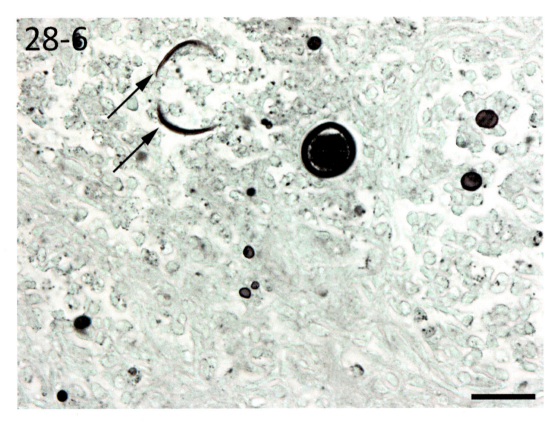

Figure 28.6 Pulmonary coccidioidomycosis. Fragments of empty spherules ("yeast-shells") are visible (arrows) together with *C. immitis* at different stages of development, including a minor spherule. GMS. Bar = 40 μm.

In difficult cases, molecular techniques such as *in situ* hybridization and polymerase chain reaction may be used to diagnose coccidioidomycosis. However, the reagents/primers necessary for these techniques are not widely available (1, 18).

REFERENCES

1. Kollath DR, Miller KJ, Barker BM. 2019. The mysterious desert dwellers: *Coccidioides immitis* and *Coccidioides posadasii*, causative fungal agents of coccidioidomycosis. Virulence, 10, 222–233.
2. Johnson RH, Sharma R, Kuran R, Fong I, Heidari A. 2021. Coccidioidomycosis: A review. J Investig Med, 69, 316–323.
3. Diep AL, Hoyer KK. 2020. Host response to *Coccidioides* infection: Fungal immunity. Front Cell Infect Microbiol, 10, 1–15.
4. Kirkland TN, Fierer J. 2018. *Coccidioides immitis* and *posadasii*; A review of their biology, genomics, pathogenesis, and host immunity. Virulence, 9, 1426–1435.
5. Reyes-Montes MDR, Pérez-Huitrón MA, Ocana-Monroy JL, Frias-De-León MG, Martinez-Herrera E et al. 2016. The habitat of *Coccidioides* spp. and the role of animals as reservoirs and disseminators in nature. BMC Infect Dis, 16, 550–557.
6. Abukamleh H, Heidari A, Petersen G, Natarajan P, Yakoub G et al. 2018. Erythema sweetobullosum: A reactive cutaneous manifestation of coccidioidomycosis. J Invest Med, 6, 1–6.
7. Cordeiro R, Moura S, Castelo-Branco D, Rocha MF, Lima-Neto R et al. 2021. Coccidioidomycosis in Brazil: Historical challenges of a neglected disease. J Fungi, 7, 85–98.
8. Bæk O, Astvad K, Serizawa R, Wheat LJ, Brenøe PT et al. 2017. Peritoneal and genital coccidioidomycosis in an otherwise healthy Danish female: A case report. BMC Infect Dis, 17, 105–508.
9. Parish JM, Blair JE. 2008. Coccidioidomycosis. Mayo Clin Proc, 83, 343–349.
10. Brennan-Krohn T, Yoon E, Nishino M, Kirby JE, Riedel S. 2018. Arthroconidia in lung tissue: An unusual histopathological finding in pulmonary coccidioidomycosis. Human Pathol, 71, 55–59.
11. Pisaraei PA, Tabsh K, Lentz J. 2016. Rare dysuria: Prostatic abscess due to disseminated coccidioidomycosis. Urol Case Rep, 9, 12–14.
12. Crum-Cianflone NF, Truett AA, Teneza-Mora N, Maves RC, Chun HM et al. 2006. Unusual presentations of coccidioidomycosis: A case series and review of the literature. Medicine, 85, 263–277.
13. Sarosi GA, Davies SF. 1996. Endemic mycosis complicating human immunodeficiency virus infection. West J Med, 164, 335–340.
14. D'Avino A, Giambenedetto S, Fabbiani M, Farina S. 2012. Coccidioidomycosis of cervical lymph nodes in an HIV-infected patient with immunologic reconstitution on potent HAART: A rare observation in a nonendemic area. Diag Microbiol Infect Dis, 72, 185–187.
15. Toomey CB, Gross A, Lee J, Spencer DB. 2019. A case of unilateral coccidioidal chorioretinitis in a patient with HIV-associated meningoencephalitis. Case Rep Ophthalmol Med. doi: 10.1155/2019/1475628.
16. Jensen HE. 2021. Animal models of invasive mycoses. APMIS, 1–9. doi: 10.1111/apm.13110.
17. Mendez LA, Flores SA, Martinez R, Paes de Almeida O. 2017. Ulcerated lesion of the tongue as manifestation of systemic coccidioidomycosis. Case Rep Med, 1–3. doi: 10.1155/2017/1489501.
18. Garcia SCG, Flores MG, Cabrera LV, Alanis JCS, Gonzalez SEG et al. 2015. Coccidioidomycosis and the skin: A comprehensive review. An Bras Dermatol. 90, 610–621.
19. Bajwa AK, Rongkavilit C. 2020. Update on coccidioidomycosis in the United States and beyond. Glob Pediatr Health, 1–8. doi: 10.1177/2333794X20969282.
20. Russell DH, Ager E, Wohltman CW. 2017. Cutaneous coccidiomycosis masquerading as an epidermoid cyst: Case report and review of the literature. Mil Med, 182, 1665–1668.
21. Kusne S, Taranto S, Covington S, Kaul DR, Blumberg EA et al. 2016. Coccidioidomycosis transmission through organ transplantation: A report of the OPTN ad hoc disease transmission advisory committee. Am J Transplant, 16, 3562–3567.
22. Jensen HE, Chandler FW. 2007. Histopathological diagnoses of mycoses. In: Topley and Wilson' Microbiology & Microbial Infections. Medical Mycology. 10th ed. Merz WG, Hay RJ, Eds. Hodder Arnold. pp 121–143.
23. Nosanchuk JD, Snedeker J, Nosanchuk JS. 1998. Arthroconidia in coccidioidoma: Case report and literature review. Int J Infect Dis, 3, 32–35.

29

Adiaspiromycosis

INTRODUCTION

Adiaspiromycosis is caused by *Emmonsia crescens* (*Chrysosporium parvum* var. *crescens*) and *E. parva* (*C. parvum* var. *parvum*; *Blastomyces parvus*), which are soil saprophytes (1–3). Despite the absence of adiaspores, a third species *E. pasteuriana* was included later and recently reclassified as a new genus *Emergomyces* including different species: *Emergomyces pasteuriana*, *E. africanus*, *E. orientalis*, *E. canadensis*, and *E. europaeus* (3). Because the *Emergomyces* species are present in tissues by the presence of yeast cells (3–7 µm), they are dealt with in the chapter on rare mycoses. Infections are rare in humans. However, small mammals such as rodents and rabbits are more frequently infected and may function as zoonotic reservoirs (1–9).

EPIDEMIOLOGY

Adiaspiromycosis infections occur worldwide. Infections occur via the airway, and lesions develop after inhalation of conidia (spores), which enlarge to form adiaconidia/adiaspores (Figs. 29.1 and 29.2) (3, 10, 11). In humans, the disease is generally self-limiting. In rare cases, there is dissemination to other organs and lesions may be produced on the skin; this happens most frequently in immunosuppressed individuals, such as patients with acquired immune deficiency syndrome (AIDS) (4, 9–12).

PATHOLOGY

Because infections occur via the airways, the lungs are frequently affected. Here, granulomatous pneumonia may develop (solitary to diffuse) (Figs. 29.2 and 29.3) (9, 10).

Sometimes, lesions may also be infiltrated by neutrophils (9). In the lung tissue, the adiaconidia are encircled by macrophages, epithelioid cells, and multinucleate giant cells, surrounded by an outermost layer of fibrous tissue (Figs. 29.2 and 29.3) (3, 8–10). Interstitial pneumonia has also been associated with adiaspiromycosis (13). Experimentally, both localized and systemic infections have been established in animal models (Figs. 29.4–29.6) (14).

FUNGAL HISTOMORPHOLOGY

The inflammatory reaction and the morphology of *Emmonsia* spp. adiaconidia exhibit distinctive characteristics. The fungal elements are spherical in tissue sections and measure 200–400 µm in diameter (Figs. 29.1 and 29.2), or even larger (3, 6, 7, 13, 15). The adiaconidia have thick (22–25 µm) bi- or tri-laminar walls (Fig. 29.5) and do not replicate in tissues (2, 3, 8). Cells are strongly stained by haematoxylin and eosin, but periodic acid-Schiff and Grocott's methenamine silver stains also highlight cellular morphology (8, 15, 16). In lesions, cells often reach their maximal size and then degrade to create granulomatous fibrotic areas (Fig. 29.3).

DIFFERENTIAL DIAGNOSIS

The large adiaconidia associated with adiaspiromycosis do not contain endospores. Therefore, these should not be confused with the large cyst-forming elements of *Coccidioides* spp. or *Rhinosporidium seeberi*. In addition, the adiaconidia walls are much thicker than those of *Coccidioides* spp. and *R. seeberi* (see chapters on coccidioidomycosis and rhinosporidiosis, respectively).

204

DOI: 10.1201/9781003306177-29

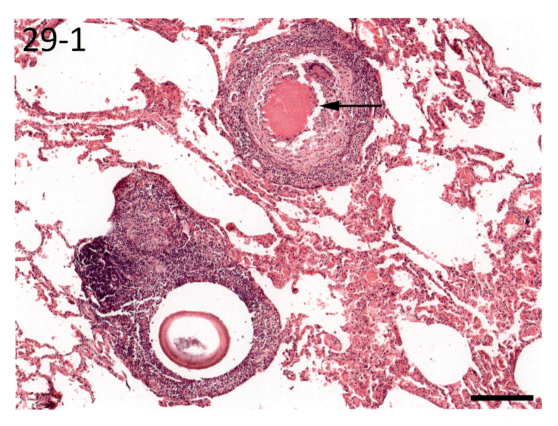

Figure 29.1 Chronic, granulomatous pulmonary adiaspiromycosis. Two adiaconidia are visible, one of which is undergoing degradation (arrow). The pathogens are surrounded by granulomatous inflammation. HE. Bar = 300 μm.

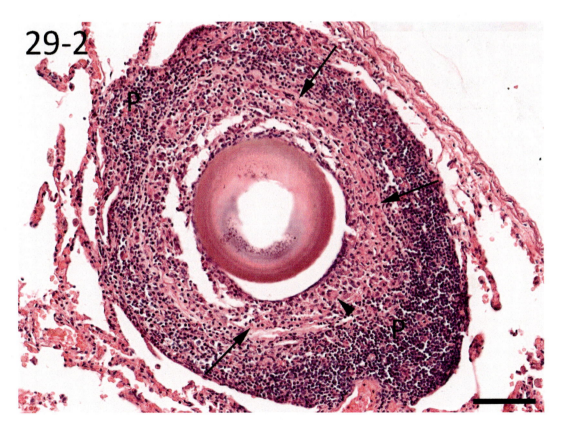

Figure 29.2 Chronic, granulomatous pulmonary adiaspiromycosis. Macrophages (arrows) and a multinucleate giant cell (arrowhead) surround the adiaconidium. Other mononuclear cells are visible at the periphery (P). HE. Bar = 180 μm.

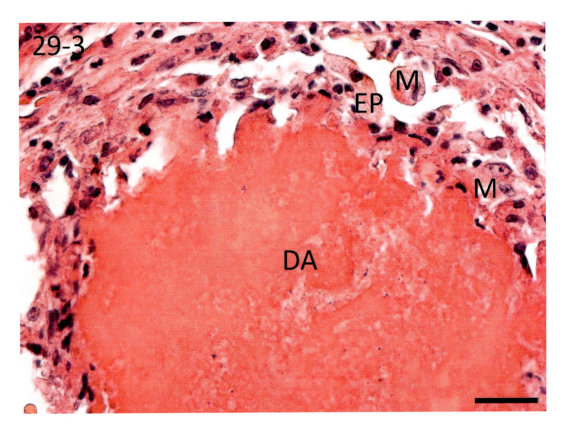

Figure 29.3 Pulmonary adiaspiromycosis. A dead adiaconidium (DA) is being cleared away by macrophages (M) located at the periphery. An epithelioid cell (EP) is also visible. HE. Bar = 25 μm.

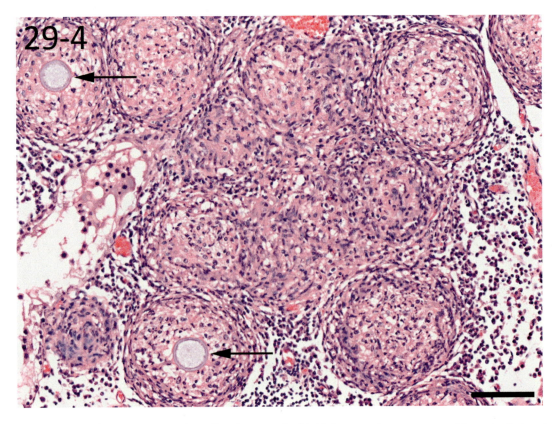

Figure 29.4 Chronic, granulomatous testicular adiaspiromycosis. Multiple granulomas, some with centrally located adiaconidia (arrows), are visible following experimental inoculation of a hamster testicle. HE. Bar = 150 μm.

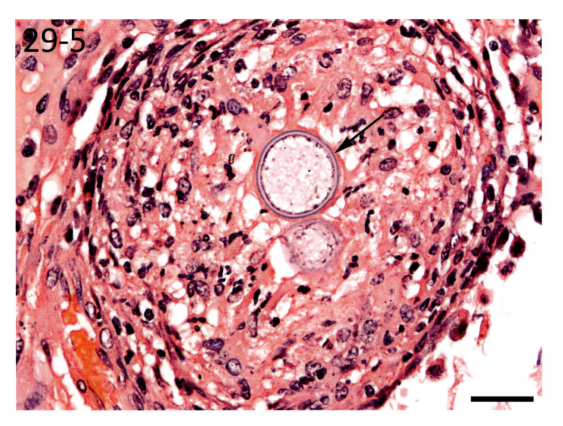

Figure 29.5 Chronic, granulomatous testicular adiaspiromycosis. An adiaconidium with its typical tri-laminar wall (arrow) is visible within a granuloma. Experimental inoculation of a hamster testicle. HE. Bar = 150 μm.

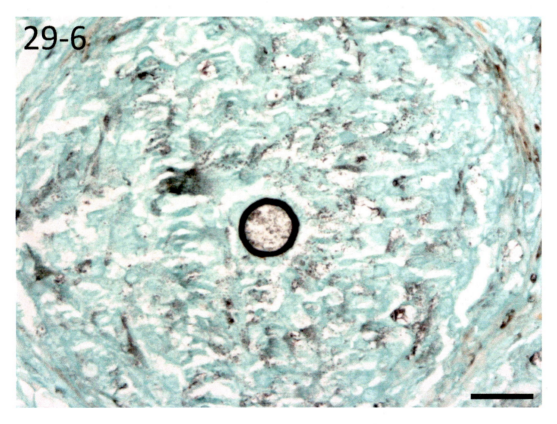

Figure 29.6 Chronic, granulomatous testicular adiaspiromycosis. The outline of an adiaconidium is clearly shown by applying Grocott's methenamine silver stain. Experimental inoculation of a hamster testicle. GMS. Bar = 50 μm.

REFERENCES

1. Malatesta D, Simpson VR, Fusillo R, Marcelli M, Bongiovanni L et al. 2014. First description of adi-aspiromycosis in an Eurasian otter (*Lutra lutra*) in Italy [Prima descrizione di un caso di adiaspiromicosi in lontra eurasiatica (*Lutra lutra*) in Italia]. Vet Ital, 50, 199–202.

2. Matsuda K, Niki H, Yukawa A, Yanagi M, Souma K et al. 2015. First detection of adiaspiromycosis in the lungs of a deer. J Vet Med Sci, 77, 981–983.

3. Borman AM, Jiang Y, Dukik K, Sigler L, Schwartz IS et al. 2018. Adiaspiromycosis and diseases caused by related fungi in Ajellomycetaceae. In: Emerging and Epizootic Fungal Infections in Animals. Seyedmousavi S, de Hoog GS, Jacques GP, Verweij E, Eds. Springer. pp 147–158.

4. Pfaller MA, Diekema DJ. 2005. Unusual fungal and pseudofungal infections of humans. J Clin Microbiol, 43, 1495–1504.

5. Chantrey JC, Borman AM, Johnson EM, Kipar A. 2006. *Emonsia crescens* infection in a British water vole (*Arvicola terrestris*). Med Mycol, 44, 375–378.

6. Kim T, Han J, Chang S, Kim D, Abdelkader TS et al. 2012. Adiaspiromycosis of an *Apodemus agrarius* captured wild rodent in Korea. Lab Anim Res, 28, 67–69.

7. Matos AC, Figueira L, Martins MH, Matos M, Pires MA et al. 2012. Pulmonary lesions consistent with disseminated adiaspiromycosis in Egyptian mongooses (*Herpestes Ichneumon*) from Portugal. J Comp Pathol, Poster 115. doi: 10.1016/j.jcpa2012.11.166.

8. Hughes K, Borman AM. 2018. Adiaspiromycosis in a wild European rabbit, and a review of the literature. J Vet Diagn Invest, 30, 614–618.

9. Santos VMD, Fatureto MC, Saldanha JC, Adad SJ. 2000. Pulmonary adiaspiromycosis: Report of two cases. Rev Soc Bras Med Trop, 33, 483–488.

10. Buyuksirin M, Ozkaya S, Yucel N, Guldaval F, Ceylan K et al. 2011. Pulmonary adiaspiromycosis: The first reported case in Turkey. Respir Med CME, 4, 166–169.

11. Naab T, Khan F. 2016. Adiaspiromycosis presenting with left wrist tenosynovitis and hyperpigmented verrucous skin lesions. Am J Clin Pathol, 146, 89–93.

12. Dot JM, Debourgogne A, Champigneulle J, Salles Y, Brizion M et al. 2009. Molecular diagnosis of disseminated adiaspiromycosis due to *Emmonsia crescens*. J Clin Microbiol, 47, 1269–1273.

13. Morandi F, Galuppi R, Delogu M, Lowenstine LJ, Benazzi C et al. 2012. Disseminated pulmonary adi-aspiromycosis in a crested porcupine (*Hystrix cristata* Linnaeus, 1758). J Wildl Dis, 48, 523–525.

14. Jensen HE, Barington K. 2021. Animal models in mycology. In: Handbook of Laboratory Animal Science. Hau J, Schapiro SJ, Eds. CRC Press. pp 695–722.

15. Jensen HE, Chandler FW. 2007. Histopathological diagnoses of mycoses. In: Topley and Wilson's Microbiology & Microbial Infections. Medical Mycology. 10th ed. Merz WG, Hay RJ, Eds. Hodder Arnold. pp 121–143.

16. Guarner J, Brandt ME. 2011. Histopathologic diagnosis of fungal infections in the 21st century. Clin Microbiol Rev, 24, 247–280.

30

Rhinosporidiosis

INTRODUCTION

The cause of rhinosporidiosis is *Rhinosporidium seeberi*, which has been assigned to the order mesomycetozoans, a heterogeneous group at the boundary of animals and fungi (1). In tissue, this organism produces endoconidia (i.e., endospores/spores) within large sporangia (i.e., cysts) (2, 3). Rhinosporidiosis diagnoses are based on histopathology because *R. seeberi* cannot be cultured on standard cell-free fungal or bacterial media, although it may grow in cell culture (4, 5).

EPIDEMIOLOGY

Infections are most frequently diagnosed in India, Sri Lanka, and Latin America, but may occur worldwide (4, 6–10). In addition to humans, several animal species have been diagnosed with rhinosporidiosis, especially dogs and horses (5–7, 11–14). Infections are due to trauma, occur typically in younger males, and are associated with a wet environment. However, *R. seeberi* spores may also survive in dry areas (15–17). The eyes and upper respiratory system (i.e., the nostrils and nasopharynx) are often affected, but the skin, urogenital organs, and bones may also become infected (9, 18–31). *R. seeberi* is probably host specific. This may explain why attempts to generate experimental laboratory animal models for this disease have proved unsuccessful (4).

PATHOLOGY

The *R. seeberi* pathogens are readily identified in haematoxylin and eosin-stained sections of rhinosporidiosis polypoidal masses. The tissue reaction is dominated by hyperplasia and granulomatous inflammation, with macrophages, multinucleate giant cells, lymphocytes, and plasma cells (23, 32, 33). The multinucleate giant cells may be bloated with sporangia (32, 33). Eosinophils and neutrophils may also be present within the inflamed area and microabscesses may form (6, 10). Lesions typically exhibit marked vascularity and haemorrhage (3, 11). Interestingly, the Splendore-Hoeppli phenomenon has not been associated with rhinosporidiosis (20).

ETIOLOGICAL HISTOMORPHOLOGY

The presence of large sporangia, containing endospores, at different stages of development may be used to diagnose rhinosporidiosis (Figs. 30.1–30.6). Because the infective elements are strongly stained in haematoxylin and eosin sections, it is usually unnecessary to use Grocott's methenamine silver or periodic acid-Schiff stains, although these are also effective (5, 6). The inner layer of the bilaminar sporangia wall (Fig. 30.3) is mucicarmine positive, as is the outer layer of the recently released endoconidia (5). The globose cysts, also called sporangia, may measure up to 100–400 µm in diameter and are filled with numerous endoconidia, each 6–10 µm in diameter (Figs. 30.1–30.6) (2–5, 10, 11, 21). After the endoconidia are released from the periphery of the sporangia, they grow and mature, adopting different shapes and sizes (Figs. 30.2, 30.4, and 30.6) (2, 10, 34). After releasing their contents, the sporangia collapse. Collapsed sporangia are detected histologically as sickle-shaped elements (Fig. 30.6).

DIFFERENTIAL DIAGNOSIS

The spherules produced by *Coccidioides* spp. also contain spores and may be confused with *R. seeberi* sporangia. However, *Coccidioides* spherules tend to be much smaller (20–200 µm in diameter) than the cysts/sporangia produced by *R. seeberi*. In addition, the spores within the *Coccidioides* spherules tend to be small (2–5 µm). However, the collapsed elements that occur in rhinosporidiosis may resemble the empty "yeast-shells" of *Coccidioides* spp. (see chapter on coccidioidomycosis). The large cells present in adiaspiromycosis may also be mistaken for rhinosporidiosis pathogens. However, the cells present in adiaspiromycosis do not contain endoconidia, and their walls consist of multiple layers (see chapter on adiaspiromycosis).

DOI: 10.1201/9781003306177-30

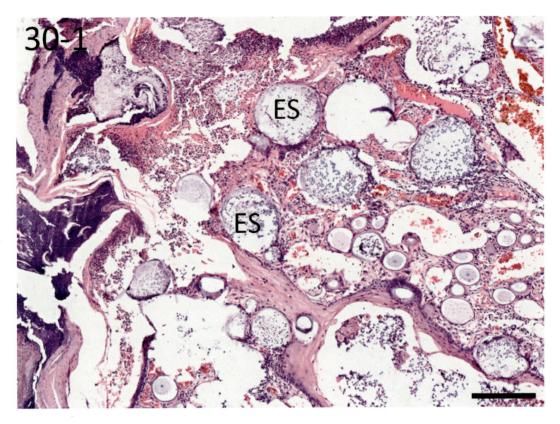

Figure 30.1 Nasal rhinosporidiosis. In rhinosporidiosis lesions, the presence of large *R. seeberi* sporangia (cysts) at different stages of development is of diagnostic importance. The sporangia contain endospores (ES). HE. Bar = 225 μm.

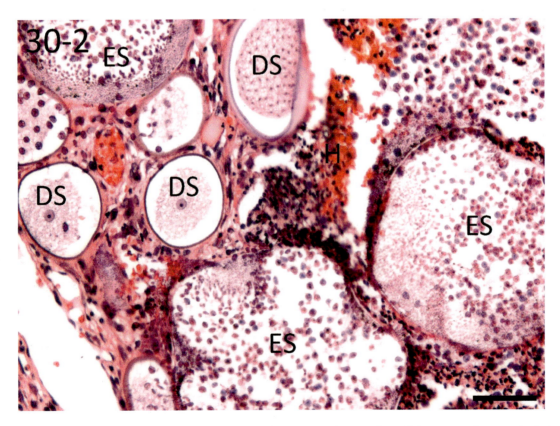

Figure 30.2 Nasal rhinosporidiosis. Heavy vascularization of rhinosporidiosis polypoidal masses often results in hemorrhage (H). The sporangia contain endospores (ES) and exhibit different stages of development (DS). HE. Bar = 75 μm.

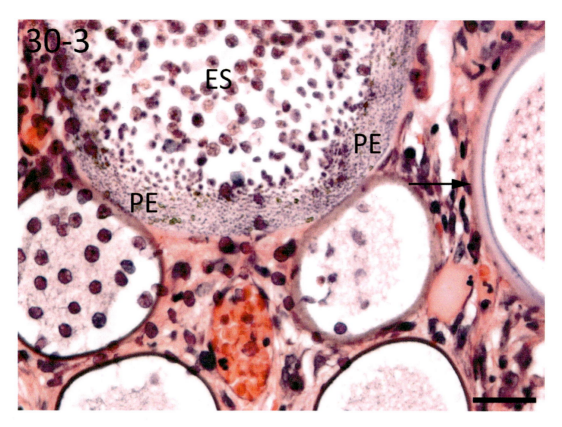

Figure 30.3 Nasal rhinosporidiosis. The double-layered wall of the sporangium (arrow) is visible next to an endospore (ES). The proliferation of endospores occurs at the periphery (PE) of the sporangium. HE. Bar = 35 μm.

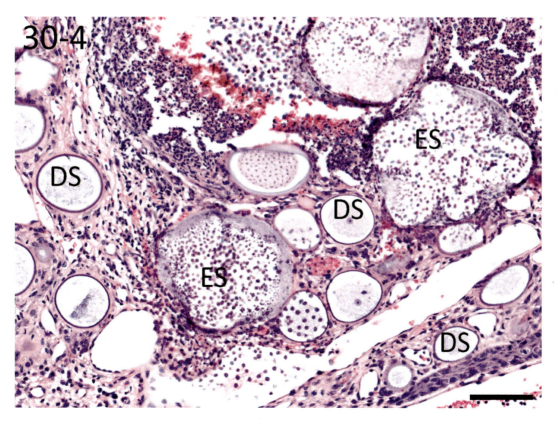

Figure 30.4 Nasal rhinosporidiosis. Different development stages of sporangia (cysts) containing endospores (ES) are present together with different development stages of sporangia (DS). HE. Bar = 100 μm.

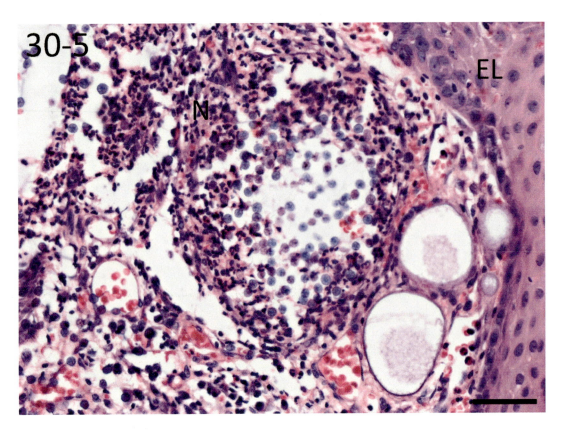

Figure 30.5 Nasal rhinosporidiosis. A ruptured cyst with released endoconidia (endospores/spores), located beneath the epithelial lining (EL), has been infiltrated by neutrophils (N). HE. Bar = 50 μm.

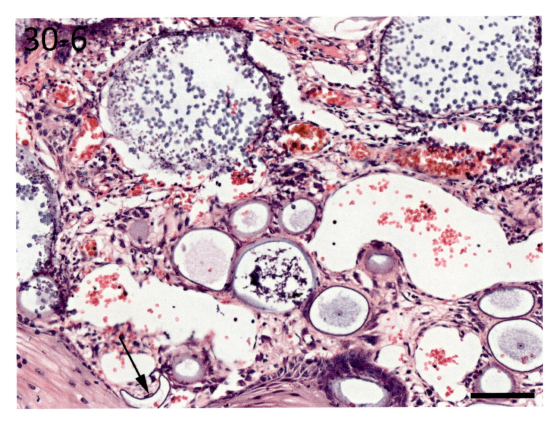

Figure 30.6 Nasal rhinosporidiosis. Within the polypoidal mass, heavy vascularization is visible together with sporangia at different stages of development. A collapsed sickle-shaped sporangia (arrow) is also visible. HE. Bar = 100 μm.

REFERENCES

1. Mendoza L, Taylor JW, Ajello L. 2002. The class Mesomycetozoea: A heterogeneous group of micro-organisms at the animal-fungal boundary. Annu Rev Microbiol, 56, 315–344.

2. Bader G, Grueber H. 1970. Histochemical studies of *Rhinosporidium seeberi*. Virchows Arch A Pathol Anat, 350, 76–86.

3. Jensen HE, Chandler FW. 2007. Histopathological diagnoses of mycoses. In: Topley and Wilson's Microbiology & Microbial Infections. Medical Mycology. 10th ed. Merz WG, Hay RJ, Eds. Hodder Arnold. pp 121–143.

4. Guarner J, Brandt, ME. 2011. Histopathologic diagnosis of fungal infections in the 21st century. Clin Microbiol Rev, 24, 247–280.

5. Easley JR, Meuten J, Levy MG, Dykstra MJ, Breitschwerdt EB et al. 1986. Nasal rhinosporidiosis in the dog. Vet Pathol, 23, 50–56.

6. Caniatti M, Roccabianca P, Scanziani E, Finazzi M, Mortellaro CM et al. 1998. Nasal rhinosporidiosis in dogs: Four cases from Europe and a review of the literature. Vet Rec, 142, 334–338.

7. Miller RI, Baylis R. 2009. Rhinosporidiosis in a dog native to the UK. Vet Rec, 164, 210.

8. Ray MS, Datta A, Sarkar P. 2011. Rhinosporidiosis of lacrimal sac: A rare case report from northeast India. Indian J Med Sci, 65, 40–42.

9. Thappa D, Kumari R, Nath A, Rajalakshmi R, Adityan B. 2009. Disseminated cutaneous rhinosporidiosis: Varied morphological appearances on the skin. Indian J Dermatol Venereol Leprol, 75, 68–71.

10. Azadeh B, Baghoumian N, el-Bakri OT. 1994. Rhinosporidiosis: Immunohistochemical and electron microscopic studies. J Laryngol Otol, 108, 1048–1054.

11. Berrocal A, López A. 2007. Nasal rhinosporidiosis in a mule. Can Vet J, 48, 305–306.

12. Hill SA, Sharkey LC, Hardy RM, Wilke VL, Smith MA et al. 2010. Nasal rhinosporidiosis in two dogs native to the upper Mississippi river valley region. J Am Anim Hosp Assoc, 46, 127–131.

13. Hoff B, Hall D. 1986. Rhinosporidiosis in a dog. Can Vet J, 27, 231–232.

14. Nollet H, Vercauteren G, Martens A, Vanschandevijl K, Schauvliege S et al. 2008. Laryngeal rhinosporidiosis in a Belgian warmblood horse. Zoonoses Pub Health, 55, 274–278.

15. Rameshkumar A, Gnanaselvi UP, Dineshkumar T, Raghuram PH, Bharanidharan R et al. 2015. Rhinosporidiosis presenting as a facial swelling: A case report. J Int Oral Health, 7, 58–60.

16. Shrestha SP, Hennig A, Parija SC. 1998. Prevalence of rhinosporidiosis of the eye and its adnexa in Nepal. Am J Trop Med Hyg, 59, 231–234.

17. Sengupta A, Pal S, Biswas BK, Jana S, Biswas S et al. 2015. Clinico-pathological study of 273 cases of rhinosporidiosis over a period of ten years in a tertiary care institute catering predominantly rural population of tribal origin. Bangladesh J Med Sci, 14, 159–164.

18. Basu SK, Bain J, Maity K, Chattopadhyay D, Baitalik D et al. 2016. Rhinosporidiosis of lacrimal sac: An interesting case of orbital swelling. J Nat Sci Biol Med, 7, 98–101.

19. Campos MCS, Surka J, Jardon MG, Bustamante N. 2005. Ocular rhinosporidiosis. South African Med J, 95, 950–952.

20. Chowdhury AR, Dey R, Bhattacharya P, Basu S. 2012. An unusual case of urethral polyp. Ann Trop Med Public Health, 5, 530–531.

21. Jamison A, Crofts K, Roberts F, Gregory ME. 2016. Educational report: A case of lacrimal sac rhinosporidiosis. Orbit, 35, 254–257.

22. Kundu AK, Phuljhele S, Jain M, Srivastava RK. 2013. Osseous involvement in rhinosporidiosis. Indian J Orthop, 47, 523–525.

23. Madana J, Yolmo D, Gopalakrishnan S, Saxena SK. 2010. Rhinosporidiosis of the upper airways and trachea. J Laryngol Otol, 124, 1139–1141.

24. Mallick AA, Majhi TK, Pal DK. 2012. Rhinosporidiosis affecting multiple parts of the body. Trop Doct, 42, 174–175.

25. Mishra LK, Gupta S, Pradhan SK, Baisakh M. 2015. Lacrimal sac rhinosporidiosis. Plast Aesthet Res, 2, 353–356.

26. Mukherjee B, Mohan A, Sumathi V, Biswas J. 2013. Infestation of the lacrimal sac by *Rhinosporidium seeberi*: A clinicopathological case report. Indian J Ophthalmol, 61, 588–590.

27. Nayak S, Acharjya B, Devi B, Sahoo A, Singh N. 2007. Disseminated cutaneous rhinosporidiosis. Indian J Dermatol Venereol Leprol, 73, 185–187.

28. Nerurkar NK, Bradoo RA, Joshi AA, Shah J, Tandon S. 2004. Lacrimal sac rhinosporidiosis: A case report. Am J Otolaryngol, 25, 423–425.

29. Pal DK, Moulik D, Chowdhury M. 2008. Genitourinary rhinosporidiosis. Indian J Urol, 24, 419–421.

30. Suryawanshi PV, Rekhi B, Desai S, Desai SM, Juvekar SL et al. 2011. Rhinosporidiosis isolated to the distal clavicle: A rare presentation clinicoradiologically mimicking a bone tumor. Skeletal Radiol, 40, 225–228.

31. Thappa DM, Venkatesan S, Sirka CS, Jaisankar TJ, Gopalkrishnan RC. 1998. Disseminated cutaneous rhinosporidiosis. J Dermatol, 25, 527–532.

32. Ghorpade A. 2008. Rhinosporidiosis: Gigantic cells with engulfed sporangia of *Rhinosporidium seeberi* in the case of dermosporidiosis. Int J Dermatol, 47, 694–695.

33. Ghorpade A. 2011. Gigantic cutaneous rhinosporidiosis with giant cells bloated with sporangia. Indian J Dermatol Venereol Leprol, 77, 517–519.

34. Pfaller MA, Diekema DJ. 2005. Unusual fungal and pseudofungal infections of humans. J Clin Microbiol, 43, 1495–1504.

31

Rare mycoses

INTRODUCTION

With an increase in the number of immunocompromised persons around the world, it is not surprising that rare mycoses are also becoming increasingly diverse. New mycoses are regularly added from case studies, and molecular studies frequently result in updates to the nomenclature and new classification of pathogens. However, in addition to the pathogens described in the chapter on minor hyalohyphomycosis, the following genera may be associated with rare invasive mycoses (1): *Malassezia, Sporobolomyces, Rhodotorula, Pseudozyma* (renamed *Moesziomyces*), *Saccharomyces, Saprochaete, Kodamaea,* and the invasive forms of the two dematiaceous fungi *Alternaria* and *Phialemonium*. These invasive forms of *Alternaria* and *Phialemonium* often exhibit hyaline hyphae in tissues, and their melanin content may only be highlighted by applying particular stains, such as Fontana-Masson stain (2–6). A novel thermally dimorphic fungal pathogen described in 2013 caused disseminated disease in persons living with advanced human immunodeficiency virus (HIV)/acquired immune deficiency syndrome (AIDS), particularly in South Africa. Although this pathogen was initially described as an *Emmonsia*-like fungus, it has now been assigned to a new genus of thermally dimorphic fungi and was recently named *Emergomyces africanus*. Five species of the genus *Emergomyces* are now known to cause emergomycosis, and cases of the disease have been reported globally, although those caused by *E. africanus* occur most frequently (7, 8).

EPIDEMIOLOGY

Similar to the pathogens that cause minor hyalohyphomycoses and many other opportunistic fungi, pathogens that cause rare mycoses occur worldwide. However, some infections are associated with particular geographic areas (1, 7). Moreover, the pathogens that cause rare mycoses are often ubiquitous throughout the environment, and several exhibit commensalism within the gastrointestinal tract and/or on the skin and mucous membranes (1). Invasive mycoses that are caused by the genera described above and other opportunistic fungal infections generally affect patients with primary or acquired immunosuppression, but other risk factors include hematologic malignancy, chemotherapy, diabetes,

and prolonged corticosteroid treatment (5, 6, 9–12). Some infections may occur via skin trauma, such as those caused by the coelomycetes, which contain a number of pigmented plant pathogenic fungi (e.g., *Phoma* spp. and *Colletotrichum* spp.), and the subcutaneous phaeohyphomycosis infections caused by *Alternaria* spp. (Figs. 31.1–31.7) (5, 6, 13). Similar to several other dimorphic fungi, *Emergomyces* spp. typically disseminate after primary pulmonary infection. Most patients infected by these fungi develop widespread cutaneous lesions, but various other organs may also be affected (7).

PATHOLOGY

Invasive forms of rare infections are histopathologically similar to infections by other fungi. Acute lesions are usually necrotic and may be infiltrated by neutrophils. Chronic lesions frequently exhibit granulomatous or pyogranulomatous inflammation, with many macrophages, epithelioid cells, and multinucleate giant cells (Figs. 31.1–31.3).

FUNGAL HISTOMORPHOLOGY

As the literature on several of the rare mycoses is sparse, and because in many reports histopathology has not been carried out, the experience with the histomorphology of several of the genera causing the rare mycoses is not well understood. However, a few descriptions are available. *Saprochaete* spp. have thin, hyaline hyphae with narrow-angle branches and pleomorphic yeast-like cells (1, 14). In invasive lesions caused by *Malassezia* spp., pseudohyphae are interspersed with budding yeast cells, and macrophages, lymphocytes, and neutrophils are present (15, 16). In acute lesions caused by *Pseudozyma* spp., there are dichotomous branching hyphae with septa and clusters of yeast cells (17, 18). In invasive lesions, *Saccharomyces* spp. form pseudohyphae and yeast cells are present in tissues (1). *Sporobolomyces* spp. has been associated with granulomatous encephalitis showing branching and septate pseudohyphal elements that were 1–4 μm in diameter and up to 15 μm in length (19). Histologically, *Emergomyces* closely resembles *Histoplasma capsulatum* var. *capsulatum*, with small (2–5 μm) intracellular and extracellular oval-to-round narrow-based budding yeast cells (7, 8). In invasive infections caused by *Alternaria*

DOI: 10.1201/9781003306177-31

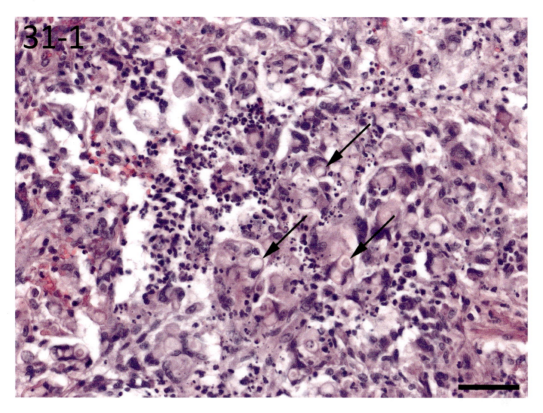

Figure 31.1 Chronic, subcutaneous alternariosis due to *A. infectoria*. In chronic lesions, pyogranulomatous inflammation is typically present with infiltration by neutrophils and multinucleate giant cells that contain fungal elements (arrows). HE. Bar = 50 μm.

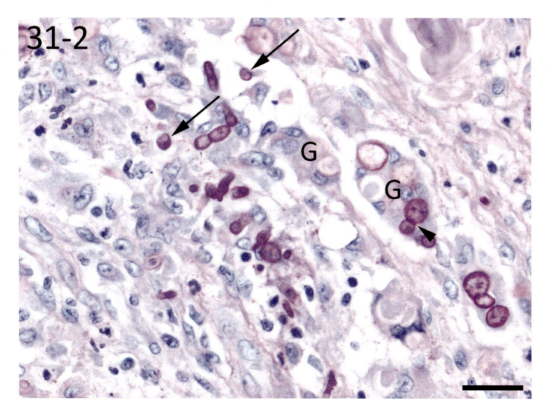

Figure 31.2 Chronic, subcutaneous alternariosis due to *A. infectoria*. Within the lesion, round-shaped fungal cells with thick walls are visible both extracellularly (arrows) and within multinucleate giant cells (G). These are different sizes due to sprouting (arrowhead). PAS. Bar = 25 μm.

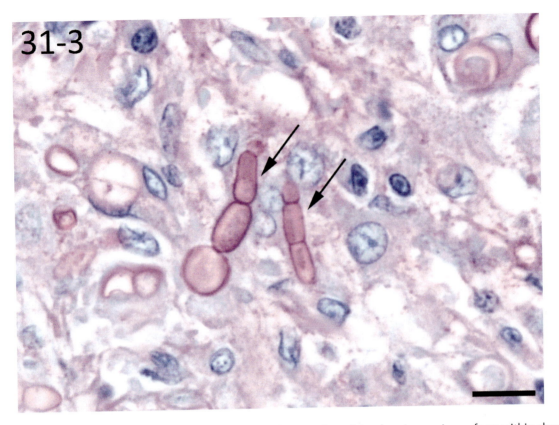

Figure 31.3 Chronic, subcutaneous alternariosis due to *A. infectoria*. Pseudohyphae (arrows) may form within chronic alternariosis lesions. PAS. Bar = 12 μm

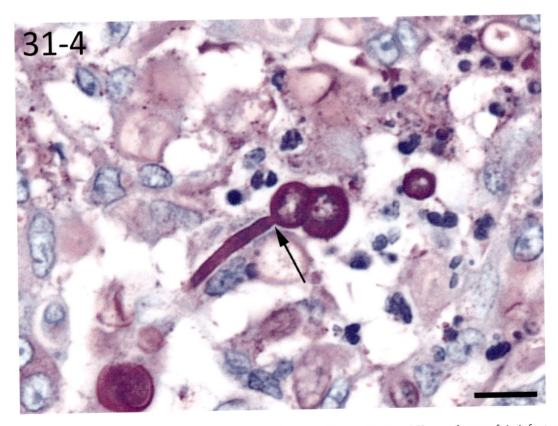

Figure 31.4 Chronic, subcutaneous alternariosis due to *A. infectoria*. Along with the different forms of *A. infectoria* in subcutaneous lesions, there may be "sprouting forms" that produce new hyphae (arrow). PAS. Bar = 12 μm.

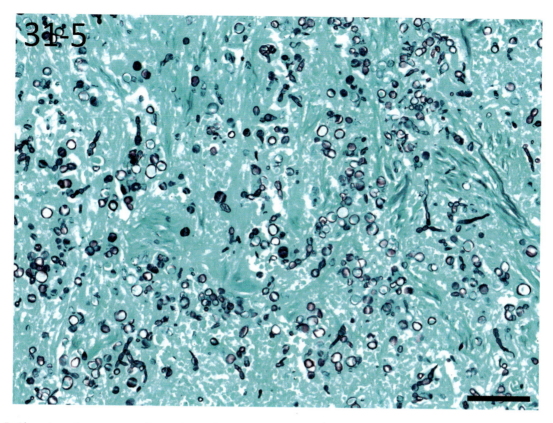

Figure 31.5 Chronic, subcutaneous alternariosis due to *A. infectoria*. The widespread occurrence of *Alternaria* elements is highlighted in Grocott's methenamine silver-stained sections. GMS. Bar = 75 μm.

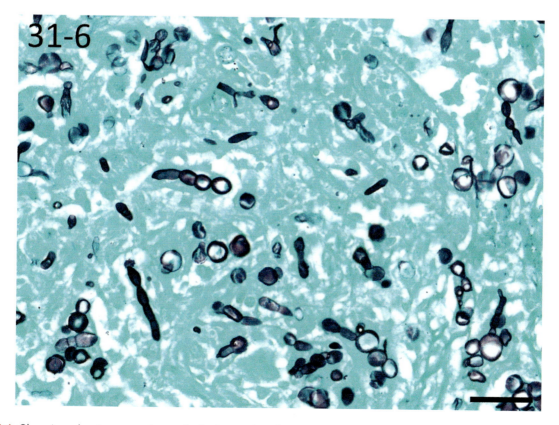

Figure 31.6 Chronic, subcutaneous alternariosis due to *A. infectoria*. Hyphal elements with dilatations are typically found in subcutaneous lesions caused by *A. infectoria*. GMS. Bar = 25 μm.

(*A. infectoria* and *A. alternata*), the hyphae appear hyaline in sections stained with haematoxylin and eosin, despite the dematiaceous nature of the fungus (5, 6). However, these hyphae are strongly highlighted by both periodic acid-Schiff and Grocott's methenamine silver stains (Figs. 31.2–31.7). Moreover, Fontana-Masson stain may be used to highlight the melanin in some of these elements. *Phialemonium* spp. (Figs. 31.8–31.12) as *Alternaria* spp. are the cause of phaeohyphomycosis, although the hyphae of the *Phialemonium* spp. as for the *Alternaria* spp. are hyaline when seen in haematoxylin and eosin-stained sections (2, 4). In invasive lesions, the fungal elements occur as septate hyphae with multiple vesicles and pseudohyphae (Figs. 31.8–31.12).

DIFFERENTIAL DIAGNOSIS

As for all opportunistic fungal infections, the gold standard for making diagnoses is recovering the fungus in culture or identification using molecular techniques together with histopathological documentation of typical, invasive fungal elements within lesions. As described above, histopathological analyses of *Emergomycosis* reveal small (2–5 μm) yeast cells that exhibit narrow-based budding and are best visualized by applying periodic acid-Schiff and Grocott's methenamine silver stains (7, 8). However, these observations are insufficiently distinct from those documented for *H. capsulatum* to enable definitive identification from histopathological appearance alone (7). Because *Rhodotorula* spp. in tissues form round/oval budding yeast cells (3 μm in diameter) and the accompanying inflammatory reaction resembles necrotizing granulomas, *Rhodotorula* spp. elements are easily confused with those of *Cryptococcus* spp. (1, 20, 21). The etiologies of other rare mycoses are also not specific. Therefore, various techniques may be necessary to accurately diagnose these infections. In addition, histopathological identification of typical fungal elements may be necessary to exclude both colonization and contamination.

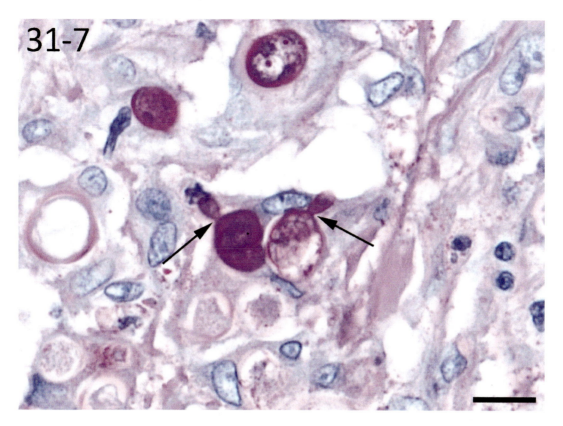

Figure 31.7 Chronic, subcutaneous alternariosis due to *A. infectoria*. Budding of cells may also be visible (arrows) in lesions caused by *A. infectoria*. PAS. Bar = 12 μm.

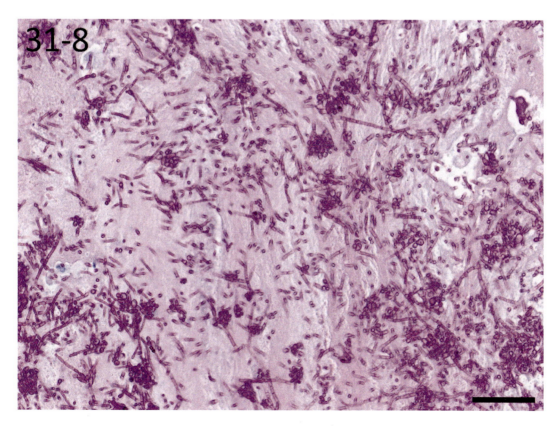

Figure 31.8 Chronic, endocardial *Phialemonium* infection. *Phialemonium* hyphae may be abundant in entrenched infections. PAS. Bar = 90 μm.

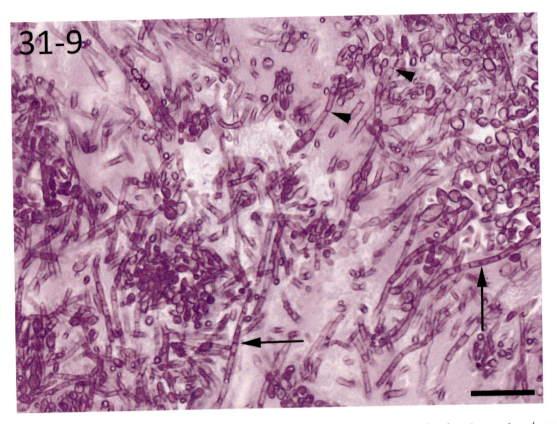

Figure 31.9 Chronic, endocardial *Phialemonium* infection. At high magnification, septate hyphae (arrows) and pseudohyphae (arrowheads) are visible. PAS. Bar = 50 μm.

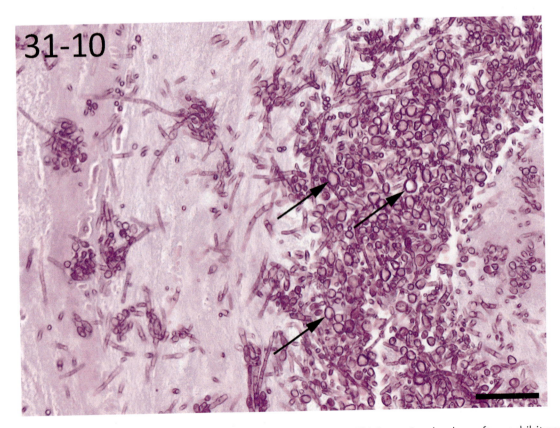

Figure 31.10 Chronic, endocardial *Phialemonium* infection. Within lesions, *Phialemonium* hyphae often exhibit vesicular dilatations (arrows). PAS. Bar = 50 μm.

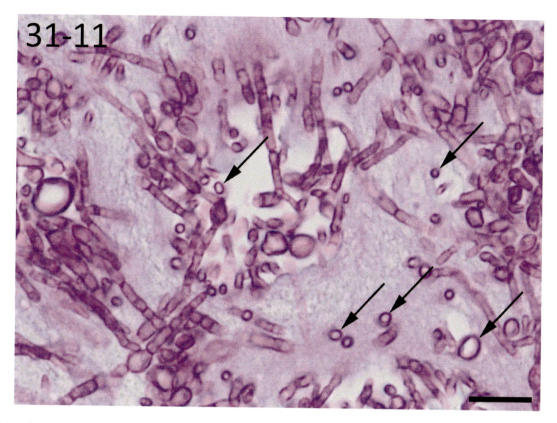

Figure 31.11 Chronic, endocardial *Phialemonium* infection. In lesions, cross-sections of hyphae and, in particular, hyphal dilatations may resemble yeast cells (arrows). PAS. Bar = 35 μm.

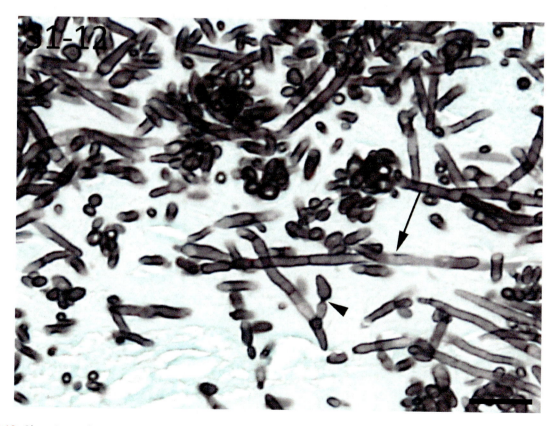

Figure 31.12 Chronic, endocardial *Phialemonium* infection. Hyphae (arrow) and pseudohyphae (arrowhead) are clearly visible in Grocott's methenamine silver-stained sections. GMS. Bar = 35 μm.

REFERENCES

1. Chen SCA, Perfect J, Colombo AL, Cornely OA, Groll AH et al. 2021. Global guideline for the diagnosis and management of rare yeast infections: An initiative of the ECMM in cooperation with ISHAM and ASM. Lancet Infect Dis, 21. doi: 10.1016/S1473-3099(21)00203-6.

2. Heins-Vaccari EM, Machado CM, Saboya RS, Silva RL, Dulley FL et al. 2001. *Phialemonium curvatum* infection after bone marrow transplantation. Rev Inst Med Trop Sao Paulo, 43, 163–166.

3. Proia LA, Hayden MK, Kammeyer PL, Ortiz J, Sutton DA et al. 2004. *Phialemonium*: An emerging mold pathogen that caused 4 cases of hemodialysis-associated endovascular infection. Clin Infect Dis, 39, 373–379.

4. Perdomo H, Sutton DA, García D, Fothergill AW, Gené J et al. 2011. Molecular and phenotypic characterization of *Phialemonium* and *Lecothophora* isolates from clinical samples. J Clin Microbiol, 49, 1209–1216.

5. Dubois D, Pihet M, Clec'h CL, Croué A, Beguin H et al. 2005. Cutaneous phaeohyphomycosis due to *Alternaria* infectoria. Mycopathologia, 160, 117–123.

6. Halaby T, Boots H, Vermeulen A, Ven AVD, Beguin H et al. 2001. Phaeohyphomycosis caused by *Alternaria infectoria* in a renal transplant recipient. J Clin Microbiol, 39, 1952–1955.

7. Schwartz IS, Govender NP, Sigler L, Jiang Y, Maphanga TG et al. 2019. Emergomyces: The global rise of new dimorphic fungal pathogens. PLoS Pathog, 15. doi: 10.1371/journal.ppat.1007977.

8. Schwartz IS, McLoud JD, Berman D, Botha A, Lerm B et al. 2018. Molecular detection of airborne *Emergomyces africanus*, a thermally dimorphic fungal pathogen, in Cape Town, South Africa. PLoS Negl Trop Dis, 12. doi: 10.1371/journal.pntd.0006174.

9. Kpodzo DS, Calderwood MS, Ruchelsman DE, Abramson JS, Piris A et al. 2011. Primary subcutaneous *Alternaria alternate* infection of the hand in an immunocompromised host. Med Mycol, 49, 543–547.

10. Pastor FJ, Guarro J. 2008. *Alternaria* infections: Laboratory diagnosis and relevant clinical features. Clin Microbiol Infect Dis, 14, 734–746.

11. Lopes L, Borges-Costa J, Soares-Almeida L, Filipe P, Neves F et al. 2013. Cutaneous alternariosis caused by *Alternaria infectoria*: Three cases in kidney transplant patients. Healthcare, 1, 100–106.

12. Morrison VA, Weisdorf DJ. 1993. *Alternaria*: A sinonasal pathogen of immunocompromised hosts. Clin Infect Dis, 16, 265–270.

13. Guarner J, Brandt ME. 2011. Histopathologic diagnosis of fungal infections in the 21st century. Clin Microbiol Rev, 24, 247–280.

14. El Zein S, Hindy J-R, Kanj SS. 2020. Invasive *Saprochaete* infections: An emerging threat to immunocompromised patients. Pathogens, 9. doi: 10.3390/pathogens9110922.

15. de St Maurice A, Frangoul H, Coogan A, Williams JV. 2014. Prolonged fever and splenic lesions caused by *Malassezia restricta* in an immunocompromised patient. Pediatr Transplant, 18, 283–286.

16. Chai FC, Auret K, Christiansen K, Yuen PW, Gardamet D. 2000. Malignant otitis externa caused by *Malassezia sympodialis*. Head Neck, 22, 87–89.

17. Joo H, Choi Y-G, Cho S-Y, Choi J-K, Lee D-G et al. 2016. *Pseudozyma aphidis* fungaemia with invasive fungal pneumonia in a patient with acute myeloid leukaemia: Case report and literature review. Mycoses, 59, 56–61.

18. Chen B, Zhu L-Y, Xuan X, Wu L-J, Zhou T-L et al. 2011. Isolation of both *Pseudozyma aphidis* and *Nocardia otitidiscaviarum* from a mycetoma on the leg. Int J Dermatol, 50, 714–719.

19. Saey V, Vanhaesebrouck A, Maes S, Van Simaey L, Van Ham L et al. 2011. Granulomatous meningoencephalitis associated with *Sporobolomyces roseus* in a dog. Vet Pathol, 40, 83–86.

20. Simon MS, Somersan S, Singh HK, Hartman B, Wickes BL et al. 2014. Endocarditis caused by *Rhodotorula* infection. J Clin Microbiol, 52, 374–378.

21. Tsiodras S, Papageorgiou S, Meletiadis J, Tofas P, Pappa V et al. 2014. *Rhodotorula mucilaginosa* associate meningitis: A subacute entity with high mortality. Case report and review. Med Mycol Case Rep, 6, 46–50.

32

Algoses

INTRODUCTION

Algal infections occur only rarely in humans and animals, and they may be caused by either chlorophyllic or achlorophyllic algae. Infections with chlorophyll-containing algae (*Chlorella* spp.) are very rare, and these are characterized by green discolouration of the tissue on gross examination (1). Therefore, only infections caused by achlorophyllic algae are described in this chapter. The genus *Prototheca* has been revised several times over the last few years to accommodate new molecular, chemotaxonomic, and phenotypic data, and 14 species are now recognized (2–4). Based on 18S rDNA sequence analysis, the former *Prototheca zopfii* has been separated into three distinct genotypes (1–3), which are now called *P. ciferrii* (genotype 1), *P. bovis* (genotype 2), and *P. blaschkeae* (genotype 3); these are the most important dairy-associated species of *Prototheca* (3, 5). The most important human-associated algae include *P. wickerhamii*, *P. cutis*, and *P. miyajii* (3, 4). In addition to dairy cattle and humans, other animals may become infected, including dogs, cattle, cats, and horses (6–14).

EPIDEMIOLOGY

Prototheca spp. occur ubiquitously throughout the environment (3, 7, 15), and immunocompromised individuals and patients with underlying diseases are particularly susceptible to infections (16–18). The skin is the organ that is most frequently infected by *Prototheca* spp.; however, the mammary glands of cattle are also frequently infected (2, 5, 19–22). The algae may spread from sites of infection to local lymph nodes (15, 20). Systemic infections may also occur (7).

PATHOLOGY

Lesions exhibit granulomatous inflammation with numerous macrophages, but multinucleate giant cells may also be present together with epithelioid cells; there may be various levels of suppuration (23–25). The *Prototheca* organisms are often abundant in lesions and may be found within macrophages and multinucleate giant cells (Figs. 32.1 and 32.2) (9, 20, 23). Systemic animal models of protothecosis have also been described (13, 26).

HISTOMORPHOLOGY OF ALGAE

The algae are visible as empty cells, forming morula-like structures in haematoxylin and eosin-stained sections (15, 23, 24). They are strongly highlighted by both periodic acid-Schiff and Grocott's methenamine silver stains (Figs. 32.1–32.4) (15, 25, 27, 28). The morphology of infectious *Prototheca* species is similar. However, *P. bovis* (serotype 2) and *P. blaschkeae* (both formerly named *P. zopfii*) cells may be slightly larger (7–30 µm) than *P. wickerhamii* cells (3–15 µm) (8). Moreover, the spherical, oval, or polyhedral cells, which are surrounded by a 2–3 µm clear halo, often measure 8–21 µm in size (6). The cells do not bud and are surrounded by a thick capsule (Fig. 32.2) (15). Because algae reproduce by fission (i.e., intracellular cleavage) to produce endospores, intracellular septations are typically present and these may facilitate diagnoses (Figs. 32.3, 32.4) (6, 15, 23). Both collapsed and degenerate cells may also be found in lesions (6). The collapsed cells are formed following the rupture of the mother cells (sporangia, i.e. elements containing endospores) liberating the endospores (Figs. 32.2–32.4) (7).

DIFFERENTIAL DIAGNOSIS

A lack of characteristic endospores in protothecosis lesions causes *Prototheca* spp. to resemble non-sporulating elements of *Blastomyces dermatitidis*, *Cryptococcus neoformans*, *Paracoccidioides* spp., and some stages of *Coccidioides* spp., *Pneumocystis jirovecii*, and *Rhinosporidium seeberi* (7, 15, 23). Morphologically, *Prototheca* spp. are similar to green algae; however, the absence of chloroplasts in *Prototheca* spp. clearly distinguishes *Prototheca* spp. from *Chlorella* spp. (15, 23). Several studies have used specific antibodies to identify *Prototheca* spp. *in situ* (6, 10, 20, 22).

DOI: 10.1201/9781003306177-32

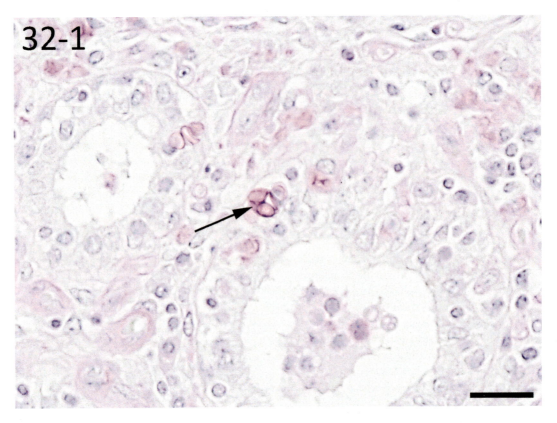

Figure 32.1 Chronic, mammary protothecosis due to *P. bovis*. Periodic acid-Schiff staining shows a characteristic algal cell, with intracellular septation, within a macrophage that is located between the alveolar epithelial cells (arrow). PAS. Bar = 20 μm.

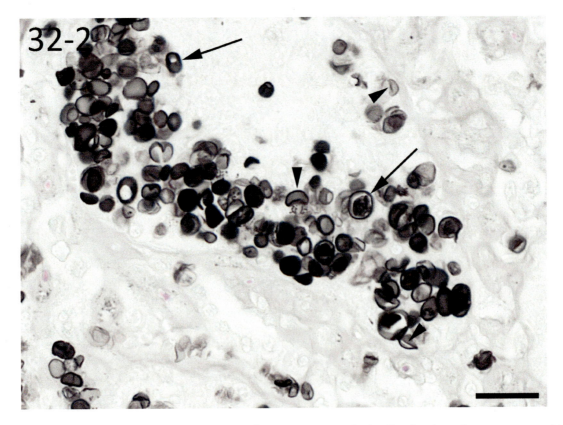

Figure 32.2 Chronic, mammary protothecosis due to *P. bovis*. Numerous algal cells of various sizes may occur within lesions. The algal elements are strongly highlighted by Grocott's methenamine silver stain. The thick cell wall of *Prototheca* is clearly visible (arrows). Some collapsed cells are also visible (arrowheads). GMS. Bar = 20 μm.

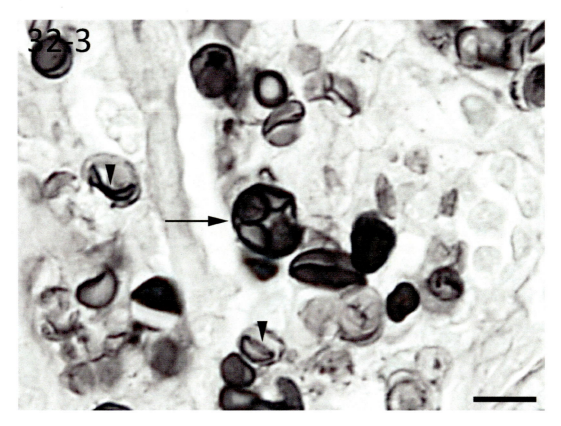

Figure 32.3 Chronic, dermal protothecosis due to *P. wickerhamii*. Intracellular cleavage figures (arrow) must be identified to make a diagnosis of protothecosis when chlorophyll is absent. Several collapsed cells are also visible (arrowheads). GMS. Bar = 10 μm.

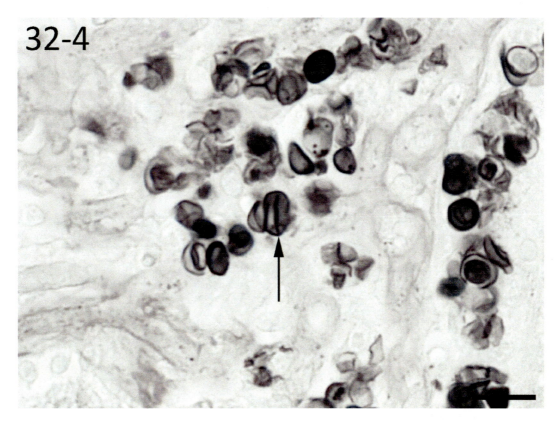

Figure 32.4 Chronic, mammary protothecosis due to *P. bovis*. Intracellular septation (arrow) within sporangia in protothecosis lesions may facilitate a diagnosis. GMS. Bar = 15 μm.

REFERENCES

1. Salfelder K. 1990. Atlas of Fungal Pathology. Kluwer Academic Publishers.

2. Jagielski T, Krukowski H, Bochniarz M et al. 2019. Prevalence of *Prototheca* spp. on dairy farms in Poland – a cross-country study. Microbial Biotechnol, 12, 556–566.

3. Jagielski T, Bakula Z, Gawor J et al. 2019. The genus *Prototheca* (Trebouxiophyceae, Chlorophyta) revisited: Implications from molecular taxonomic studies. Algal Res, 43, 101639.

4. Bakula Z, Siedlecki P, Gromadka R et al. 2021. A first insight into the genome of *Prototheca wickerhamii*, a major causative agent of human protothecosis. BMC Genomics, 22, 168.

5. Fidelis CE, Franke M, de Abreu LCR et al. 2021. MALDI-TOF MS identification of *Prototheca* algae associated with bovine mastitis. J Vet Diagn Invest, 33, 1168–1171.

6. Huth N, Wenkel RF, Roschanski N, Rösler U, Plagge L et al. 2015. *Prototheca zopfii* genotype 2-induced nasal dermatitis in a cat. J. Comp. Pathol, 152, 287–290.

7. Leimann BCQ, Monteiro PCF, Lazera M, Candanoza ERU, Wanke B. 2004. Protothecosis. Med Mycol, 42, 95–106.

8. Macedo JTSA, Riet-Correa F, Dantas AFM, Simoes SVD. 2008. Cutaneous and nasal protothecosis in a goat. Vet Pathol, 45, 352–354.

9. Salvadori C, Gandini G, Ballarini A, Cantile C. 2008. Prothecal granulomatous meningoencephalitis in a dog. J Small Anim Prac, 49, 531–535.

10. Schöniger S, Roschanski N, Rösler U, Vidovic A, Nowak M et al. 2016. *Prototheca* species and *Pithomyces chartarum* as causative agents of rhinitis and/or sinusitis in horses. J Comp Pathol, 155, 121–125.

11. Shank AMM, Dubielzig RD, Teixeira LBC. 2015. Canine ocular protothecosis: A review of 14 cases. Vet Ophthalmol, 18, 437–442.

12. Stenner VJ, Mackay B, King T, Barrs VRD, Irwin P et al. 2007. Protothecosis in 17 Australian dogs and a review of the canine literature. Med Mycol, 45, 249–266.

13. Jensen HE, Aalbæk B. 1993. Pathogenicity of yeast and algae isolated from mastitis secretions in a murine model. Mycoses, 37, 101–107.

14. Ginel PJ, Pérez J, Molleda JM, Lucena R, Mozos E. 1997. Cutaneous protothecosis in a dog. Vet Rec, 140, 651–653.

15. Lass-Flörl C, Mayr A. 2007. Human protothecosis. Clin Microbiol Rev, 20, 230–242.

16. Zhang QQ, Li L, Zhu LP, Zhao Y, Wang YR et al. 2012. Cutaneous protothecosis in a patient with diabetes mellitus and review of published case reports. Mycopathologia, 173, 163–171.

17. Cooper JD, Tyler W, Hoyos CMJ, Medina RA. 2016. *Prototheca wickerhamii* in a patient with chronic hepatitis C. Infect Dis Clin Pract, 24, 283–285.

18. Figueroa CJ, Camp BJ, Varghese GI, Miranda E, Querfeld C et al. 2014. A case of protothecosis in a patient with multiple myeloma. J Cutan Pathol, 41, 409–413.

19. Aalbæk B, Jensen HE, Huda A. 1998. Identification of *Prototheca* from bovine mastitis in Denmark. APMIS, 106, 483–488.

20. Jensen HE, Aalbæk B, Bloch B, Huda A. 1998. Bovine mammary protothecosis due to *Prototheca zopfii*. Med Mycol, 36, 89–95.

21. Benites NR, Guerra JL, Melville PA, da Costa EO. 2002. Aetiology and histopathology of bovine mastitis of spontaneous occurrence. J Vet Med, 49, 366–370.

22. Corbellini LG, Driemeier D, Cruz CEF. 2001. Immunohistochemistry combined with periodic acid-Schiff for bovine mammary gland with prothecal mastitis. Biotech Histochem, 76, 85–88.

23. Hillesheim PB, Bahrami S. 2011. Cutaneous protothecosis. Arch Pathol Lab Med, 135, 941–944.

24. Humphrey S, Martinka M, Lui H. 2009. Cutaneous protothecosis following a tape-stripping injury. J Cutan Med, 13, 273–275.

25. Da Silva PCG, Lima RB, Lupi O. 2013. Cutaneous protothecosis – case report. An Bras Dermatol, 88, 183–185.

26. Jensen HE, Barington K. 2021. Animal models in mycology. In: Handbook of Laboratory Animal Science. 4th ed. Hau J, Schapero SJ, Eds. CRC Press. pp 695–722.

27. Seok JY, Lee Y, Lee H, Yi SY, Oh HE et al. 2013. Human cutaneous protothecosis: Report of a case and literature review. Korean J Pathol, 47, 575–578.

28. Walsh SV, Johnson RA, Tahan SR. 1998. Protothecosis: An unusual cause of chronic subcutaneous and soft tissue infection. Am J Dermatopathol, 20, 379–382.

Index

Note: Locators in *italics* represent figures and **bold** indicate tables in the text.

Trichosporon spp., **14**, 138, 147, 149
    T. asahii, **36**, 149, *150–151*
    T. beigelii, **46**
    T. inkin, **36**, 149
Trophozoites, 189
Trypanosoma spp., 184

U

Uvitex 2B brightener, 22

V

Vasculitis, *140–141*
Vesicle, 52

W

Wade-Fite stain, 123
Wright stain, 22

Y

Yeast-like cells, 8, 13, **14**, 27
"Yeast-shells", 209

Z

Ziehl-Neelsen (ZN) stain, *23*, 123
Zygomycosis, 96
Zygospore, 52